AF323017

Laryngectomee Rehabilitation

Laryngectomee Rehabilitation

Second Edition

Edited by

Robert L. Keith, M.S.
Speech Pathologist, Mayo Clinic
Associate Professor, Mayo Medical
  School

and

Frederic L. Darley, Ph.D.
Emeritus Staff, Speech Pathology, Mayo
  Clinic
Professor, Mayo Medical School

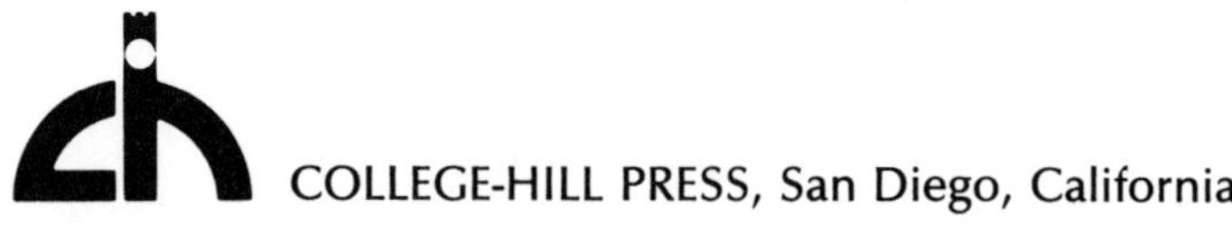

COLLEGE-HILL PRESS, San Diego, California

College-Hill Press, Inc.
4284 41st Street
San Diego, California 92105

Library of Congress Cataloging-in-Publication Data
Main entry under title:

Laryngectomee rehabilitation.

  Papers presented at the Laryngectomee Rehabilitation
Seminars held in 1980-1984.
  Includes index.
  1. Laryngectomees—Rehabilitation—Congresses.
2. Speech, Alaryngeal—Congresses.   I. Keith,
Robert L.   II. Darley, Frederic L.   II. Laryngectomee
Rehabilitation Seminar.   [DNLM: 1. Laryngectomy—
rehabilitation—congresses.   2. Speech, Alaryngeal—
congresses.   W3 LA301 1980-84 / WV 540 L3357 1980-84]
RF540.L36   1986   617'.53301   85-24313

ISBN 0-88744-104-1

Printed in the United States of America

CONTENTS

Contents

Preface

The first volume was a record of the proceedings of the Fifth Laryngectomee Rehabilitation Seminar held June 10–15, 1979, at Mayo Clinic in
Rochester, Minnesota. The revised edition is an update as a result of the
seminar from 1980, 1981, 1982, 1983, 1984.

The need for such an assemblage of information arose from realization that although each participant had made significant contributions
to the understanding of laryngectomee rehabilitation, no attempt had
been made to integrate this information into a coherent volume of collected papers. This volume contains historical reviews of various aspects
of laryngectomy rehabilitation as well as of current research and
research considerations.

It was the intent of the editors to collate and organize rather than
modify the content of the contributed papers. The papers were prepared
by the faculty members and were presented by them essentially as they
appear in this volume.

If reference in a paper is made to a slide used during a presentation
at the Seminar, the content of the slide is now represented as a figure,
numbered to correspond with the textual reference. Also, if there are
references to audiotapes, their content has not been added to the text
except where interest is in the words spoken rather than in the type of
sound produced, and note has been made that a tape was used.

The sequence in which papers appear in this book does not necessarily reflect the order of steps in treatment of the laryngectomized
patient but rather the order in which they were presented.

All royalties from the proceeds of this book are directed to the
Mayo Foundation and are designated for continued laryngectomee rehabilitation programs or research.

Acknowledgments

The Laryngectomee Rehabilitation Seminar from which this edition was derived was supported by various groups, whose contributions are gratefully acknowledged:

The Section of Speech Pathology, Mayo Clinic
The Cancer Rehabilitation Program, Mayo Clinic
The Department of Otorhinolaryngology, Mayo Clinic
The American Cancer Society, Minnesota Division

We also want to extend a special thanks to all private contributors who helped support this Seminar financially and to those who donated freely of their talent and time.

A special thanks to all the laryngectomees and their spouses who devoted the week to attending and allowing therapy to be conducted with observation in order that methods of teaching by speech pathologists in training might be improved.

All proceeds from this volume are designated for future programs in laryngectomee rehabilitation at the Mayo Clinic.

Contributors

Walter Amster, Ph.D.
Chief, Audiology and Speech
  Pathology Service
Veterans Administration Medical
  Center
Syracuse, NY 13210

Eric D. Blom, Ph.D.
Head and Neck Surgery Associ-
  ates
Suite 780 Medical Tower Inn
1633 North Capital Avenue
Indianapolis, IN 46202

Zilpha T. Bosone, Ph.D.
Speech Pathologist
Veterans Administration Medical
  Center
Washington, DC 20422

P. Helbert Damsté, M.D.
Foniatrist, Academisch
  Ziekenhius Utrecht
Utrecht, Netherlands

Lawrence W. DeSanto, M.D.
Consultant, Department of
  Otorhinolaryngology
Mayo Clinic
Rochester, MN 55905

Marshall J. Duguay, Ph.D.
Professor of Communication
  Disorders
State University College
Buffalo, NY 14222

Douglas E. Fox, M.S.
Director of Speech Pathology
North Memorial Medical Center
3220 Lowry Avenue South
Minneapolis, MN 55422

Stuart I. Gilmore, Ph.D.
Professor, Department of
  Speech, Communication,
  Theatre, and Communication
  Disorders
College of Arts and Sciences
Louisiana State University
Baton Rouge, LA 70803

Melvin Hyman, Ph.D.
Professor Emeritus
Bowling Green State University
Codirector Hyman Speech, Lan-
  guage, and Hearing Services
Maumee, OH 43537

Robert L. Keith, M.S.
Associate, Speech Pathology
Mayo Clinic
Rochester, MN 55905

Dan Kelly, Ph.D.
Associate Professor
Speech and Hearing Institute
Health Science Center
Houston, TX 77030

Daniel E. Martin, Ph.D.
Director, Speech and Language
  Pathology
Lakeshore Ear, Nose and Throat
  Center, P.C.
19501 East Eight Mile Road
St. Clair Shores, MI 48080

Nancy Morozink, R.N.
Medical College at Ohio
C.S. 10008
Toledo, OH 43699

Bryan Neel, III, M.D., Ph.D.
Professor and Chairman,
    Department of Otorhinolary-
    ngology
Mayo Clinic
Rochester, MN 55905

Bruce W. Pearson, M.D.
Associate Professor, Department
    of Otorhinolaryngology
Mayo Clinic
Rochester, MN 55905

Shirley J. Salmon, Ph.D.
Speech Pathologist
Veterans Administration Medical
    Center
Kansas City, MO 64128

Ann Schutt, M.D.
Department of Physical Medi-
    cine and Rehabilitation
Mayo Clinic
Rochester, MN 55905

James C. Shanks, Ph.D.
Professor and Director, Speech
    Pathology Services
Indiana University School of
    Medicine
702 Barnhill Dr. A-56
Indianapolis, IN 46223

Paula A. Square, Ph.D.
Graduate Department of Speech
    Pathology
88 College Street
Toronto, Ontario
Canada M5G 1L4

Frances M. Stack, M.A.
Supervisor, Speech and Hearing
    Department
Christ Hospital
Oak Lawn, IL 60454

R. E. (Ed) Stone, Jr., Ph.D.
Associate Professor, Department
    of Otolaryngology—Head and
    Neck Surgery
Indiana University
School of Medicine
702 Barnhill Dr. A-56
Indianapolis, IN 46223

Bernd Weinberg, Ph.D.
Professor and Chairman
Department of Audiology and
    Speech Science
Purdue University
Lafayette, IN 47901

Daniel H. Zwitman, Ph.D.
Assistant Professor
Private practice/Hospital con-
    sultant
Los Angeles, CA 90024

Chapter **1**

Introduction: Self-Assessment of and Discussion Questions on Laryngectomee Rehabilitation

R. E. (Ed) Stone, Jr.

For the Florida Laryngectomee Association, 1984 was a significant year. It marked the end of many years of planning for and the initiation of a semiannual speech institute sponsored by that organization and the Florida Unit of the American Cancer Society. It is operated not only for speech pathologists but also for members of the Association with high degrees of speaking proficiency. Thus, it provides opportunity for members to demonstrate the culmination of their own rehabilitation by preparing to serve others in need of developing speech following laryngectomy.

Its greatest uniqueness possibly involves the two-phase nature of the program. The first half of the seminar is conducted in May, the second in October; both halves are similar to other speech seminars in format and curriculum. The instructional pace, however, is more comfortable for those not accustomed to classroom and clinical instruction. Expanded time for clinical observation and supervised practicum is permitted. The hiatus between the two sessions affords opportunity for observation of clinicians in the participants' own geographic areas and for self-instruction through assigned readings. The completion of the course is marked by the participants' individual demonstration of speaking acceptability and proficiency through the group's evaluation of their own videotaped performance of speaking and by their successful completion of a written test.

The assigned readings included the 1979 edition of the current text. Questions were developed for most of the chapters to help the readers focus and maintain reading interest. The answers submitted to the staff also served as assurance of the completion of the activity. Many participants felt that the questions additionally served as stimulus to meet with local clinicians for additional learning through discussion. Because of the perceived benefits derived from access to the questions, the participants of the institute encouraged their inclusion in the current edition of this text; they appear at the end of each chapter. The author of these questions and the editors do not claim that the items necessarily highlight only the most significant contributions of the writers of the various chapters. It is hoped, however, that readers will refer to the questions for a given chapter as preparation for their reading of that particular section. Then upon completion of the section the reader may return to the questions and compose their answers, rereading appropriate parts of the section if they choose in order to derive a response.

The final examination presented at the Florida Institute also appears at the end of the book. Previewing the test may help provide direction for study for someone being introduced to the field of laryngectomee rehabilitation. It also may be found helpful in preparing for tests such as that required for the Certificate of Clinical Competence by the American Speech-Language-Hearing Association and the International Association of Laryngectomees for listing of an individual in their directory of instructors. This current test, however, is not intended to reflect the breadth, depth, or format of examinations given by such organizations. Yet, seasoned clinicians taking the test have found it to be comprehensive and stimulating and have found that a few of the indicated answers may be suitable for debate. Whereas many of the answers to the questions will be found in this text, the reader may find need to refer to other sources of information in order to answer all the questions.

Chapter **2**

Historical Highlights: Laryngectomee Rehabilitation

Robert L. Keith and James C. Shanks

THE HISTORY OF LARYNGECTOMY*

Medical history sometimes does not do justice to those who have made important contributions to medical science. Perhaps this is due to the complexity involved in reviewing, analyzing, and differentiating the influences of those who have contributed, in some way, to a specific topic, such as the history of the laryngectomy procedure. It is not the intent of this article to give a detailed account of each historical event that has contributed to current laryngectomy surgical procedures but rather to illustrate a brief historical sketch of the most significant events that have led to the present day techniques.

A Review

In 1829, Albers, while conducting experiments on the physiology of the larynx, removed the entire larynx from a dog. The dog lived for 9 days. Schemes for human laryngectomy were allegedly proposed by Baron Bernard R.K. von Langenbeck (1875) and Eugene Keberle in 1856 (Rosenberg, 1971). However, it was not until 1866 that the actual operation was pioneered by Patrick H. Watson of Edinburgh. Below is an account of the earliest clinical case of a laryngectomy, reported by Watson (1881):

---

*The history of laryngectomy has been adapted from Keith, R. L., and Shanks, J. C. (1983). Laryngectomee rehabilitation: Past and present. In N. J. Lass (Ed.), *Speech and language: Advances in basic research and practice, Volume 9*. New York: Academic Press.

The first case was a gentleman, age 36, suffering from tertiary syphilis, with the destruction of the laryngeal cavity. I had previously, about a year before, opened his trachea to relieve him from the ulcerative condition. The larynx then healed, but the puckering gave rise to a condition of matters by which some portion of all fluid nutriment and saliva made its way into the trachea, and occasioned fits of spasmodic cough. Feeding by the tube did not prevent the saliva from passing down, and in almost every instance on its withdrawal some fluid regurgitated, and some of it passed into the trachea, etc. I operated by a linear incision, clearing the trachea, first above the tracheotomy opening, I cut it right across, introduced a gum elastic tube (a full-sized lithotomy tube) and tied the trachea upon it by a piece of silk ligature. I then cleared the soft parts from the larynx by means of the points of probe-pointed scissors, using them to pull away the structures when one could, and clipping with them when it was necessary. The patient rallied from the operation, but died some weeks afterward from pneumonia. (p. 255)

Since the patient operated on by Watson died, the procedure was generally condemned; nevertheless, the idea had been instilled in the literature. The fundamentals were grasped by Vincenz Czerny (1870), of Heidelberg, who executed effective laryngectomies on dogs. Czerny was a young surgical assistant of Billroth (Donagan, 1965).

Early efforts at laryngectomy, therefore, were discouraging and until 1900 progress was very slow. Glück and Soerensen (1920, 1922) in Berlin probably did the most to improve and develop the technical details of laryngectomy. Starting with and abandoning a two-stage operation, they developed an approach on a wide-field basis with open exposure of the neck. They developed the plan of removing the larynx from above and downward and of closing the pharyngeal defect before amputation of the larynx (Jesberg, 1960).

The illustrious Theodore Billroth was born at Bergen on an island in the Baltic Sea on April 26, 1829. Billroth showed little early brilliance and needed coaching from tutors, one of whom described him as being slow to comprehend and as having stumbling speech. Encouraged to study medicine by his family, Billroth enrolled at the University of Gottingen, where he became interested in surgical pathology and physiology. He graduated in 1852, his thesis being, "The nature and cause of pulmonary affections produced by bilateral vagal section" (Weir, 1973).

Billroth, then 25 years old, was appointed to an assistantship at the Langenbeck Clinic. He remained there for 6 years, during which time he became engrossed in surgical pathology and published many papers. After many unsuccessful bids for surgical posts, he was eventually appointed to the Chair of Surgery at Zurich on Christmas Eve, 1859.

Billroth's pupils at first numbered but ten, and it has been said that his private practice was insufficient to pay for his morning cups of coffee. However, his reputation as a teacher at Zurich continued to grow. As part of his interest in music he studied the viola, which enabled him to take part in a variety of string quartets. He also wrote music critiques for the "Neue Aurische Zeitung." Through this budding musical talent, he met Johannes Brahms, who later became his close friend.

In 1867 Franz Shuh retired and vacated the Chair of Surgery in Vienna. Billroth applied for the position with some hesitation, as histories on both sides of his family indicated a strong likelihood of pulmonary tuberculosis, and Vienna at that time was certainly less sanitary than Zurich. However, his desire and ambition for the surgical post overruled his fears of family illness. Thus, Billroth and his family moved to Vienna to accept the position vacated by Shuh. A few years after he began his post, tragedy struck when his second daughter died of tuberculosis.

In the beginning, the Viennese were not favorably disposed to Billroth's ambitious nature. Students complained that he did not teach surgery as a complete science but rather that there was much that was indefinite and unknown. Because Billroth tried to chart the unknown, his clinic became a surgical mecca during the 26 years that he worked in Vienna. He performed the first excision of the esophagus in 1872, the first successful laryngectomy for cancer in 1873, the first subtotal colectomy in 1879, and the first gastrectomy in 1881.

For historical interest, here is a review of the case of the first successful laryngectomy as reported by Carl Gussenbauer, Billroth's assistant (Schechter and Morfit, 1965).

> The entire procedure of total laryngectomy took Billroth one hour and 45 minutes.
>
> The patient, a 36-year-old teacher with a tumor below the true vocal cords, was first treated with multiple cauterizations and biopsies (microscopic report: epithelial carcinoma of the larynx). On November 21, 1873 (after a preliminary tracheotomy), Dr. Billroth performed a laryngofissure and removed the tumor with scissors and sharp curette. The main tumor was situated on the left side, so the surgeon was able to preserve the right vocal cord; the wound edges were approximated with tape. On the second postoperative day the patient began to have septic temperatures, and infection developed in the wound, which was treated with a preparation containing silver nitrate; on the seventh postoperative day the patient was up and about, and two days later a high degree of dyspnea developed. The wound was reopened and examination revealed that the growth had recurred.
>
> In an attempt to curette the larynx, Dr. Billroth reopened the wound, but discovered that the malignant growth had invaded the cartilage. The patient was awakened, informed of the necessity to remove the larynx and again anesthetized. The technique consisted mainly in dull dissection of the larynx on both sides while the assistant exerted a pull on the larynx. The trachea was divided just below the cricoid, the larynx was pulled forward and up, and dissected from the anterior wall of the esophagus; the thyrohyoid membrane was divided last. The anesthesia was not sufficient, and the operative procedure was frequently interrupted by strong coughing

spells during which blood in rather large amounts was expelled from the trachea. The bleeding was controlled by pressure with large sponges.

The growth must have been quite large since, after examining the specimen, Dr. Billroth decided to remove most of the epiglottis and the first two tracheal rings. The tracheal stoma was fixed to the skin with one suture on each side and the opening into the pharynx was made smaller by applying three sutures. Four hours later, during a bout of coughing, a profuse hemorrhage developed from the left superior laryngeal artery which required a ligature. Dr. Gussenbauer remarked about the large amounts of coagulated blood which the patient had coughed up without having had great signs of dyspnea. Three days after the operation the sutures and the ligatures were removed. The wound represented a groove with the tracheal stoma in the lower end and the opening into the pharynx on the upper end.

Fortunately, the patient escaped all secondary complications, such as shock, aspiration, pneumonia, mediastinitis, sepsis, meningitis, tetanus and large abscess. The pharyngeal fistula began to close early, and the patient was started on a soft diet on the eighth post-operative day; the gastric feeding tube was removed on the eighteenth day. The patient was dismissed on March 3, 1874, after he had learned how to use the artificial larynx designed by Dr. Gussenbauer. . . . Unfortunately, a recurrence of the lesion with metastatic nodes developed, and the patient died approximately one year after the operation. (p. 465)

The second recorded total laryngectomy for carcinoma of the larynx was performed in April, 1874, by Heine of Prague (Schüller, 1880). The patient survived for six months; in June of the same year Maas (1876a) of Breslau performed the third laryngectomy. Pneumonia developed, and the patient died 2 weeks after the operation. Schmidt (1875) of Frankfurt performed the fourth laryngectomy on August 12, 1874, but the 56 year old patient survived only 4 days and died of collapse. Billroth performed his second total laryngectomy combined with removal of a small goiter on November 11, 1874, on a 54 year old man. The patient suffered preoperatively of bronchitis and died of bronchopneumonia on the fourth day after operation.

The first successful laryngectomy with many years of survival was performed on a 24 year old man in 1875 in Italy by Bottini (Schüller, 1880). The lesion was a mixed round and spindle cell sarcoma. The patient lost a large amount of blood and erysipelas developed; but he survived, and for years he was able to continue his work as a mail carrier in a mountainous region.

Notable advance in the technique of total laryngectomy was reported by von Langenbeck (1875). On July 28, 1875, he presented an unusual specimen during the meeting of the Medical Society in Berlin. It included the entire larynx with epiglottis, hyoid, a third of the tongue, the anterior and lateral portion of the pharynx, a portion of the esophagus, both submaxillary glands, and lymphatic tissue from the submaxillary triangle. A 57 year old man with carcinoma of the larynx had undergone tracheotomy but refused to have a laryngectomy. He returned 7 months after the operation and on July 21 was operated on by von Langenbeck. The incision was T-shaped. The dissection was performed from above so that the trachea was severed last. The time involved was a little more than 2 hours. It is recorded that the operation was done as exactly as an anatomic dissection, and in spite of the extensive region involved, the blood loss was unusually small because each vessel was ligated prior to being cut. Forty-one ligatures were made, including both external carotid arteries, lingual, facial, superior thyroids, and so on. The patient survived for 4 months but died on November 23, 1875, of collapse during an attempt to remove the metastatically involved glands of the left side of the neck. This operation of von Langenbeck could be considered the forerunner of the combined wide-field laryngectomy and neck dissection.

The *Journal of Laryngology and Rhinology* in December 1887 published a review of the first 103 total laryngectomies for cancer. Of these, at least 40 (39 per cent) patients died of the immediate effects of the operation within a period varying from a few hours to 8 weeks, over half of them as a result of pneumonia. Recurrence was noted in 21 (20 per cent) patients, the shortest time being in 2 months, the average being 6 months. One patient died suddenly of suffocation 8 months after his laryngectomy. There was no evidence of recurrence at postmortem, but a feather used to clean the tracheostomy cannula was found in the trachea (Newman, 1886a).

Although Billroth was credited with the first total laryngectomy for cancer, he personally operated on only four patients out of the reported 103. He said, "At my years I can be regarded only as a useful direction pointer—and who can point in the direction of the right way?" (Newman, 1886b).

Billroth drew some conclusions from the experience of the total laryngectomy: first, it should have been performed at an earlier stage of the disease; and second, to prevent recurrence the epiglottis should be removed with the tumor. He believed strongly in the value of meticulous documentation of cases and pioneered the importance of accurate statistics. Billroth published 140 papers, and his major work, "Allgemeine chirurgische Pathologie und Therapie," was translated into nine languages.

Billroth laid the foundations on which present-day surgery is built, and his teachings were furthered by his pupils, some of whom were Czerny, Gussenbauer, Mikulicz, and Woeffler; these men were later to hold Chairs of Surgery throughout Europe (Weir, 1973).

Following a severe attack of pneumonia in 1887, Billroth became increasingly troubled with congestive heart failure. He went to Italy in December of 1893 in the hopes of regaining his health, but he never was to return to his adopted Vienna. He died at Abbazia on the Adriatic on February 5, 1894.

Total laryngectomy was not regarded as successful unless the patient's life was extended at least 12 months. It was believed that this length of survival could be achieved by tracheotomy alone. Only 9 (8.5 per cent) of the 103 cases fulfilled these criteria, the longest length of survival being 5 years. The surgeon in one third of the successful cases was Carl Gussenbauer.

The unusually high mortality rate and the minimal incidence of cures provoked a number of physicians to question seriously whether surgery for cancer of the larynx was justified. Such skepticism spread throughout Europe, painting a gloomy future for laryngectomy surgery. As Paul Kock, a noted authority then put it, "The surgeon's skill is sometimes shown by the patient not dying under his knife" (Schechter and Morfit, 1965, p. 467).

Some of the comments made portrayed an inauspicious beginning. Solis-Cohen in one survey made the statement: "Laryngectomy has not tended to the prolongation of life; and the prolonged existence of a very few cases seemed purchasable only at the sacrifice of the remnant of existence of many others" (Schechter and Morfit, 1965, p. 467).

These issues were discussed at a meeting of the International Medical Congress, where opinions were sharply divided on the merits of laryngectomy. Solis-Cohen again reiterated: "I am afraid that there is a tendency to the operation being overrated, if we do not appreciate the usually miserable conditions of the patients who have undergone it successfully, for there is an important difference between 'recovery' and mere 'survival after operation' " (Schechter and Morfit, 1965, p. 467).

The renowned Sir Felix Semon of London remarked:

> I cannot help feeling that in the whole question one important fault is committed by a good many members of the profession, namely, that of confounding the two very different ideas of the "possibility" and of the "justifiability" of an operation. I am astonished to hear . . . taken for granted that as the diagnosis of carcinoma of the larynx is established, under all circumstances extirpation should forthwith be proceeded with. . . . I desire to say that I have no theoretical objections against the operation as such . . . but that I consider it a duty to protest against its indiscriminate recommendation in all cases of carcinoma, a recommendation which, I think, is with difficulty theoretically justifiable, and which is certainly practically not justified. I wish to protest still stronger against the operation in cases of recurrent papillomata, a subject on which I shall have to say more on a future occasion.
>
> (Schechter and Morfit, 1965, p. 467)

Remarks made by Professor K. Burow refer not only to the choice of treatment but to information given the patient:

> In my opinion it is better not to perform total extirpation on patients with carcinoma of the larynx, but if the case be a suitable one, to make endolaryngeal, even if only partial, excision, and to tracheotomize if dyspnea makes its appearance. Such patients live on the average of two and a half years from the beginning of the affection, and one and a half after tracheotomy, and are frequently able to follow their vocation for a considerable time. If the operation of extirpation is to be performed at all in such cases, it certainly ought to be done at a very early period; but will we in such an early period, when the symptoms are still slight, get the patient's permission, unless we tell them the malignant nature of their affection? By doing so, we make the rest of their existence miserable, and deprive them of the desirable self-deception in which we can keep them for a long time if we only temporize—i.e., tracheotomize. These are my present views, but it is, of course possible that new observations in coming years may lead me to modify them.
>
> (Schechter and Morfit, 1965, p. 467)

Czerny's statements probably were as complete and encompassing as any made:

> The question of extirpation of the larynx presents such difficulties that I have come here not to teach but to learn. Fully as I recognize the right of existence of the skeptical party which has to separate the chaff from the grain, yet I must pertinently claim for my less skeptical party the recognition that we ask, quite as conscientiously as the other side, in every individual case: "What would you wish to be done unto yourself under the circumstances of the case?" If we look at Dr. Foulis' tables, it is true that we should come to the conclusion the extirpation of the larynx was but of little value, only five of all who had been operated on being alive now. But let us be true to ourselves, and confess that of all patients operated on for carcinoma but few have been permanently cured. As long as we do not possess a treatment as efficient against malignant tumors as the knife, we really must be consistent, and not refuse the patient, who is irreparably lost through his laryngeal carcinoma, the possible advantage of the operation. As to the permissibility of the extirpation of the larynx, the state of the patient after the operation is, it is true, of decisive importance, and we have just heard that an American patient was very, very miserable after its performance. I have performed the operation three times on men, and do not consider it so very dangerous, but the after-treatment is one of the most difficult tasks that could be given to the surgeon, and the functional results vary very much according to the stage of the disease. But even in my first two cases, in which I was only able to operate late, as the diagnosis was for a long time uncertain, yet there is the advantage that the pains, which before the operation rendered taking of food almost impossible, ceased afterwards. It is necessary to remove much skin, the cicatricial contraction is not sufficient to cover completely the space around the artificial larynx; under these circumstances, taking food, especially fluid, is often impeded. In my last case, which unfortunately is only of three months date, the state of affairs is so favorable, and the artificial vocal apparatus

answers so admirably, that the patient is about to resume his duties as to superior judge. Let us hope that he may fulfill them for a long time! The question, in functional respects, as to the preservation of the epiglottis, is not yet decided. The results vary much according to the case and according to the patient's individuality, which as the greatest influence upon the functional success. For all this it follows that the whole question is a most difficult one, and which will not be ripe for decision for a long time to come. I believe that extirpation of the larynx, apart from other indications, is demanded as soon as the diagnosis of a malignant new formation, be it by means of the laryngoscope or by microscopic examination of removed particles, is attained, and as soon as it becomes visible that after failure of other remedies the malady irresistibly progresses, and unquestionably endangers the life of the patient.

(Schechter and Morfit, 1965, p. 468)

The principle of the postoperative treatment in those early days was to leave the wound wide open and to pack it with sponges soaked in carbol solution to soak up wound secretions. The outer dressing produced counterpressure to eliminate dead space. The trachea was secured to the skin with silk sutures and the tracheal cannula was inserted. The dressings were changed daily and the wound was irrigated with carbol solution.

The oral cavity was washed out several times daily with disinfectant solutions, and the patient was fed by a gastric tube. A steam kettle evaporating turpentine oil with carbolic acid and glycerine was placed in the room.

In January 1887, when he was 58 years old, the Emperor Frederick III developed the first symptoms of gradually increasing hoarseness following a common cold. Examination of the larynx was carried out in March by Professor Gerhardt of Berlin. His findings indicated a polypoid swelling on the edge of the left vocal cord, slightly anterior to the vocal process. There was also redness of both cords, but the motility was unimpaired. Galvanocautery was used several times without improvement. After many biopsies, and many problems with increasing obstruction and continued hoarseness, a tracheotomy became necessary on February 8, 1888. On June 15, 1888, he died from complications with the tracheostomy, metastases, aspiration pneumonia, and pulmonary gangrene. In this case the necessity for biopsy was argued. For the next 50 years arguments for and against biopsy continued with the contention that biopsy contributed to the spread of cancer. This controversy influenced the course of laryngology through the first quarter of the twentieth century (Holinger, 1975).

It can be seen from the aforementioned review that the first laryngectomy was not an isolated event in the history of laryngology. Therapy was hampered by lack of adequate understanding of the pathology of laryngeal lesions, and it should also be remembered that direct laryngoscopy and biopsy postdated the first laryngectomy by approximately 20 years. The first laryngectomy was really the culmination of nearly half a century of groping toward an understanding of the pathology, its natural history, and a more effective management regimen of cancer of the larynx. And so the question continues today ever-increasing knowledge of the larynx and its diseases is pursued.

Predicting the future of laryngectomy in terms of surgical procedures and the nature of cancer at a fundamental and etiological level is probably hazardous at this time. It would seem that for the predictable future, fundamental advances will continue. It is noteworthy that the earliest operations were not applied to malignant neoplastic disease, but were originally performed for nonmalignant conditions. It may be that the need for partial and total laryngectomy will outlast the application to carcinoma (Jesberg, 1960).

The historical data given are as accurate as possible but inevitably are incomplete; any attempt at completeness would necessitate extensive research and be astoundingly expensive, and this book would become impractical and unwieldy. With the aid of a brief historical outline and an extensive bibliography (see References and Additional Readings) the individual who desires more information may delve into the topic in greater depth.

Historical Highlights before 1900

400 B.C.   Hippocrates said, in effect, "A tumor is a tumor, a superabundance of tissue, and therefore should be removed" (Jackson and Jackson, 1939, p. 214). Though many great clinicians of the time recognized differences in tumors when opened and during the clinical course, they did not have microscopes and thus histological evaluation was impossible (Jackson and Jackson, 1939).

1743   The first authenticated attempt at examining the larynx was by Leveret, a French accoucheur, who devised a bent mirror for examination of the throat (Albers, 1829).

1829   H. Albers (1829) did experimental laryngectomies, partial and total on dogs, but there seems to be no record of his attempting the operation on human beings.

1829   Babington (1829) presented the first effective invention that could be called a laryngoscope to the Hunterian Society of London.

1833   The first laryngofissure was performed for tumor treated with cautery (Rosenberg, 1971).

1837   A. Trousseau (1837), the great clinician and observer of diseases of the passage, reported a case of "carcinomatous laryngeal phthisis," making a distinction between tuberculosis and carcinoma.

1851   The first laryngofissure was performed for excision of tumor (Rosenberg, 1971).

1854   The indirect laryngoscopy was discovered by a Spanish singing teacher, Manuel Garcia (Rosenberg, 1971).

1858   Virchow's (1858) *Cellular Pathology* established the modern era of distinguishing tumors by their cellular structure.

1858   Krackowizer, an Austrian immigrant, introduced the art of laryngoscopy to North America when he came to New York (Delavan, 1912).

1866   A laryngectomy was done by Patrick Heron Watson (1881) of Edinburgh because of syphilis.

1867   Joseph Lister (1867) founded antiseptic surgery and laid the foundation for aseptic surgery. Although not generally accepted until about 1884, it soon thereafter had a marked effect on the results of laryngectomy as on every other operation. Surgeons of today to whom asepsis and use of sterile gloves are a routine, nerve-cell habit shudder to read of an operation done in 1886 and described in a standard textbook of the time: "Laryngectomy was affected by (a) further careful and thorough separation of the attachments to the pharynx by raspatory, knife-handle, and fingernail; (b) division" and so on. That "fingernail" is haunting (Jackson and Jackson, 1939).

1870   V. Czerny (1870), interested in the total extirpation done by Patrick Watson, experimented with total laryngectomy on dogs and assisted Billroth in the first recorded laryngectomy for cancer.

1871   Morrell MacKenzie (1880), indirect laryngeal biopsy.

1873   C. A. T. Billroth (Billroth and Gussenbauer, 1874). Laryngectomy, male patient, aged 36, carcinoma. Recurrence fatal 7 months later.

1874   C. Heine (1876). Laryngectomy, male patient, aged 50, carcinoma. Recurrence fatal 6 months later.

1874   Morris Schmidt (1875). Laryngectomy, male patient, aged 56, carcinoma. Operative death fifth day.

1875   E. Bottini (1875). Laryngectomy, male patient, aged 24, sarcoma. Two years later well and at work as a mail carrier on a long rural route.

1875   C. A. T. Billroth (Billroth and Gussenbauer, 1874). Laryngectomy, male patient, aged 54, carcinoma. Death from pneumonia 2 days later.

1875   Karl W. E. J. Schönborn (1875). Laryngectomy, male patient, aged 72, carcinoma. Death a few days later.

1875   B. R. K. von Langenbeck (1875). Laryngectomy, male patient, aged 57, carcinoma. Recurrence, cervical lymphatics, fatal 4 months later.

1876   C. Reyher (1877). Laryngectomy, male patient, aged 60, carcinoma of vocal cords. Death eleventh day, hypostatic pneumonia.

1876   H. Gerdes (1877). Laryngectomy, male patient, aged 76, carcinoma. Death, collapse, fourth day.

1876   H. Maas (1876b). Laryngectomy, male patient, aged 50, epithelioma. Recurrence, base of tongue, 3 months later. Fatal, 6 months. In another case the patient died on the fourteenth day (Maas, 1876a).

1877   E. Bottini (1878). Laryngectomy, male patient, aged 48, epithelioma. Death third day, double pneumonia.

1877   D. F. Foulis (1877a). Laryngectomy, male patient, aged 28, mixed papilloma and spindle-cell sarcoma. Death, phthisis pulmonalis, a year and a half later.

1877   J. K. Kosinski (1877). Laryngectomy, female patient, aged 36, epithelioma involving skin. Recurrence, death, 9 months after operation.

1878   Billroth performed the first conservative hemilaryngectomy (Rosenberg, 1971).

1878   Paul von Bruns (1878). Laryngectomy, male patient, aged 54, epithelioma. Recurrence fatal 9 months later.

1878   E. Bottini reported a bloodless laryngectomy by means of galvanocautery. The patient died on the third day from double pneumonia (Jackson and Jackson, 1939).

1879   Lange (1880) became the first to perform laryngectomy in America.

1879   The American Laryngological Association was founded, inaugurating the study of the larynx as a specialty. Jackson and Jackson (1939) reported that during the 60 years (to 1939) that elapsed, almost every meeting contributed something to the study of the great problem of cancer of the larynx.

1880   H. Schüller (1880) described his technique of laryngectomy from above downward, which included placing his finger in the patient's mouth to guide the point of the knife so as to include the epiglottis with the exsected larynx.

1880   Morell Mackenzie (1880) summarized results of laryngectomy by various operators. Of 19 patients, 1 died of passage of a bougie into the mediastinum, 8 died of collapse or pneumonia within a fortnight, 7 had recurrence within a few months, and 1 lived 18 months. Two cases out of 19 were lasting cures. Mackenzie thought this good work and quoted Koch, "The skill of the surgeon is, in some cases, shown by the patient not dying under his knife."

1881   D. F. Foulis (1881), collective research. Of the first 25 laryngectomized patients none survived a year.

1887   Morell Mackenzie and Crown Prince Frederick of Germany. Biopsy by indirect laryngoscopy benign, but the patient soon died of this malignancy (Rosenberg, 1971).

1892   George Crile (1947) performed the first laryngectomy in the United States; 34 surgeries were performed in the next 20 years (Crile, 1913).

1892   Solis-Cohen (1892a, 1892b, 1892c) of Philadelphia performed the first successful laryngectomy in America.

1880–   The operative mortality of total laryngectomy was nearly 50
1900   per cent (Rosenberg, 1971).

1925   After half a century, laryngectomy became accepted (Rosenberg, 1971).

HISTORY OF THE ARTIFICIAL LARYNX

Not surprisingly, the era of the artificial larynx coincides with the period when the larynx was removed surgically to preserve life. What may be rather surprising is that the early versions of an artificial larynx also sought to preserve life. For example, laryngeal extirpation opened paths communicating upward into the hypopharynx and downward into the respiratory tree. To restore voice early laryngologists tried to dam the air stream up from the lungs. To block the route down from the throat was to prevent aspiration of food and liquid. The hazard of aspiration still remains to threaten efforts to establish connections between the respiratory and alimentary systems.

The forms of artificial larynxes have varied. At least three variables are involved: (1) What is the sound source? (2) How does generated sound get delivered into the vocal tract? (3) What problems of health are created by the particular artificial larynx in question?

In the past 1¼ centuries the engineer and the surgeon have collaborated in the pursuit of life and voice. The quest continues. The following account highlights some of the more memorable efforts.

The artificial larynx is a prosthesis meant to replace the diseased or damaged larynx when it has been surgically removed or when, as a result of a disease process, it can no longer produce phonation. As far as is known, the first description of a laryngeal prosthesis was given by the Czech physiologist Johann Nepomuk Czermak (1859). In 1859 Czermak reported in the Imperial Academy of Sciences in Vienna on an 18 year old girl who had been tracheotomized because of a complete laryngeal stenosis. Czermak provided her with an artificial larynx. In the tube there was a reed, that is, a small flexible tongue of metal that could be set into vibration by blowing air through the tube. And so began the history of the artificial larynxes. In 1859, while studying a case of complete laryngeal stenosis, Czermak conceived the idea that the expiratory current of air issuing from the tracheal cannula that the patient carried could be used to produce voice and speech if it were conducted into the mouth through a tube containing a reed capable of vibrating. Brucke (Czermak, 1859) constructed an apparatus based on Czermak's idea. Using it the patient could, with sufficient effort, produce single syllables. A few years later Czerny (1870), experimenting with animals, contrived several different machines. Billroth, who in 1873 performed the first successful total extirpation of the larynx, following Czerny's lead, worked out with Eiselberg a laryngeal prosthesis in which the tone was conducted through the tracheal opening into the pharyngeal cavity. His artificial larynx consisted of three parts: a tracheal, a pharyngeal, and a phonation cannula. The phonation cannula was set inside the pharyngeal cannula. The tone-producing reed, which was thrown into vibration by the expiratory breath, was set in the phonation cannula. The tone, when projected into the resonating space above, could be transformed into the sounds of articulate value (Billroth and Gussenbauer, 1874).

Foulis (1877a) developed a device for a patient (Fig. 2–1). He used a vulcanite laryngeal tube that was fitted, and by means of a simple arrangement, a vibrating reed was introduced that took the place of the vocal cord. The patient spoke in a resonant, loud, and clear but monotonous voice.

Within the year this device was further improved. Bruns (1881), trying to make the artificial tone sound like the natural voice, discarded the rigid laryngeal tube and replaced it with a flexible semirubber membrane. Stoerk (1880, 1887, 1896) used an ordinary reed pipe placed between the teeth and connected to the tracheal cannula by means of a rubber tube through which the expiratory breath current went to the reed. The patient articulated at the same time that he produced the tone.

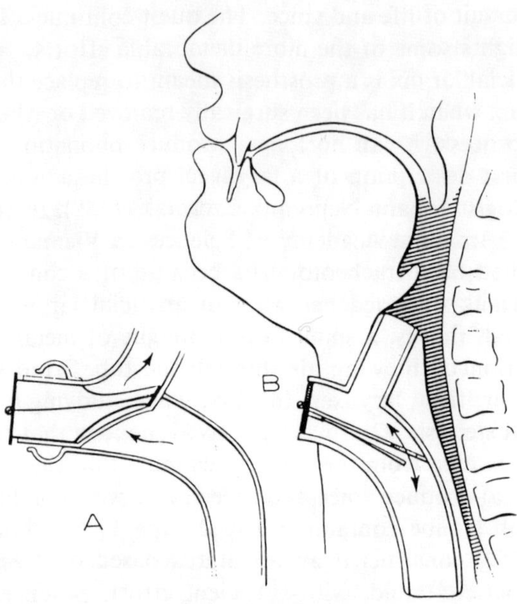

Figure 2–1. *A,* Gussenbauer's "artificial larynx" with a metal membrane. *B,* Modification by Foulis. (Adapted from M. Schuller, 1880).

If he wished, he could sound the reed by means of a double balloon bulb specially adapted for it. The purpose of other improvements, such as Wolff's (1893a, 1893b), was to prevent the accumulation of secretions and particles of food. Other improvements reduced irritation by the machine. Cases of recurrence had been reported in which the irritation of tissue in contact with the apparatus was suspected as a contributing etiological factor.

With this in mind, Gottstein (1900) took up the ideas of Czermak and Stoerk again. His apparatus had an accessory piece adapted for the trachea that was connected to a flexible rubber tube. The wall of the tube was held rigid by means of a spiral wire within it. To the free end of this rubber tube was attached a metal piece placed as to lie behind the last molar. Air from the trachea reached the pharyngeal cavity by this route. The voice-producing mechanism was placed in the rubber tube.

Without any knowledge of Stoerk's apparatus, which had already been described, Hochenegg (1892), after some experiments, prepared an apparatus similar to it but differing primarily in the manner of application. The artificial breath stream for activation of the reed was placed through the nose into the oropharynx, and its source, instead of being a small balloon, consisted of a bellows fastened to the left side of the patient's thorax. Hochenegg had to abandon his first idea of activating the reed by the use of pulmonary air itself. The patient was found to lack force of breath sufficient to initiate a tone and, in addition, the instrument made him cough violently. When Glück and his co-workers appeared on the scene, they established for themselves a place in the history of laryngeal surgery. They made fundamental modifications of the technique used in total extirpation of the larynx and invented and constructed laryngeal prostheses ingenious enough to influence radically the patient's postoperative social status. Glück (1904, 1908, 1913, 1921) constructed a whole series of cannulas and artificial larynges activated by bellows. His later models, however, were made to depend on the lungs for the air, the vibrating mechanism being placed within an endonasal or endo-oral metal olive. He also prepared tiny voice boxes connected with bellows and compression chambers, which could be activated mechanically or electrically. These voice boxes permitted the production of speech by means of a similar sensitive vocal olive. Later, he prepared gramophone records on which was registered a sustained tone beautifully sung by a good singer; these gramophones were capable of amplification by means of a diaphragm. This tone, conducted through a tube in the patient's mouth, could be articulated and used for the purposes of speech. Interruption of the tone was controlled by special adjustments. Tests with this method showed much promise, but its further development seems to have met some obstacle. Perhaps the increasing evidence of the possibility of developing a vicarious voice physiologically influenced its demise.

The problem of producing an artificial voice varied with the technique of laryngectomy. As it is now performed, laryngectomy excludes any communication between the trachea and the pharynx. Some of the laryngeal prostheses are remarkably skillfully contrived. Onodi (1918) constructed a model in which tone was carried by means of a microphone into the nasopharynx. The devices of Mackenty (Fletcher, 1929), Leyro Diaz (1924), Casadesus (1923), Tapia (1914), and Hinojar (1923) are based on the same fundamental idea, but naturally each man considered his own device to be the best. Detailed descriptions of all these devices were given in the respective articles as they were published.

The disadvantages of the older laryngeal prostheses appeared to be many. Some of the devices were believed to irritate the tissue and to account for occasional cases of recurrence, according to Kallen (1931). Many produced shrill and squeaky sounds. Others caused respiratory complications. All increased salivation unpleasantly. The actual speaking situations were rather painful and trying. Although later apparatuses made things easier for the patient, the cost was, for many patients, prohibitive and was one obstacle in the lack of widespread use. As noted by Kallen, even if the patient could afford one, it often failed to work and caused him much anxiety and excitement.

The prime reason for not using even the best of these devices, however, is that there is hardly a patient who, within a relatively short time, cannot be taught to learn to use a fair voice capable of a degree of modulation. This, when articulated, becomes a speech more natural and "human," more clearly enunciated. Kallen (1931) goes on to note that for psychological reasons, the mastery of a vicarious voice is of great importance in maintaining the health of the laryngectomized person's psyche. A mechanical device can never have the same psychological significance as a living organ with a newly developed function; such a function becomes entirely identified with the individual personality. However, this is not as likely when a mechanical device is used.

In 1920, the first notable improvement in this country was made by J. E. Mackenty of New York (Fletcher, 1929). He used the rubber band as a reed transversely but discovered that a soft rubber mouth piece was a great aid in improving the quality of the voice. The case of his instrument was made of hard rubber.

In 1924, Mackenty enlisted the cooperation of the Western Electric Company in the development of a larynx that overcame to a great extent the defects of the other devices. This device delivered a low-pitched, somewhat guttural but strikingly human voice. His ideas on the best way to accomplish this, namely, by a transverse rubber band, were not at first accepted because the Western Electric Company felt that a better voice could be developed with reeds. Dr. Mackenty had tried reeds and had failed, and he indicated that the reed requires too strong a current of air to vibrate it, consequently tiring the patient, and the voice it produces is a musical and singing tone, thought to be disagreeable to the ear. His plans were adopted and partially worked out. The result was a very useful instrument, not embarrassing, burdensome, impractical, delicate, or difficult to repair (Fletcher, 1929). In the hands of any one of ordinary mechanical ability it worked well.

Pollock and Lederer (1922) described an artificial larynx: "An artificial larynx was presented, which consisted in the main of a trachea cannula and a pharyngeal cannula, the latter being made of flexible rubber in order to prevent irritation of the epiglottis that results when a metallic tube, which does not give, is used. A diaphragm arrangement between the two allows for phonation" (p. 480).

McKesson (1927) described a mechanical larynx in the *Journal of the American Medical Association*. This artificial larynx employed the reed element, which was a thin rubber band inserted transversely in the container.

In 1931, Charles Sheard of the Mayo Clinic presented a new artificial larynx. He claimed that it could operate at all times and under all circumstances, would permit ordinary or loud speaking, would possess a given fundamental pitch or frequency that could be made as high or as low as desired, and could be reproduced by replacement of the reed in case the reed was broken or damaged in cleaning (Sheard, 1931).

Goldstein (1932) described the modification of an artificial larynx to the American Laryngological Association. He also presented metal disks for the permanent recording or reproduction of speech of a patient. He presented a new terminal on the rubber connecting tube to be applied to the larynx after the tracheal cannula has been removed; it consisted of a half a rubber sponge ball with the center punched out, adapted to a tracheal fistula. He removed the rubber flange underneath the metallic reed and substituted a small fiberlike flange with small holes in it in order to avoid having the reed adhere to the base by moisture.

In 1936, Iglauer presented a new artificial larynx, with a patient demonstrating its use. It was much the same as that made by the Bell Telephone Company except that a thumb screw regulated the movements of the reed (Iglauer, 1936).

The first instrument made for the Bell Telephone Laboratories was made by George W. Burchett of Peekskill, New York and patented in December 1931 (Hanson, 1940). The second instrument was invented by Robert R. Riesz (1930) of New York. In 1932 and 1933, Bell modified the instrument with reed-adjusting devices.

The Laboratories' initial efforts resulted in an instrument that employed rubber bands stretched in a manner to simulate the vocal cords and was designated Type 1A. These rubber bands deteriorated rapidly and were a source of considerable dissatisfaction. Consequently, during 1929 a new larynx, designated Type 2A, was developed that incorporated several refinements, including the substitution of a vibrating metallic reed for the elastic bands. This model, with minor changes, was manufactured by Western Electric Company for many years (Barney, Haworth, and Dunn, 1959).

In 1923, Brown (1925) made an attempt to fashion an artificial larynx by means of a "tube flap." A very good voice resulted; however, the difficulty caused by the escape of saliva made him discard the method. This also required that the patient have both the pharyngeal opening and the tracheal opening. With considerable experimentation he was able to control the leakage of saliva, and the patient could wear the device up to 3 hours at a time.

The principles of the electronic larynx can be demonstrated by mouthing words while placing any vibrator source on the neck. The vibrator is the sound source, which is activated electrically. In 1942, Wright (Rigrodsky, Lerman, and Morrison, 1971), using this principle with the Aurex Corporation and later the Kett Engineering Corporation, developed and manufactured instruments. The Aurex Model M 410 used a cord connecting the battery and the vibrator unit, whereas the Aurex Model M 520 eliminated the cord by encasing the battery into the instrument. Kett Mark I required a cord and C-2 batteries; Mark II and Mark III were cordless. The Mark III utilized a nickel cadmium battery capable of being recharged. In 1960, the Bell Telephone Company developed a cordless, transistorized electronic larynx that has an octave pitch when the "on" switch is depressed completely (Haworth, 1960).

Cooper, a dentist, developed two variations of the electronic larynx (Cooper and Millard, 1959). The Cooper-Rand Speech Aid combines the principle of electrically generated sound with the sound being conducted via a tube inserted in the mouth. The other Cooper instrument used the principle of battery power carried by wire to a transducer located on a denture. Tait and Tait (1959) came out with a similar instrument, known as the Oral Vibrator. Ticchioni used an electromagnet fitted into the bowl of a pipe and powered with a battery source so that sound could be delivered through the pipe to the mouth.

Since this is not a text on the artificial larynx but rather is an article on the use of the artificial larynx (Martin, 1963), its history will not be belabored. Highlights are given in the following section. It is important, however, to know about the evolution of this device. Today there are many devices with many modifications that can effectively serve the laryngectomee. The reader is referred to an excellent booklet edited by Lebrun (1973) for a detailed history of the development of the artificial larynx.

Historical Highlights of Artificial Larynxes

1859   Czermak described a laryngeal prosthesis used for an 18 year old girl who had been tracheotomized because of laryngeal stenosis. A reed device used air from the lungs directed into the corner of the mouth via a thin tube.

1873   First successful laryngectomy by Billroth (1874). Josef Leiter, an instrument maker, devised for Billroth's patient an artificial larynx that could be inserted between the trachea and the pharynx. Actually, it was an internal pneumatic laryngeal prosthesis.

1874   Carl Gussenbauer (Billroth, 1874) improved on Leiter's prosthesis (Fig. 2–1A). Gussenbauer replaced Leiter's fixed phona-

tory cannula with a reed case placed nearer to the tracheostoma and easily withdrawn.

1877   David Foulis (1877b) had a new voice tube designed with the help of Dr. Irvine and the assistance of a dentist named Fould. It was based on Gussenbauer's plan but had essential modifications (Fig. 2–1B).

1877   Carl Stork in Vienna contrived an external prosthesis that was driven by air from a bulb that the patient, a tracheotomized girl with a laryngeal stenosis, had to squeeze with her hand. As the bulb did not produce enough air, Stork suppressed the bulb and connected the artificial larynx to the patient's tracheal cannula (Hochenegg, 1892).

1880s   Themistocles Glück recommended that in laryngectomized patients the bottom of the pharynx be completely sewn up in order to obviate the greatest hazard of laryngectomy, aspiration pneumonia (Glück and Zeller, 1881).

1881   Paul Bruns (1881) substituted a flexible cannula for the rigid laryngeal cannula and discarded the artificial epiglottis, which had proved to be of little help. In order to prevent food from falling into the lungs a plug fitted on a curved rod had, as in the Irvine-Fould prosthesis, to be introduced before each meal into the laryngeal cannula through the tracheostoma.

1885   Two French physicians, Leon Labbe (1886) and Cadier, made a prosthesis seemingly modeled on Gussenbauer's artificial larynx.

1892   Julius Hochenegg (1892) reduplicated Stork's appliance. The patient was unable to exhale with sufficient strength to cause the reed to vibrate. Moreover, the buccal tube interfered with articulation. Consequently, he designed an artificial larynx powered by air from a pair of bellows that the patient held under his armpit. The puffs of air were delivered into the pharynx through a nasal tube.

1893   Julius Wolff (1893a, 1893b) felt that the Bruns-Beurle device had several drawbacks. During speech saliva dripped into the device. The voice was monotonous and the valve did not admit enough air. Wolff tried to remedy these flaws by shortening the laryngeal cannula and lengthening the phonatory cannula so that they were of equal length. According to Wolff, these changes improved the quality of the voice.

1896   Anderson-Stuart, a professor of physiology at the University of Sydney, developed an artificial larynx with a tracheal butt that could be inserted into the rubber cannula, which the patient wore permanently. This short tube was attached to a voice box provided at its base with a large opening for breathing. When the patient occluded this opening with a thumb and exhaled, air was forced into the superior part of the voice box, which contained a metallic reed taken from a mouth organ. The puffs of air delivered by the reed left the voice box through a wired rubber tube that entered the pharynx through a fistula cut below the hyoid bone. In order to prevent saliva and food from falling into the prosthesis, the top of the pharyngeal tube was provided with a valve made of kid leather. This valve, Anderson-Stuart wrote (1897), "is absolutely efficient, for while wet it readily permits the sound-bearing air to pass into the pharynx, it prevent anything from passing down into the artificial larynx, so that the patient wore the apparatus the livelong day."

1900   Taptas (1900) wrote a paper in which he described an artificial larynx. The device comprised a tracheal cannula, a pharyngeal cannula, and a flexible tube. The pharyngeal cannula was inserted into a pharyngostoma and was connected with the tracheal cannula by the flexible tube. The upper end of the pharynageal cannula had a valve that prevented food and saliva from entering the prosthesis. By this device pulmonic air could be led to the vocal tract and the patient could produce an audible, whispered voice. However, no regular voice could be generated.

1902   The French phonetician Rousselot (1902) reported on an artificial larynx made by Dr. Claude Martin. The appliance consisted of a tracheal cannula, a phonatory cannula, and a hood. The front part of the tracheal cannula was closed by an emergency valve that could be opened in case the artificial larynx should become obstructed. The bottom of the phonatory cannula communicated with the tracheal cannula. It resulted a truncated pyramid capped by a flat rubber tube.

1910   At the turn of the century, Themistocles Glück was experimenting with various types of external artificial larynges. In some of them the reed was a bead placed in the patient's nose, and a small tube delivered air puffs to the pharynx. In others the reed was attached to an upper denture (Glück, 1910). In still others the rubber reed and the inhalatory valve sat in a cylindrical box just outside the patient's tracheostoma (Tapia, 1914).

1914   Tadeo Pereda, a Spanish laryngectomee, attempted to remedy the flaws noted by Glück: He discarded the cylinder containing the reed and the inhalatory valve. The tracheal tube was left open and provided with a side butt. A rubber tube linked this butt with a voice box carried in the patient's pocket or held in a hand. Another rubber tube conducted puffs of air from the voice box to the mouth. When the patient wanted to speak, he had to close the opening in the front of his tracheal cannula with his finger (Tapia, 1914).

1918   Onodi and Stockman (Onodi, 1918) constructed a device similar to the one used by Glück in which the bellows were driven by an electromotor powered by batteries.

1920s   John Mackenty, senior surgeon of the Manhattan Eye, Ear, and Throat Hospital in New York, together with Harvey Fletcher and Charles Lane, two scientists of the Western Electric Company, developed an artificial larynx consisting of a soft-rubber tracheal pad and a flexible tracheal connection that could be strapped over the tracheostoma; a silver cylinder containing a hard-rubber tube across which a rubber band was stretched; a thumb nut to adjust the tension of the membrane and, consequently, the pitch of the voice; and a mouthpiece that fitted in the metal stem in the top of the reed box. The cylinder had an inhalatory hole that the user occluded with a finger during speech (Barney, 1958).

1924   Jorge Leyro Diaz (1924) used a tube connecting the trachea with the nasopharynx. Near the lower end the tube had a lateral opening through which the patient could breathe. When the patient communicated, he had to exhale, close the breathing hole with a finger, and turn the pulmonic airstream into an audible whisper.

1925   The Australian surgeon Graham Brown (1925) reported on an artificial larynx that resembled Stuart's appliance of 1896. Brown had cut a pharyngostoma in his patient's neck just below the hyoid bone. An aural speculum made of gold and containing a violin pitch pipe was fitted into the pharyngostoma and held in position by two tapes tied round the head. The patient was further provided with a thin shield of vulcanite that closely fitted the front of her neck except at its superior border, where a small gap was left between it and the neck. The shield was held in position by tapes that passed around the back of the neck. The loosely applied portion at the superior border allowed breathing to take place through the tracheostoma. When speech was required, the patient brought her head forward, producing an airtight space between the neck and the shield. The expired air entered the reed, which then delivered air puffs to the pharynx.

1925   The Bell system became concerned with this area of communication. F. B. Jewett, president of Bell Telephone Laboratories at that time, suggested the development of an artificial larynx. The Laboratories' initial efforts resulted in an instrument that employed rubber bands stretched in a manner to simulate the vocal cords and was designated type 1A (Riesz, 1930).

1929   McKesson's (1927) device was christened the Vocophone. A description appeared in the *Journal of the American Medical Association:* "This instrument enables a patient whose larynx has been removed because of carcinoma to speak with a voice approaching the normal in volume and quality. A neckpiece is held in place by means of the collar, to which it is attached by an ordinary collar button. A rubber tube connects the neckpiece with the trumpet, and a tube from the trumpet conducts the sound into the mouth. To speak, the neck piece is pressed gently against the neck, and air is blown through the trumpet, setting up a sound resembling the normal voice."

1929   During 1929 a new larynx, designated type 2A, was developed that incorporated several refinements, including the substitution of a vibrating metallic reed for the elastic bands (Riesz, 1930). The metallic reed is connected by tubing to the tracheal stoma so that the user's breath can actuate the reed. The sound of the vibrating reed is conducted through another tube into the mouth to be articulated into speech. In ensuing years Riesz, a Bell Laboratory engineer, patented variations (Figs. 2–2 through 2–5). Another variation is shown with a bellows for initiating voice (Fig. 2–6), then placed beside a Western Electric No. 2 (WE2) for comparison (Fig. 2–7).*

1930s   Elias Narro-Casadesus, an instrument maker of Barcelona, designed a pneumatical artificial larynx. It consists of an adjustable metallic reed whose housing is carried in the patient's pocket. A flexible rubber tube connects the reed with the tracheal cannula and another tube connects it with the patient's mouth. The reed box is provided with an inhalatory valve. The bottom of the box can be unscrewed to remove mucus deposits.

1931   Charles Sheard (1931) designed a device (Fig. 2–8) after the Western Electric pneumatic device. The four essential parts of this new artificial larynx included a rubber tube for inser-

---

*Materials shown in Figures 2–2 through 2–7 were provided by Speech Pathologist Roberta Rauch of Cleveland, the daughter of inventor Robert Riesz.

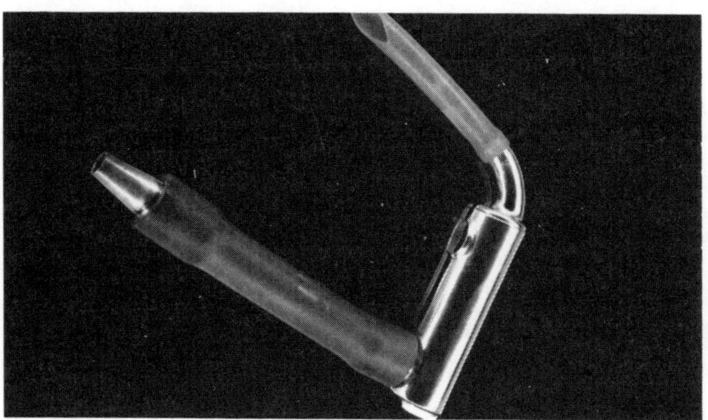

Figure 2–2. Western Electric 2A pneumatic mechanical larynx. (Courtesy of Roberta Rauch.)

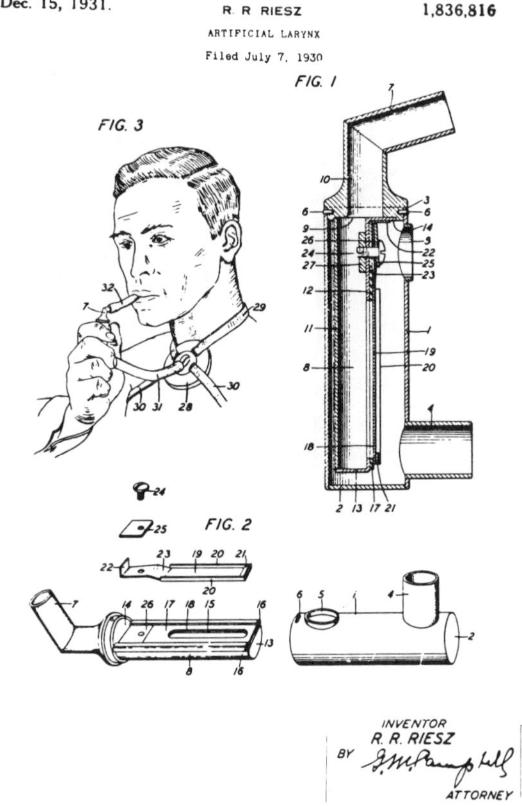

Figure 2–3. Variation of 2A mechanical larynx. (Courtesy of Roberta Rauch.)

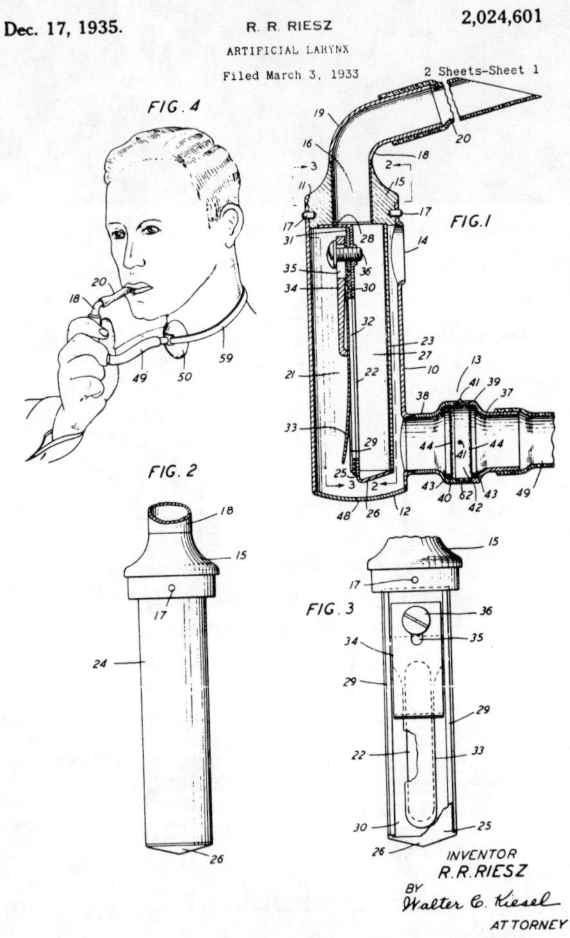

Figure 2–4. Later variation of WE2. (Courtesy of Roberta Rauch.)

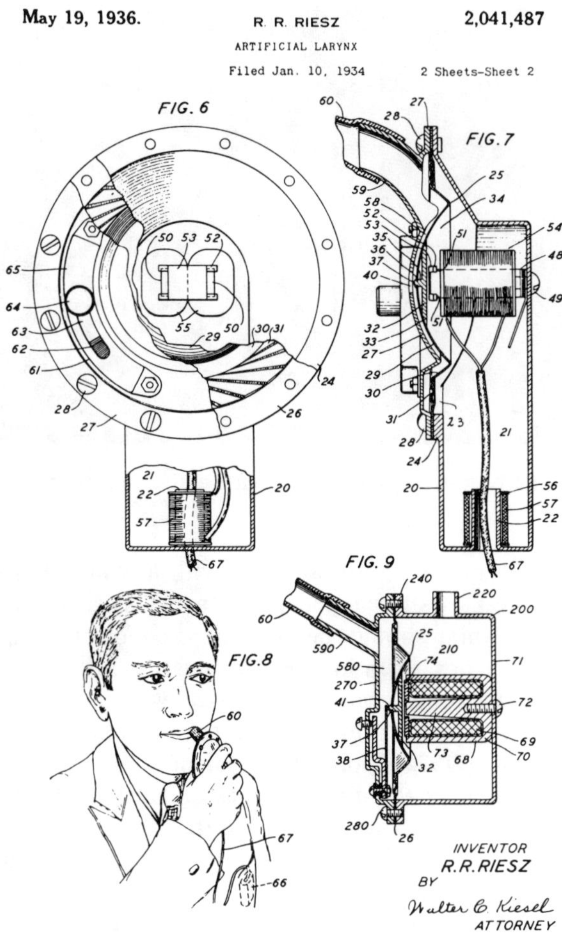

Figure 2–5. WE2 variation of pneumatic larynx by R. R. Riesz. (Courtesy of Roberta Rauch.)

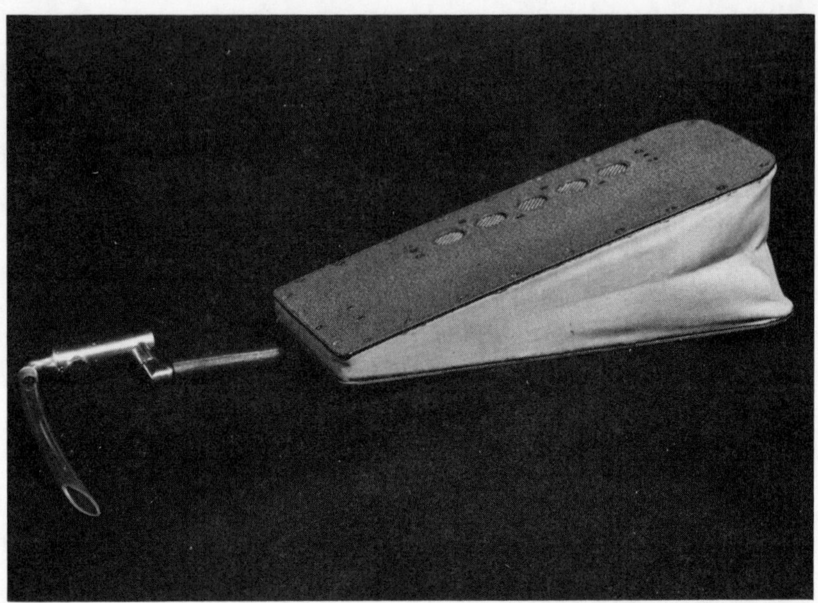

Figure 2–6. Early mechanical larynx with activating bellows. (Courtesy of Roberta Rauch.)

tion in the mouth and one with a connection to the neck. The partially cupped plate carries a valve for purposes of breathing should the user fail to remove his thumb from the voice box when he needs to breathe. Fifty years after Riesz, a workable homemade device was made using strips of radiographic film as a vibrator source (Fig. 2-9).

1932   C. E. Lane (1932) applied for a patent for an improved larynx that overcomes the disadvantages of previous devices. A trachea connection is applied to the trachea opening in the neck of the user. This connection is joined to a sound chamber through an air passageway to introduce air from the lungs into the sound chamber, which contains a vibratory element in the form of a tubular elastic member rigidly supported at one end of the chamber and having its free end slightly open. After the air passes through the element, it is led to the mouth of the user to form the sound into articulated speech.

1933   E. I. McKesson (1933) applied for a patent, which was assigned to the Vocophone Company, Toledo, Ohio. This invention relates to the air handling, especially for oral resonance control. It has utility for mouth communication from the lungs,

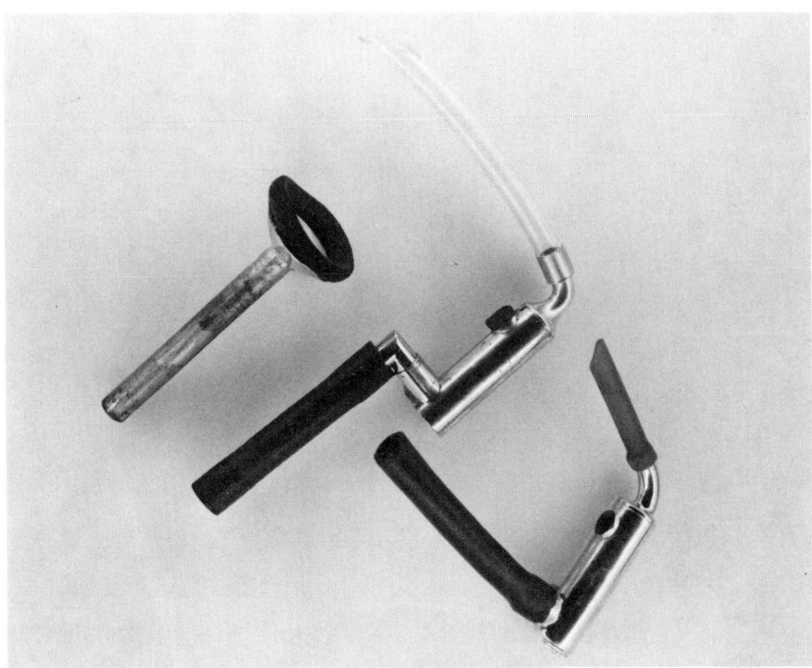

Figure 2–7.   Original WE2 and subsequent variations of pneumatic larynxes. (Courtesy of Roberta Rauch.)

bypassing the larynx and throat as in Lane's 1932 device.

1936   Snidecor (1962) noted a retired St. Louis policeman who was using a self-designed instrument: "The source of power was the hand-squeezed bulb of an old automobile horn of the type that once graced the side of a Stutz Bearcat. A tube led into the mouth where a reformed clarinet reed vibrated with ample power and complexity" (p. 149).

1936   Thomas Loring demonstrated the prosthesis he had made for himself (Iglauer, 1936). The device resembled the artificial larynx described by Riesz. The reed worked in an open slot, however, whereas in the WE2 larynx there was a reed cushion.

1937   W. F. Kellotat (1937) applied for a patent for a device consisting of a denture and a mechanism for producing voice. It included a sound chamber having outlets; a reed chamber having an inlet, the reed chamber being operatively associated with the sound chamber; a vibrating reed within the reed chamber; side extensions carried by the denture and conforming to the contour of the side of the mouth; a flexible apron disposed

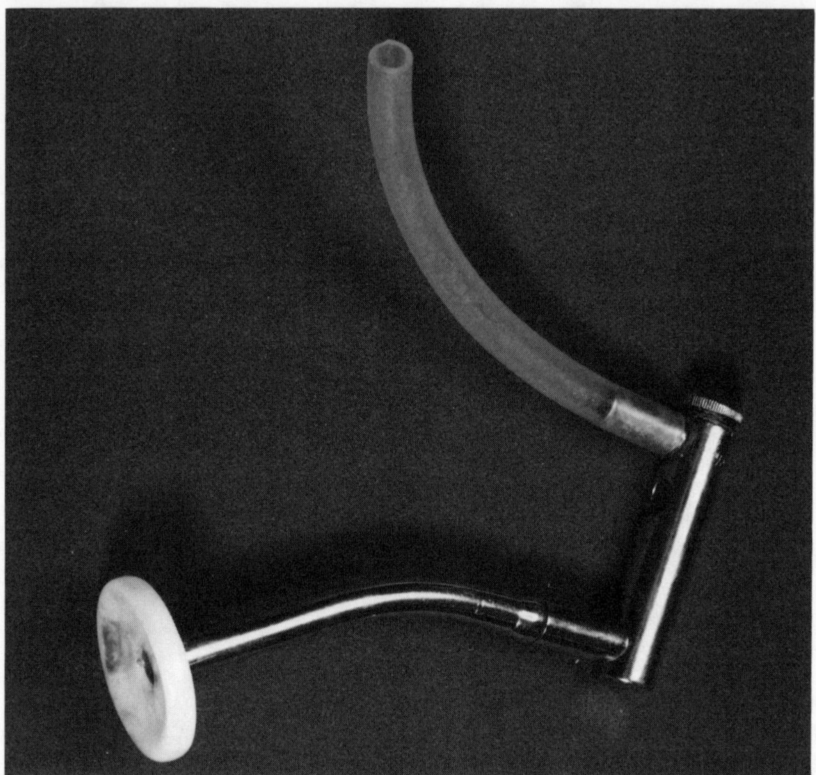

Figure 2–8. The Neher Pneumatic Larynx developed by Sheard.

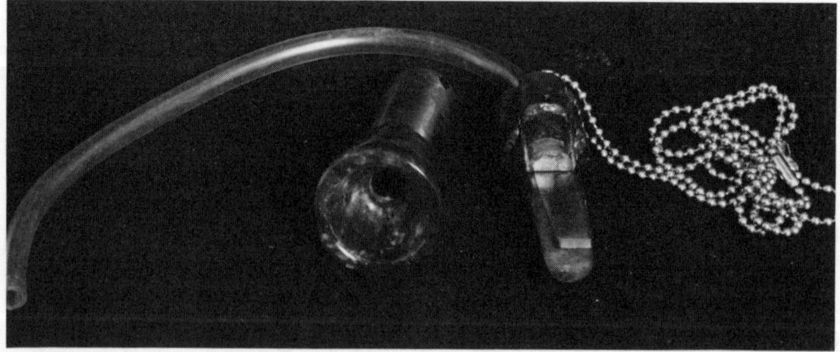

Figure 2–9. Vibrator using strips of radiographic film as sound source.

between the side extensions and functioning therewith to seal the back of the throat and direct the air of exhalation into the inlet of the reed chamber. The entire assembly was adapted to be wholly contained within the oral cavity.

1939   Hanson (1940) and a laryngectomee named Ottie Roberts made an artificial larynx out of hard rubber. By means of this prosthesis a voice could be produced that Hanson claimed was close to the natural laryngeal voice. In addition, the device was light, unbreakable, and moisture resistant.

1940   Firestone (1940) designed an instrument whereby voice could be generated by a means of a diaphragm that is exterior to the oral cavity and connected with the mouth by an air column. This device was composed of a relaxation oscillator and a receiver. The pulses delivered by the diaphragm of the receiver were introduced into the oral cavity through an air-filled glass tube. Firestone recommended that the oscillator be provided with a continuous, rapidly operable control of frequency so as to permit inflection. He also suggested the use of a pushbutton volume control for distinguishing between voiced and unvoiced consonants.

1942   Wright (1942) probably should receive credit for the first electrolarynx. With separate power pack connected by cord, sound was introduced into the throat by transmission through the neck wall. The device was known as the Sonovox (which also let the train "talk" in the Walt Disney movie, "Dumbo").

1945   Wright's (Luchsinger, 1949) artificial larynx was eventually produced by the Aurex Corporation of Chicago, Illinois, first as the Wright Electrolarynx (Fig. 2–10) and then as the Aurex Neovox M-520T (Fig. 2–11). Wright's design also inspired a similar electronic larynx (Fig. 2–12), later known as the Kett Mark III (Fig. 2–13), that was manufactured by the Kett Engineering Co.

1957   Herbert Pichler (1961b) of Vienna invented an electrolarynx consisting of four parts: a battery-powered signal generator carried in the patient's pocket, an antenna worn around the patient's neck, a tiny receiver affixed to the patient's denture, and a switch located in the patient's tracheal cannula. When the patient exhaled with sufficient energy, the switch let the generator emit radio signals, which caused the diaphragm of the receiver to vibrate.

1957   Dr. Herbert Cooper (1958), head of the Cleft Palate Clinic in Lancaster, Pennsylvania, and electronic engineers of the Rand Development Corporation manufactured a Cooper-Rand elec-

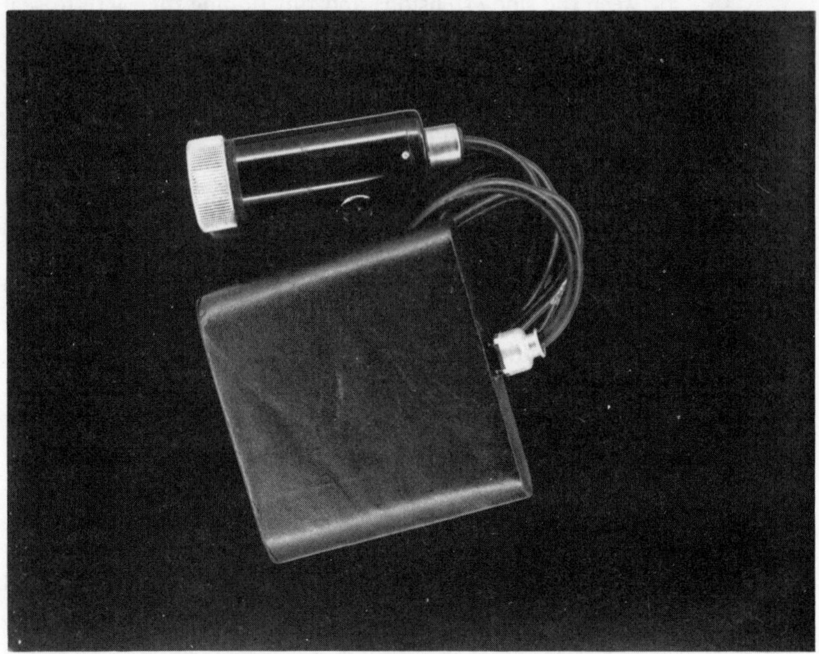

Figure 2–10.   Wright Electrolarynx produced by Aurex.

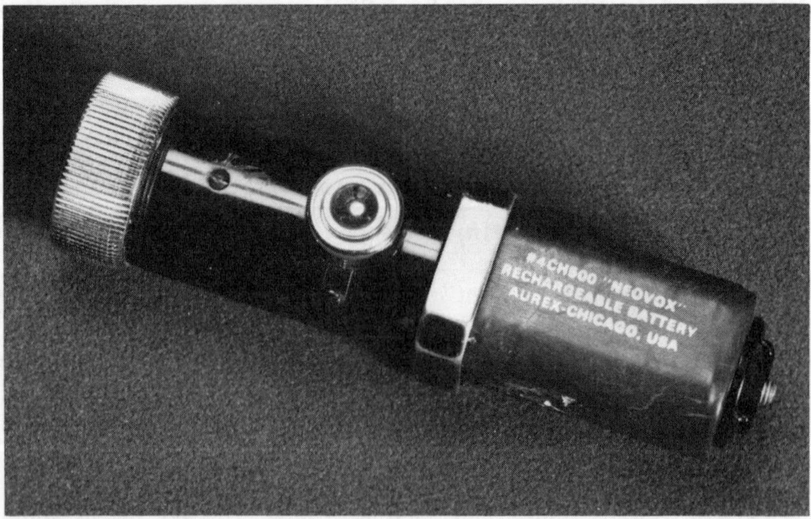

Figure 2–11.   Neovox Electrolarynx with rechargeable battery.

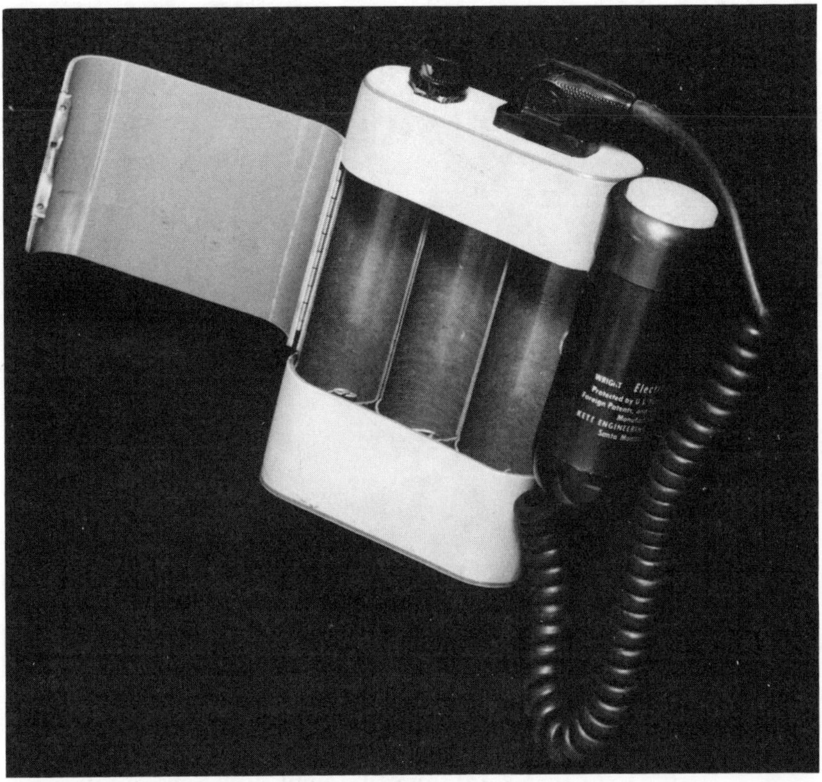

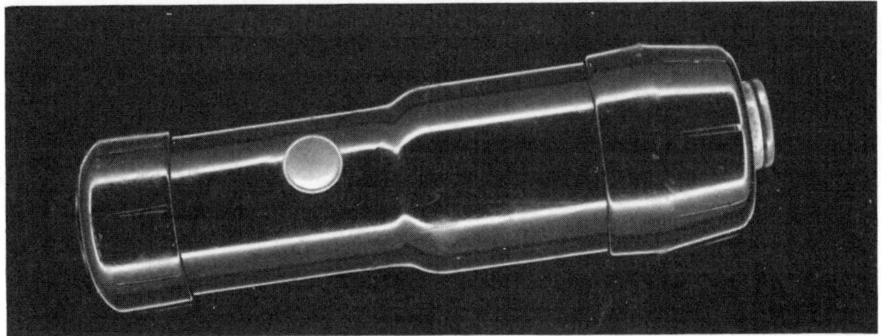

Figure 2–12. Wright Electrolarynx produced by Kett.

Figure 2–13. Cordless electrolarynx, Kett Mark III, with rechargeable battery.

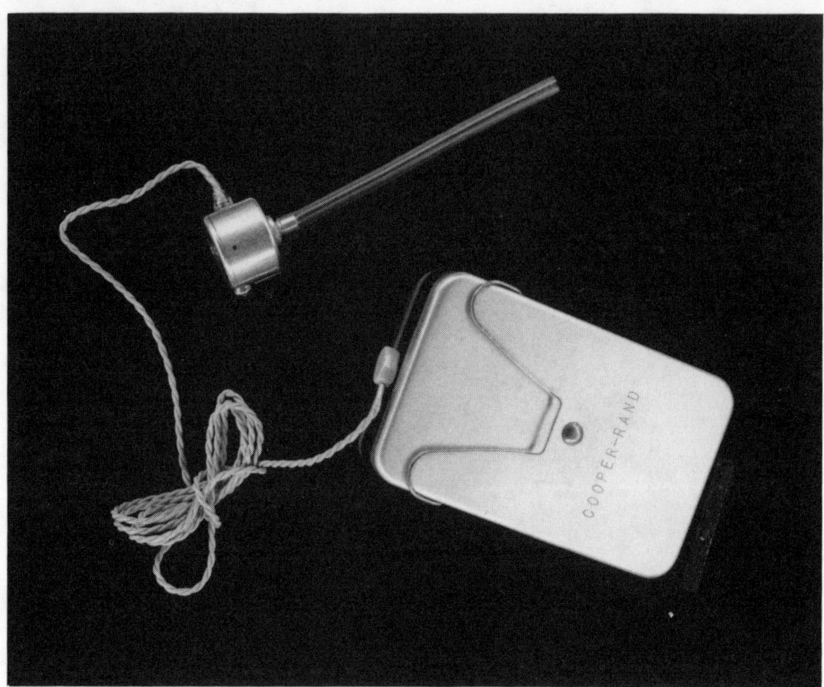

Figure 2–14. Cooper-Rand, a mouth-type electrolarynx.

trolarynx (Fig. 2–14) from 1957 until 1972. Subsequently neck-type devices utilized the Cooper-Rand feature of independent controls for levels of loudness and pitch. These European models included the Servox (Fig. 2–15), the Romet (Fig. 2–16) and the Rehaton (Fig. 2–17). The original development was initiated to meet a twofold need for a new artificial larynx: (1) To provide laryngectomees with a temporary means of speech, both in the interim period immediately following surgery and prior to esophageal speech lessons and also during the times when, due to a cold, digestive upset, or any other reason, esophageal speech becomes difficult or impossible; (2) To provide laryngectomees with a compact instrument that would introduce sound into the mouth and be easy to use, especially for those who are weak or lying down.

1957   Cooper and Millard (1959) filed a patent for a mouth-type electronic artificial larynx. The device consisted of a battery pack carried in the pocket, an on-off switch located under the armpit, and a wire leading from the battery pack to a

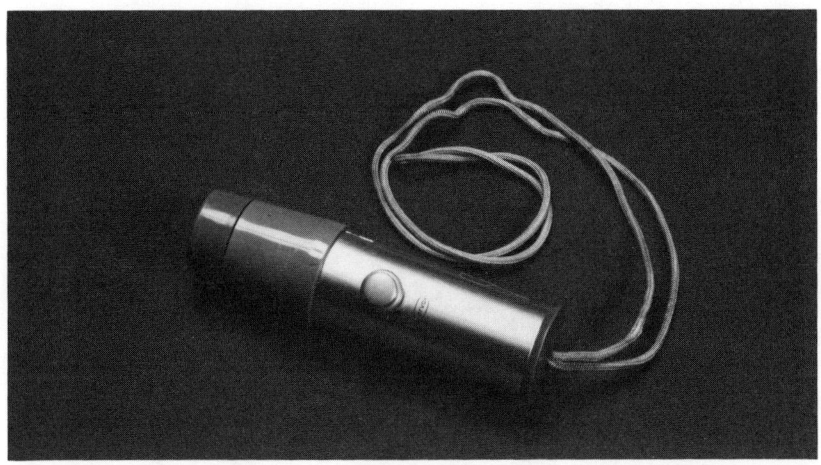

Figure 2–15. Servox Electrolarynx.

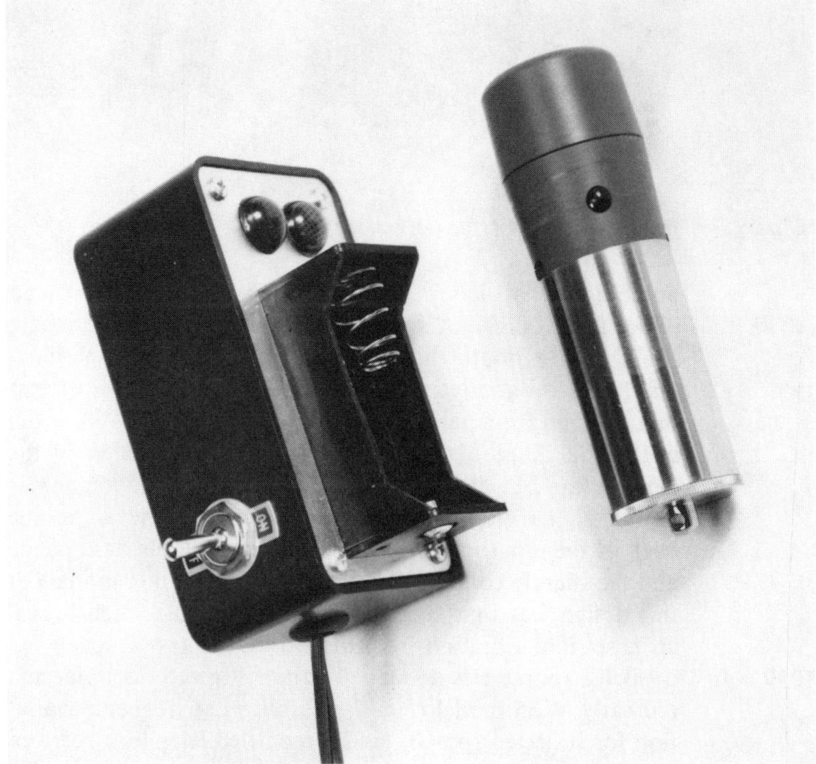

Figure 2–16. The Romet Electrolarynx, with battery charger.

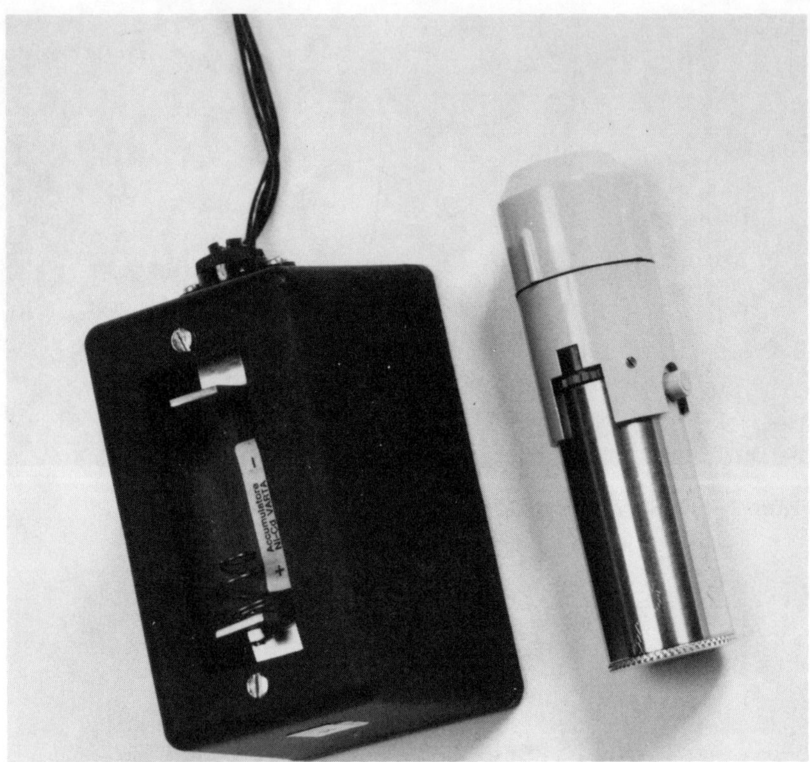

Figure 2–17.   Rehaton Electrolarynx.

diaphragm that was plugged into the lateral aspect of an upper dental plate. A slight squeeze of the arm produced a sound in the mouth that could be articulated into speech.

1958   Cooper (1958) was granted a United States patent for a prosthesis that differed from Tait's oral vibrator (Tait, 1959, 1960, 1962) in that the diaphragm was not attached to the center of the dental plate but at the side of it. When the diaphragm was energized, its vibrations were transmitted to the air at the back of the mouth by the air column between the hard palate and the slightly concave dental plate. The general rationale of this design was that speech is more intelligible when buccal air is set into vibration from behind, as in normal speakers.

1959   In 1959 Bell Laboratories developed a transistorized electrolarynx. An early WE5 model (Fig. 2–18), allowing frequency variation for inflected speech, used a modified telephone receiver. By 1964 the neck connector was reduced in size. Subsequent

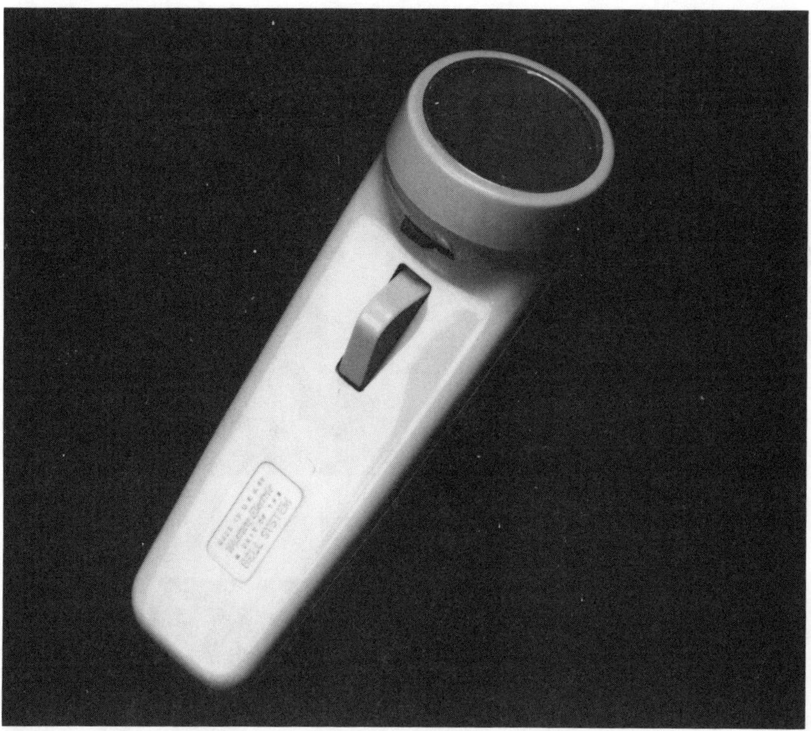

Figure 2–18.   Early WE5 electrolarynx.

efforts were made by the company to alter intensity levels
(Fig. 2–19). Additional alterations were attempted by users
for continuous frequency variation (Fig. 2–20) and to deliver
sound directly into the mouth (Fig. 2–21). In the 1980s Bell
introduced Model 5C (Fig. 2–22), using a 9-volt transistor
battery but sacrificing frequency variation.

1963   The Laryngophone was made in Belgium, partly out of metal
and partly out of flexible material. It had no inhalatory
valves. The DSP 8 artificial larynx (Fig. 2–23) was made in
Holland. It was made of nylon and weighed about 30
grams. It consisted of a flexible plastic cup with an inflated
collar, a sieve with staggered joints that prevented secretions
from entering the prosthesis, an inhalatory valve, and a thin
adjustable membrane disc that vibrated to create sound.

1964   Japanese inventors created pneumatic larynges based on a different vibrator. An inch-long strip of rubber, ½ inch wide, is

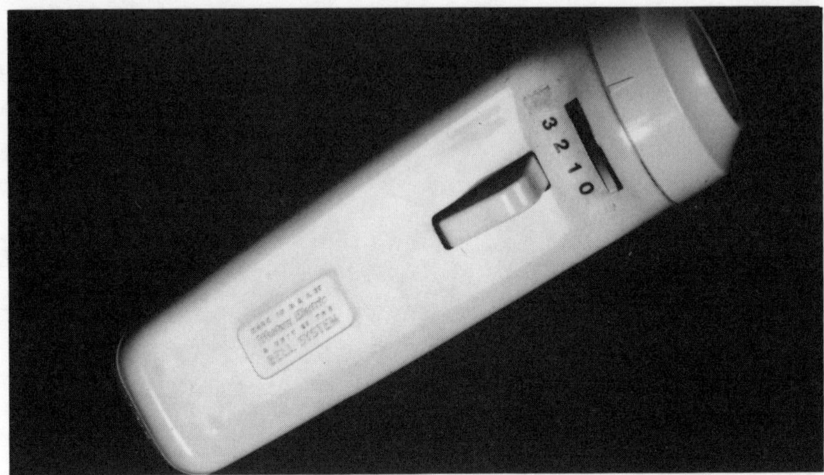

Figure 2–19. Experimental model of WE5, with variable intensity level.

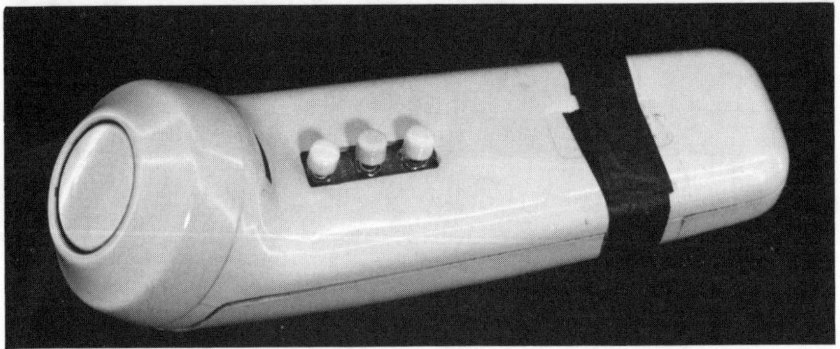

Figure 2–20. Experimental model of WE5 with continuously variable frequency.

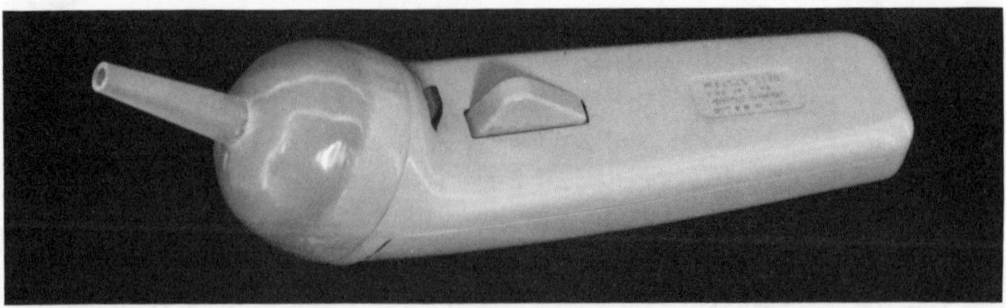

Figure 2–21. Experimental model of WE5 directing sound into the mouth.

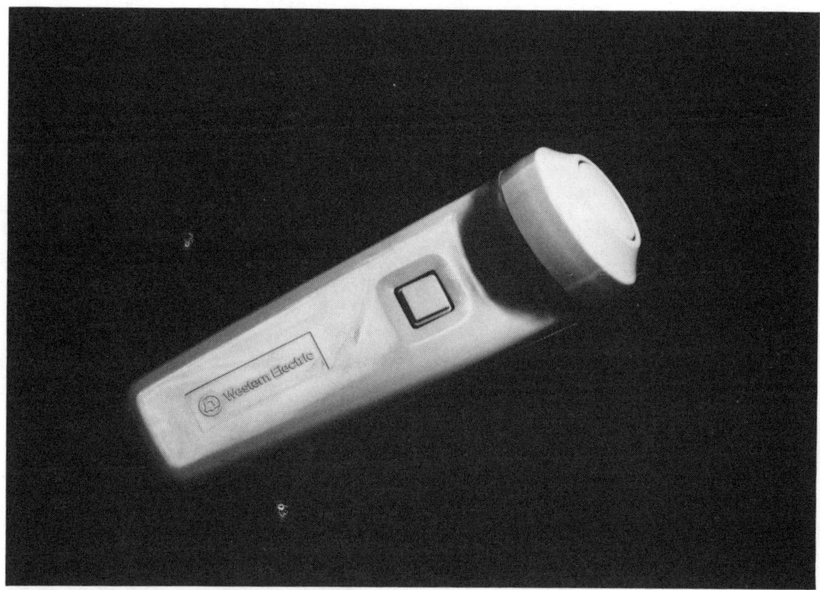

Figure 2–22. WE artificial larynx model 5C.

held taut by a rubber band. Brought to the United States by Al St. Germain, these devices (Fig. 2–24) have been popularized by "Red" Woodworth of Texas.

1965   Zerneri (1965) contrived a simple and cheap device. It consisted of a small rubber cup that was to be held over the tracheostoma and that contained a transverse rubber band stretched over the opening of a plastic tube. This tube passed through the top of the bell-like voice box and conducted puffs of air into the speaker's mouth.

1972   Taub and Spiro (1972) made a device similar to the one created by the Australian surgeon, Graham Brown. Taub used a U-shaped pneumatic prosthesis, one end of which was inserted into the trachea while the other end was introduced into the hypopharynx through a fistula surgically cut in the lateroanterior part of the neck. The tracheal butt of the artificial larynx was provided with a one-way valve for inspiration. Expiration took place through the prosthesis. The metal reed, like that in the WE2, vibrated in the U-shaped tube only when pressure was exerted on exhalation. This accorded with a physiological process; in normal speakers, quiet expiration is passive and the pressure drop through the

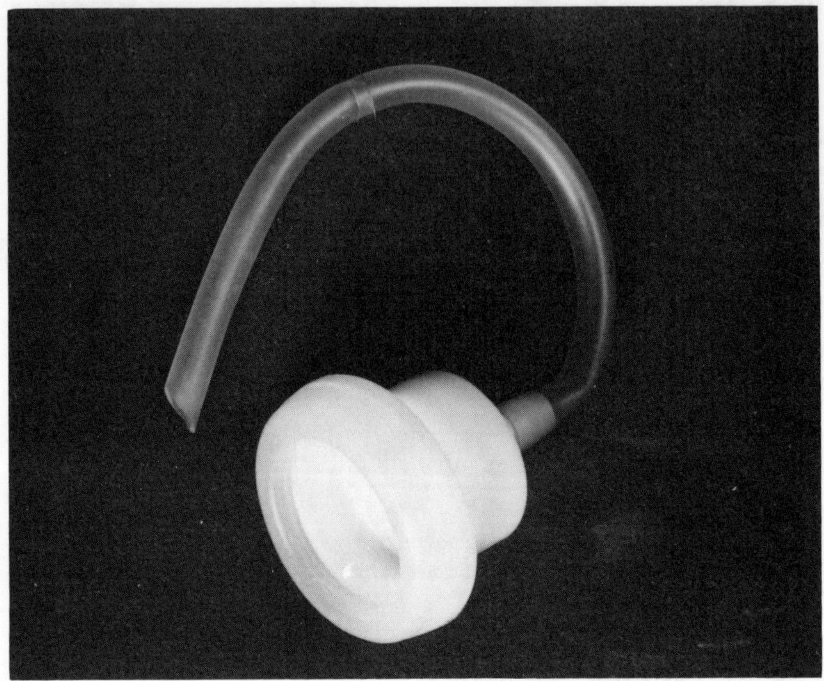

Figure 2–23. Dutch DSP 8 using a disc to create tone.

respiratory tract is small. In order to produce audible speech the pressure of exhalation had to be actively increased.

1972   The Danapipe was a Danish mouth-type electronic larynx consisting of miniaturized circuitry, a transducer, and a battery concealed in a bowl portion of a tobacco pipe. A switch on the side of the bowl activated the sound, which was transmitted through the stem of the pipe to the user's mouth. The same principle was employed earlier in the Pipa di Ticchioni (Fig. 2–25), made in Milan, and later, in the Artificial Larynx of North America (Fig. 2–26).

1983   The Speechmaster intraoral artificial larynx was developed to fit against the upper palate like a dental bridge. It operates on a 6 volt replaceable power supply. The off-on switch is controlled by the tongue (Fig. 2–27).

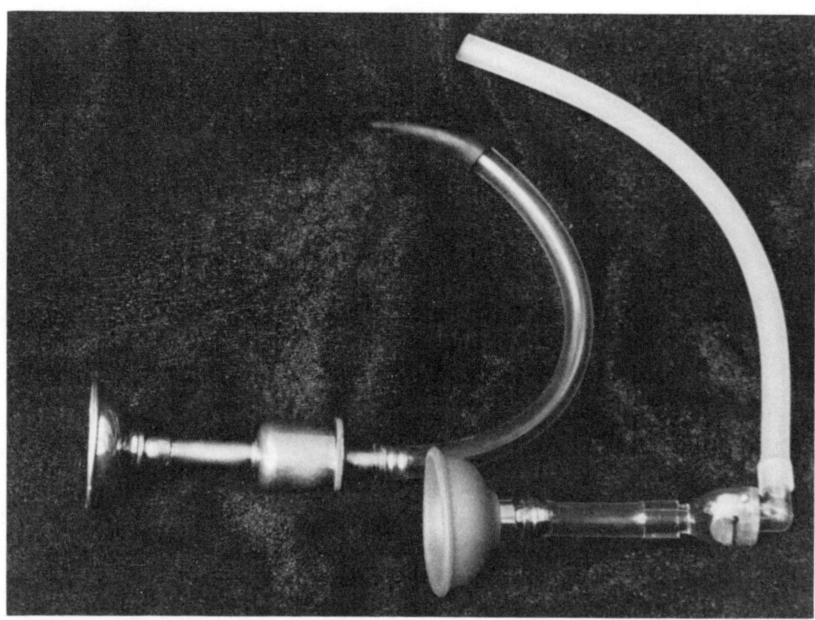

Figure 2–24. Japanese pneumatic larynxes, using strips of rubber to vibrate for tone.

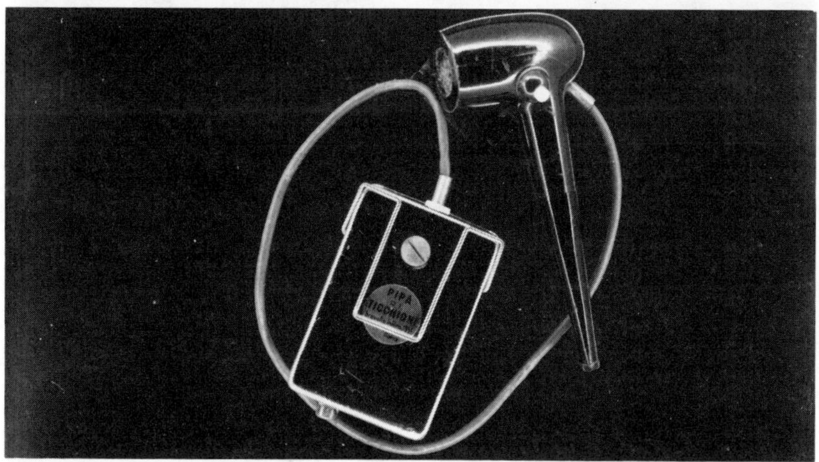

Figure 2–25. Pipa di Ticchioni electrolarynx.

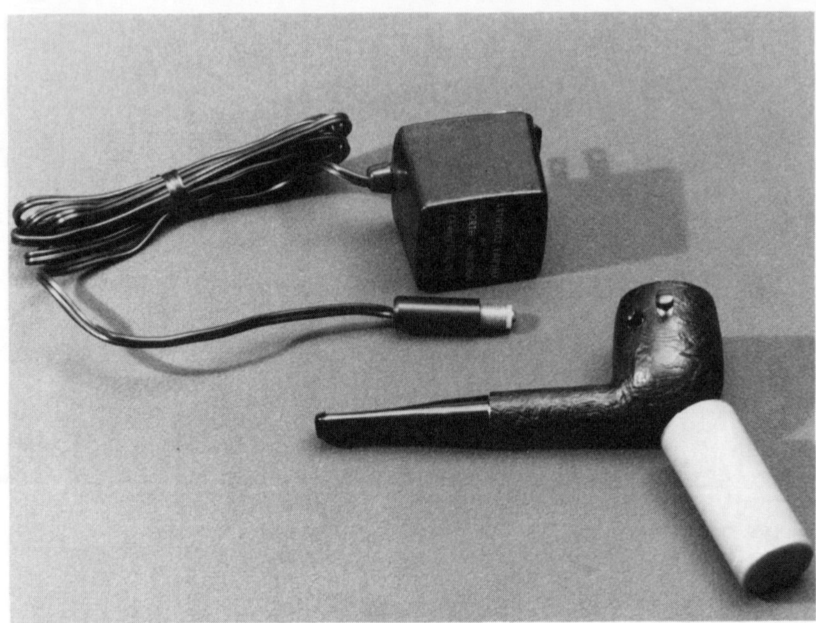

Figure 2–26. Artificial Larynx of North America.

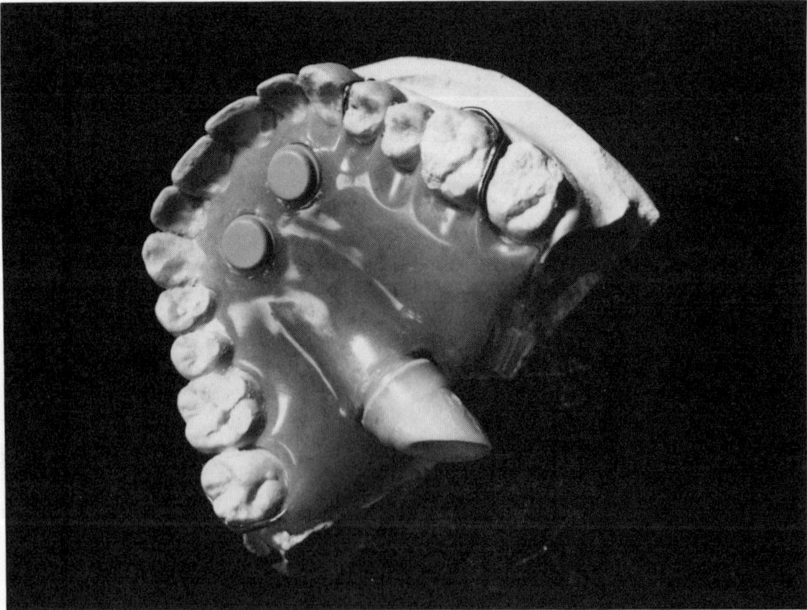

Figure 2–27. Speechmaster electrolarynx providing tone at top of oral cavity.

QUESTIONS

1. What was the profession of the patient receiving the first successful laryngectomy done by Billroth?
2. Bottin is credited for what accomplishment?
3. Why was the artificial larynx developed before the first laryngectomy was performed to remove cancer?
4. What country contributed the first electric artificial larynx?
5. What five dates in this historical review seem to be the most significant to you and why?

REFERENCES

Albers, J. F. H. (1829). Graefe und Walther jour. *Beitrage zur physiologie des kehlkops, für chirurgie und augenheilkunde, 13,* 244. Cited in C. Jackson and C. L. Jackson (1939), *Cancer of the larynx* (pp. 241 and 277). Philadelphia: Saunders.

Anderson-Stuart, T. (April 17, 1897). An artificial larynx. *The Lancet,* 1081–1084.

Babington, B. G. Cited in Proceedings of the Hunterian Society (March 18, 1829), *London Medical Gazette, 3,* 555–556; also cited in Mackenzie, M. (1880). *Diseases of the pharynx, larynx and trachea* (p. 159). New York: William Wood & Co.

Barney, H. L. (1958). A discussion of some technical aspects of speech aids for post-laryngectomized patients. *Ann. Otol. Rhinol. Laryngol., 67,* 558–570.

Barney, H. L., Haworth, F. E., and Dunn, H. K. (1959). An experimental transistorized artificial larynx. [Monograph 3395]. *The Bell System Technical Journal, 38,* 1337–1356.

Billroth, C. A. T., and Gussenbauer, C. (1874). Über die erste durch Th. Billroth am menschen ausgefuhrte kehlkopf extirpation und die anwendung eines kunstlichen kehlkopfes. *Arch. für klinische Chirurgie, 17,* 343–356.

Bottini, E. (1875). Communicazione Letta Innanzi la R. *Giornale della academia di medicina di Torino,* 418–434.

Bottini, E. (1878). Extirpation totale du larynx a l'aide du galvano-cautere. *Annales des Maladies de l'Oreille et du Larynx et des Organes, 4,* 182–186.

Brown, R. G. (1925). A simple but effective artificial larynx. *J. Laryngol., 40,* 793–797.

Bruns, P. von (1878). *Die Laryngotomie zur Entfernung intralaryngealer Neubildungen.* Berlin: A. Hirschwald.

Bruns, P. von (1881). Ueber enige Verbesserungen des kunstlichen Kehlkopfes. *Arch. klinische Chirurgie, 26,* 780–782.

Casadesus, F. (1923). Phonetic apparatus for laryngectomized. *Anales de la Academia Medico-Quirurgica Espanola, 10,* 109. Cited by Snidecor, J. C. (1968). *Speech rehabilitation of the laryngectomized* (2nd ed.) (p. 215). Springfield, IL: Charles C Thomas.

Cooper, H. K., US Patent No 2,862,209 issued December 2, 1958.

Cooper, H. K., and Millard, R. T. (1959). A dental approach to speech restoration in the laryngectomee: A preliminary report. *Dental Digest, 65,* 106–112.

Crile, G. W. (1913). Laryngectomy for cancer. *Trans. Amer. Surg. Assoc., 31,* 259–276.

Crile, G. W. (1947). *George Crile: An autobiography* (Vols. 1 and 2). Philadelphia: Lippincott.

Czermak, J. N. (1859). Über die sprache bei luftdichter verschliessung des kehlkopfs, sitzungsberichte der kaiserlichen academie der wissenschaften mathematischnaturwissenschaftliche classe. Wien, *35,* 65–72.

Czerny, V. (1870). Versuche uber kehlkopf extirpation. *Weiner medizinische Wochenschrift, 20,* 557, 591.

Delavan, D. B. (1912). Laryngology: An historical sketch. In H. A. Kelly, (Ed.), *Cyclopedia of American medical biography* (pp. lxiii-lxxi). Philadelphia: Saunders.

Donagan, W. L. (1965). An early history of total laryngectomy. *Surgery, 57,* 902–905.

Firestone, F. (1940). An artificial larynx for speaking and choral singing by one person. *J. Acous. Soc. Amer., 11,* 357–361.

Fletcher, H. (1929). Artificial larynx. In *Speech and hearing* (pp. 12–13). New York: Van Nostrand.

Foulis, D. F. (1877a). Excision of larynx, and use of artificial vocal apparatus. *Brit. Med. J.,* 811–812.

Foulis, D. F. (1877b). Extirpation of the larynx. *Lancet, 2,* 530–532.

Foulis, D. F. (1881). Indications for the complete or partial extirpation of the larynx. *Proceedings of Sub-Section for Diseases of the Throat, Transactions of 7th Session, International Medical Congress, 3,* 251–258.

Gerdes, H. (1877). Total extirpation des kehlkopfes: Tod am vierten tage. *Arch. klinische Chirurgie, 21,* 473–477.

Glück, T. (1899). Flustersprache und phonationsapparate. *Berliner klinische Wochenschrift, 36,* 215–216.

Glück, T. (1904). Der gegenwartige stand der chirurgie des kehlkopfs, pharynx, oesophagus, und der trachea. *Monatsschrift für Ohrenheilkunde, 39,* 89, 141.

Glück, T. (1908). *Verhandlungen des internationalen laryngo-rhinologen kongresses.* Wein: *1,* 66–108.

Glück, T. (1910). Patienten mit totalexstirpation des pharynx, larynx und oesophagus, denen eine kunstliche stimme durch einen automatisch arbeitenden apparat geliefert wird. *Berliner klinische Wochenschrift, 47,* 33–35.

Glück, T. (1913). Das techische und funktionelle problem bei den operationen und den obesen luft- und speisewegen. *Internationales Centrablatt für Laryngologie, Rhinologie, und verwandte Wissenschaften, 29,* 610.

Glück, T. (1921). Probleme und Zeile der Chirurgie der oberen Luftwege und Speiswege. *Monatschrift für Ohrenheilkunde, 55,* 1150–1174.

Glück, T., and Soerensen, J. (1920). Ergebnisse einer neuen Reihe von 100 total Extirpationen des Kehlkopfs. *Arch. Laryngologie und Rhinologie, 33,* 84–102.

Glück, T., and Soerensen, J. (1922). Die extirpation and resektion des kehlkopfes. *Handbuch der speziellen chirurgie des ohres und der oberen luftwege* (3rd ed.) (Vol. 4) (pp. 1–70). Würtzburg: C. Kabisch.

Glück, T., and Zeller, A. (1881). Die prophylactische resektion der trachea. *Arch. die klinische Chirurgie, 26,* 427–436.

Goldstein, M. A. (1932). Metal discs for permanent recording and reproduction of speech: Modification of the artificial larynx. *Trans. Amer. Laryngol. Assoc., 54,* 105–111.

Gottstein, G. (1900). Pseudo-stimme nach total extirpation des larynx. *Arch. klinische Chirurgie, 62,* 126–146.

Hanson, W. L. (1940). A new artificial larynx with a historical review. *IL Med. J. 78,* 483–486.

Haworth, F. E. (1960). An electronic artificial larynx. *Bell Laboratories Recordings, 38,* 362–368.

Heine, C. (1876). Resection des kehlkopfes bei laryngostenose. *Arch. klinische Chirurgie, 19,* 514–526.

Hinojar, A. (1923). Simple phonetic apparatus. *Anales de la Academia Medico-Quirurgica Espanola, 10,* 93.

Hochenegg, J. (1892). Totale kehlkopf-exstirpation and resektion des oesophagus wegen carcinoma laryngis. Oesophagoplastick. Ein neuer sprechapparat. *Weiner klinische Wochenschrift, 5,* 123–127.

Holinger, P. H. (1975). The historical development of laryngectomy. *The Laryngoscope, 85,* 287, 322–333.

Iglauer, S. (1936). Artificial larynx, with patient demonstrating its use. *Trans. Amer. Bronch. Soc., 19,* 31–32.

Jackson, C., and Jackson, C. L. (1939). *Cancer of the larynx.* Philadelphia: Saunders.

Jesberg, N. (1960). Laryngectomy: Past, present, and future. *Ann. Otol. Rhinol. Laryngol., 69,* 184–198.

Kallen, L. (1931). Vicarious vocal mechanisms. *Arch. Otolarngol., 20,* 460–503.

Kellotat, W. F., US Patent No. 2,093,453 issued Sept. 21, 1937.

Kosinski, J. K. (1877). Vollstandige extirpation des kehlkopfs. *Centralblatt für Chirurgie, 4,* 401–406.

Labbe, L. (1886). Sur un cas d'extirpation totale du larynx. *Bull. Acad. Med. 50, (2) 15,* 159–162.

Lange, F. (1880). Extirpation of the larynx and anterior wall of the oesophagus—recovery. Arch. Laryngol., *1,* 36–49.

Lane, C. E., US Patent No. 1,840,112 issued Jan. 5, 1932.

Langenbeck, B. R. K. von (1875). Total extirpation des kehlkopfs mit dem zungenbein, einem theil der zunge, des pharynx und esophagus. *Berliner klinische Wochenschrift, 12,* 453–455.

Lauder, E. M. (1980). *Self-help for the laryngectomee.* San Antonio, TX: Lauder.

Lebrun, Y. (1973). The artificial larynx. Amsterdam: Swets & Zeitlinger.

Leyro Diaz, J. (1924). Consideraciones sobre laringectomia y aparato de fonacion en los laringectomizados. *La Semana Medica, 31,* 27–30.

Lister, J. (1867). Antiseptic principle in the practice of surgery. *Lancet, 1,* 353–356.

Luchsinger, R. (1949). Voice without a larynx: Alaryngeal dysphonia. In R. Luchsinger and G. E. Arnold (Eds.), *Voice-speech-language* (p. 288). Belmont, CA: Wadsworth Publishing.

Maas, H. (1876a). Vellständige extirpation des kehlkopfes; Tod nach 14 tagen. *Arch. für klinische Chirurgie, 19,* 507–513.

Maas, H. (1876b). Extirpation des kehlkopfes; heilung. *Arch. klinische Chirurgie, 20,* 535–539.

Mackenzie, M. (1880). *Diseases of the pharynx, larynx and trachea.* New York: William Wood & Co.

Martin, H. (1963). Rehabilitation of the laryngectomee. *Cancer, 16,* 823–841.

McKesson, E. I. (1927). A mechanical larynx. *J. Amer. Med. Assoc., 88,* 645–646.

McKesson, E. I., US Patent No. 1,922,385 issued Aug. 15, 1933.

Newman, D. (1886a). Notes of a case of excision of the larynx for malignant disease. *Lancet, 2,* 159–161.

Newman, D. (1886b). Two lectures on tumors of the larynx, their pathology, symptoms and treatment; with illustrative cases. *Brit. Med. J., 1,* 579–583, 769, 813, 865.

Onodi, A. (1918). Ergebnisse der Abteilung für Hor-Sprach-Stimmstorungen und Tracheotomierte. *Monatsschrift für Ohrenheilkunde und Laryngo-Rhinologie, 52,* 85–102.

Pichler, H. (1961a). Klinische Erfahrungen mit einem neuen kunstlichen Larynx. *Monatsschrift für Ohrenheilkunde, 95,* 299–301.

Pichler, H. (1961b). Ueber ein neuartiges automatisch gesteuertes elektronisches Sprechgerät für Laryngektomierte. *Acta Otolaryngologica, 53,* 374–380.

Pollock, H. L., and Lederer, F. L. (1922). Artificial larynx. *Trans. Amer. Acad. Ophthalmol., 27,* 480.

Reyher, C. (1877). Die laryngotomie als diagnostischer und therapeutischer eingriff bei ulcerationen im kehlkopf; eine extirpation laryngis wegen karcinom der stimmbänder. *St. Petersburger medicinische Wochenschrift, 2,* 137, 149.

Riesz, R. R. (1930). Description and demonstration of an artificial larynx. *J. Acous. Soc. Amer., 1,* 273–279.

Rigrodsky, S., Lerman, J., and Morrison, E. (1971). *Therapy for the laryngectomized patient.* New York: Teachers College Press.

Rosenberg, P. J. (1971). Total laryngectomy and cancer of the larynx. *Arch. Otolaryngol., 94,* 313–316.

Rousselot, J. (1902). La parole avec un larynx artificiel. *La Parole, 12,* 65–79.

Schechter, D. C., and Morfit, H. H. (1965). The evolution of surgical treatment of tumors of the larynx. *Surgery, 57,* 457–479.

Schmidt, M. (1875). Total extirpation des Kehlkopfes mit ungümstigem Ausgange. *Arch. klinische Chirurgie, 18,* 189–194.

Schönborn, K. W. E. J. (1875). Extirpatio laryngis. *Berliner klinische Wochenschrift, 12,* 525.

Schüller, H. (1880). *Die tracheotomie, laryngotomie, und extirpation des kehlkopfes* (monograph). Stuttgart: F. Enke.

Sheard, C. (1931). A new, simple artificial voice box and its use. *Proc. Staff Meetings Mayo Clinic, 6,* 253–256.

Snidecor, J. (1962). *Speech rehabilitation of the laryngectomized.* Springfield, IL: Charles C Thomas.

Solis-Cohen, J. (1892a). Two cases of laryngectomy for adenocarcinoma of the larynx. *Trans. Amer. Laryngol. Assoc., 14,* 60–66.

Solis-Cohen, J. (1892b). Two cases of laryngectomy for adenocarcinoma of the larynx. *New York Med. J., 56,* 533–535.

Solis-Cohen, J. (1892c). A case of laryngectomy. *J. Laryngol., 7,* 285–289.

Stoerk, K. (1880). *Klinik der krankheitendes kehlkopfs der nase, und des rachens.* (pp. 546–555). Stuttgart: F. Enke.

Stoerk, K. (1887). Über larynxextirpation. *Weiner medizinische Wochenschrift, 37,* 1586–1590.

Stoerk, K. (1896). Über extirpation des larynx bei karzinom. *Arch. Laryngol. Rhinol., 5,* 22–31.

Tait, V., and Tait, R. (1959). Speech rehabilitation with the oral vibrator. *Speech Path. Ther., 2,* 64–69.

Tapia, A. G. (1914). Presentacion de un laringuectomizado hablando con un sencillismo aparato artificial. *Revista Espanola de Laringologia, Otologia y Rhinologia, 5,* 48–55.

Taptas, N. (1900). Un cas de laryngectomie totale pour sarcome; larynx artificiel externe. *Annales des Maladies de l'Oreille et du Larynx, 26,* 37–45.

Taub, S., and Spiro, R. H. (1972). Vocal rehabilitation of laryngectomees: Preliminary report of a new technic. *Amer. J. Surg., 124,* 87–90.

Trousseau, A., and Belloc, H. (1837). De la phthisie laryngee. Paris: Monograph. Cited by C. Jackson and C. L. Jackson, (1939). *Cancer of the larynx* (pp. 214, 287). Philadelphia: Saunders.

Virchow, R. L. K. (1858). *Die cellular pathologie in thren begrundung auf physiologische und pathologische gewebelehre.* Berlin: A. Hirschwald.

Watson, P. H. (1881). Laryngectomy for syphilis of the larynx. In Foulis, D. F. (Ed.), *Proceedings of the Transactions of the Seventh Session, International Medical Congress, 3,* 255. Cited by C. Jackson and C. L. Jackson, (1939), *Cancer of the larynx.* (pp. 241–287). Philadelphia: Saunders.

Weir, N. F. (1973). Theodore Billroth: The first laryngectomy for cancer. *J. Laryngol. Otol., 87,* 1161–1169.

Wolff, J. (1893a). Über den künstlichen und die pseudo-stimme. *Arch. klinische Chirurgie, 45,* 237–241.

Wolff, J. (1893b). Über den künstlichen kehlkopf und die pseudo-stimme. *Berliner klinische wochenschrift, 30,* 1009–1013.

Wright, G. M., US Patent No. 2,273,077 issued February 17, 1942.

Zerneri, L. (1965). Su un nuovo apparecchio protesico per laringectomizzati. *Archivio Italiano di Otologia, Rinologia e Laringologia, 76,* 748–754.

ADDITIONAL READINGS

Amatsu, M., Matsui, T., Maki, T., and Kanagawa, K. (1977). Voice rehabilitation after total laryngectomy: A new one-stage surgical technique. *Nippon Jibiinkoka Gakkai Kaiho, 80,* 779–785.

Amster, W. (1954). *A comparative study of the breathing and speech coordination of laryngectomized and normal subjects, and the relationships between the breathing and speech coordinations and articulatory errors of laryngectomized subjects to their speech intelligibility.* Unpublished doctoral dissertation, Syracuse University, Syracuse, NY.

Anderson, J. O. (1950). *A descriptive study of elements of esophageal speech.* Unpublished doctoral dissertation, Ohio State University, Columbus.

Arslan, M. (1975). Techniques of laryngeal reconstruction. *The Laryngoscope, 85,* 862–865.

Arslan, M., and Serafini, I. (1972). Restoration of laryngeal function after total laryngectomy: Report of the first 25 cases. *The Laryngoscope, 82,* 1349–1360.

Asai, R. (1965). *Asai's new voice production method: A substitution for human speech.* Paper presented at the Eighth International Congress of Otorhinolaryngology, Tokyo, Japan.

Asai, R. (1972). Laryngoplasty after total laryngectomy. *Arch. Otolaryng., 95,* 114–119.

Barton, R. (1965). A review of attempted physiological restoration of voice following total laryngectomy. *Proceedings of the 8th International Congress of Otorhinolaryngology* (pp. 731–734). Amsterdam: Excerpta Medica.

Berlin, C. (1965). 1. Clinical measurement of esophageal speech: III. Performance of non-biased groups. *Speech Hearing Dis., 30,* 174–183.

Blom, E. D. (1972). *A comparative investigation of acoustical and perceptual features of esophageal speech and speech with a Taub prosthesis.* Unpublished doctoral dissertation, University of Maryland, College Park.

Blom, E. D., and Singer, M. (1979). Surgical-prosthetic approaches for postlaryngectomy voice restoration. In R. L. Keith and F. L. Darley (Eds.), *Laryngectomee rehabilitation* (pp. 251–276). Houston, Texas: College-Hill Press.

Braini, A. (1958). Il ricupero sociale dei laringectomizzati attraverso un metodo personale operatorio. *Medicina Sociale, 8,* 265–269.

Brucke, E. W., cited by Czermak, J., in Lebrun, Y. (1973). *The artificial larynx* (p. 19). Amsterdam: Swets and Zeitlinger.

Bruns, P. von (1881). Über einige verbesserungen des kunstlichen kehlkopfes. *Verhandlunger der deutschen gesellschaft für chirurgie.* 10 Kongress, *10,* 51–53.

Calcaterra, T. C., and Jafek, B. W. (1971). Tracheo-esophageal shunt for speech rehabilitation after total laryngectomy. *Arch. Otolaryngol., 94,* 124–128.

Coleman, R., and Wendahl, R. (1967). Vocal roughness and stimulus duration. *Speech Monographs, 34,* 85–92.

Conley, J. J., DeAmesti, F., and Pierce, J. K. (1958). A new surgical technique for the vocal rehabilitation of the laryngectomized patient. *Ann. Otol., Rhinol., Laryngol., 67,* 655–664.

Conley, J. J. (1959). Vocal rehabilitation by autogenous vein graft. *Anals Otol., Rhinol., Laryngol. 68,* 990–995.

Conley, J. J. (1959). Vocal rehabilitation by autogenous vein graft. *Ann. Otol. Rhinol. Laryngol., 68,* 990–995.

Creech, H. B. (1966). Evaluating esophageal speech. *J. Speech Hearing Assoc. (Virginia), 72,* 13–19.

Damsté, P. H. (1958). *Oesophageal speech after laryngectomy.* Groningen: Hoitsema.

Damsté, P. H. (1975). Methods of restoring the voice after laryngectomy. *The Laryngoscope, 85,* 649–655.

DiBartolo, R. (1971). Psychological considerations in the attainment of esophageal speech. *J. Surg. Oncol., 3,* 451–466.

DiCarlo, L. M., Amster, W., and Herer, G. (1955). *Speech after laryngectomy.* Syracuse, NY: Syracuse University Press.

Diedrich, W. M. (1968). The mechanism of esophageal speech. *Ann. New York Acad. Science, 155,* 303–317.

Diedrich, W. M., and Youngstrom, K. (1961). An investigation of speech after laryngectomy. Final Report, Project 337, Office of Vocational Rehabilitation.

Diedrich, W. M., and Youngstrom, K. (1966). *Alaryngeal speech.* Springfield, IL: Charles C Thomas.

Doehler, M. (1953). *Esophageal speech.* Boston: American Cancer Society.

Duguay, M. J. (1966). Preoperative ideas of speech after laryngectomy. *Arch. Otolaryngol., 83,* 69–72.

Duguay, M. J. (1980). The speech-language pathologist and the laryngectomized lay teacher in alaryngeal speech rehabilitation. *ASHA, 22,* 965–966.

Edwards, N. (1974). Post-laryngectomy vocal rehabilitation. *J. Laryngol. Otol., 88,* 905–918.

Edwards, N. (1975). Post-laryngectomy rehabilitation by the external fistula method: Further experiences. *The Laryngoscope, 85,* 690-699.

Edwards, N. (1976). New voices for old: Restoration of effective speech after laryngectomy by the pulmonary air-shunt vocal fistula principle. *Bristol Medico Chirurgical Journal, 90,* 11–17.

Foulis, D. F. (1878). Extirpation of the larynx. *Lancet, 1,* 118–120.

Foulis, D. F. (1879). Extirpation of the larynx. *Lancet, 1,* 436–437.

Gardner, W. H. (1962). *The tenth anniversary of the International Association of Laryngectomees.* Paper presented at the eleventh annual meeting of the Voice Institute of the International Association of Laryngectomees, Memphis, TN.

Gardner, W. H. (1966). Adjustment problems of laryngectomized women. *Arch. Otolaryngol., 83,* 31–42.

Gardner, W. H. (1971). *Laryngectomee speech and rehabilitation.* Springfield, IL: Charles C Thomas.

Gardner, W. H. (1977). *Origins of the International Association of Laryngectomees, present services, and its future.* Paper presented at the seventeenth annual meeting of the Voice Institute of the International Association of Laryngectomees, Cleveland, OH.

Gardner, W. H., and Fortune, G. J. (Eds.). (1953). *Proceedings, First Institute on Voice Pathology.* Cleveland, OH: Cleveland Hearing and Speech Center.

Gates, G. A., Ryan, W., Cooper, J. C., Lawlis, G. F., Canter, E., Hayashi, M. A., Lauder, E., Welch, R. W., and Hearne, E. (1981). Current status of laryngectomee rehabilitation. San Antonio, TX: University of Texas Health Science Center. *Amer. J. Otolaryngol., 3,* 1–7 (1982).

Gilmore, S. I. (1962). *Social and vocational acceptability of esophageal speakers compared to normal speakers.* Final Project Report, RD 421, Office of Vocational Rehabilitation.

Goldberg, R. T. (1975). Vocational and social adjustment after laryngectomy. *Scand. J. Rehab. Med., 7,* 1–8.

Gonella, C., Parker, D., Hollender, J., Lowell, G., Pettersen, P., and Miller, S. (1978). Normative criteria for cancer rehabilitation. Rehabilitation and Research Monograph No. 1, Emory University Regional Rehabilitation Research and Training Center, Atlanta, GA.

Goode, R. (1973). The development of an improved artificial larynx. *Trans. Amer. Acad. Ophthalmol. Otolaryngol., 73,* 279–287.

Gussenbauer, C. (1874). Ueber die erste durch Billroth am menschen ausgeführte kehlkopf—exstirpation und die anwendung eines kunstlichen kehlkopfes. *Arch. klinische Chirurgie, 17,* 343–356.

Guttman, M. R. (1932). Rehabilitation of the voice in laryngectomized patients. *Arch. Otolaryngol., 15,* 479.

Guttman, M. R. (1935). Tracheohypopharyngeal fistulization. *Trans. Amer. Laryngol. Rhinol. Otol. Soc., 41,* 219–226.

Herzog, W., and Neumann, D. (1965). Ein künstlicher elektronischer kehlkopf. *Phonetica, 13,* 117–133.

Hodson, C. J., and Oswald, M. V. (1958). *Speech recovery after total laryngectomy.* London: Livingstone.

Horn, D. (1962). *Laryngectomy survey report summary.* Paper presented at the Eleventh Annual Meeting of the Voice Institute of the International Association of Laryngectomees, Memphis, TN.

House, A., and Fairbanks, G. (1953). The influence of consonant environment upon the secondary acoustical characteristics of vowels. *J. Acous. Soc. Amer., 25,* 105–103.

Iglauer, S. (1936). Artificial larynx with patient demonstrating its use. *Ann. Otol. Rhinol. Laryngol., 45,* 1176–1177.

Jackson, C., and Jackson, C. L. (1937). *The larynx and its diseases.* Philadelphia: Saunders.

Johnson, J. T., Casper, J., and Lesswing, N. J. (1979). Toward the total rehabilitation of the alaryngeal patient. *The Laryngoscope, 89,* 1813–1819.

Kalfuss, H. A., and Hoops, H. R. (1969). *Counseling the laryngectomee: A study of the surgeon's approach.* Paper presented at the ninth annual meeting of the Voice Institute of the International Association of Laryngectomees, Pittsburgh, PA.

Katz, R. (1960). The IAL: Voice of the voiceless. *Cancer News, 14,* 1, 2–6.

Keith, R. L., and Darley, F. L. (Eds.) (1979). *Laryngectomee rehabilitation.* San Diego, CA: College-Hill Press.

Keith, R. L., Linebaugh, C. W., and Cox, B. G. (1978). Presurgical counseling needs of laryngectomees: A survey of 78 patients. *The Laryngoscope, 88,* 1660–1665.

Keith, R. L., Shane, H. C., Coates, H. L., and Devine, K. D. (1977). *Looking forward . . . A guidebook for the laryngectomee.* Rochester, MN: Mayo Foundation.

Kelly, D. H., and Welborn, P. (1980). *Neckwear for the laryngectomee and other neck breathers.* Houston: College-Hill Press.

Kettrick, H. S. (1972). *For me—a "new" voice. I am a laryngectomee.* Dunedin, FL: S. Kett.

Kidd, N. (1962). The oral vibrator used in a case of polyomyelitis. *Dental Technician, 15,* 32–34.

King, H. (September 1, 1956). I lost my voice to cancer. *Sat. Eve. Post.,* pp. 20–21, 71–73.

Kluyskens, P., and Ringoir, S. (1970). Follow-up of a human larynx transplantation. *Laryngoscope, 80,* 1244–1250.

Komorn, R. M. (1974). Vocal rehabilitation in the laryngectomized patient with a tracheoesophageal shunt. *Ann. Otol. Rhinol. Laryngol., 83,* 445–451.

Komorn, R. M., Weycer, J. S., Sessions, R. B., and Malone, P. E. (1973). Vocal rehabilitation with a tracheoesophageal shunt. *Arch. Otolaryngol., 97,* 303–335.

Lebrun, Y., and Hasquin, J. (1971a). On the so-called dissociation between electrogram and phonogram. *Folia Phon., 23,* 225–227.

Lebrun, Y., and Hasquin, J. (1971b). Variations in vocal wave duration. *J. Laryngol. Otol., 85,* 43–56.

Leyro Diaz, J. (1924). Laryngectomy and the artificial larynx. *La Semana Medica, 31,* 27–30.

Lieberman, P. (1961). Perturbation in vocal pitch. *J. Acous. Soc. Amer., 33,* 597–603.

Mathis, J., Lehman, G. A., Shanks, J., and Blom, E. (1980). The importance of gastroesophageal reflux in acquiring esophageal speech (abstract). *Gastroenterology, 78,* 1219.

McClear, J. E. (1960). *Esophageal voice production.* New York: National Hospital for Speech Disorders.

McConnel, F. M., Sisson, G. A., and Logemann, J. A. (1977). Three years experience with a hypopharyngeal pseudoglottis after total laryngectomy. *Trans. Amer. Acad. Ophthalmol. Otolaryngol., 84,* 63–67.

McGrail, J. S., and Oldfield, D. L. (1971). One-stage operation for vocal rehabilitation at laryngectomy. *Trans. Amer. Acad. Ophthalmol. Otolaryngol., 75,* 510–512.

Miller, A. H. (1967). First experiences with the Asai technique of vocal rehabilitation after total laryngectomy. *Ann. Otolaryngol. Rhinol. Laryngol., 76,* 829–833.

Miller, A. H. (1968). Further experiences with the Asai technique for vocal rehabilitation after laryngectomy. *Trans. Amer. Acad. Ophthal. Otolaryngol., 72,* 779–781.

Miller, A. H. (1971). Four years experience with the Asai technique of vocal rehabilitation for the laryngectomized patient. *J. Laryngol. Otolaryngol., 85,* 567–576.

Montgomery, W. W., and Toohill, R. J. (1968). Voice rehabilitation after laryngectomy. *Arch. Otolaryngol., 88,* 499–506.

Moolenaar-Bijl, A., (1953). Connection between consonant articulation and the intake of air in oesophageal speech. *Folia Phon., 5,* 212–216.

Morrison, W. W. (1931). The production of voice and speech following total laryngectomy. *Arch. Otolaryngol., 14,* 413–431.

Nelson, C. R., (1949). *You can speak again; post-laryngectomy speech.* New York: Funk & Wagnalls.

Nichols, A. C. (1976a). Confusions in recognizing phonemes spoken by esophageal speakers: I. Initial consonants and clusters. *J. Comm. Dis., 9,* 27–41.

Nichols, A. C. (1976b). Confusions in recognizing phonemes spoken by esophageal speakers: II. Vowels and diphthongs. *J. Comm. Dis., 9,* 247–260.

Panje, W. R. (1981). Prosthetic vocal rehabilitation following laryngectomy—The voice button. *Ann. Otol. Rhinol. Laryngol., 90,* 116–120.

Pearson, B. W. (January 24, 1981). *Subtotal laryngectomy.* Paper presented at the Middle Section of American Laryngological, Rhinological and Otological Society, Inc., Oklahoma City. Also (1981) *The Laryngoscope, 91,* 1904–1912.

Pearson, B. W., Woods, R. D., and Hartman, D. E. (1980). Extended hemilaryngectomy for T3 glottic carcinoma with preservation of speech and swallowing. *The Laryngoscope, 90,* 1950–1961.

Peterson, G., and Barney, H. (1952). Control methods used in a study of the vowels. *J. Acous. Soc. Amer., 24,* 175–184.

Robe, E. Y., (1954). *A study of the role of three factors in the development of speech after laryngectomy: Type of operation, site of pseudoglottis, and coordination of speech with respiration.* Unpublished doctoral dissertation, Northwestern University, Evanston, IL.

Sacco, P. R., Mann, M. B., and Schultz, M. C. (1967). Perceptual confusions among selected phonemes in esophageal speech. *J. Speech Hearing Assoc., 26,* 19–33.

Salmon, S. J. (1975). *Psychological considerations.* Paper presented at the twenty-fourth annual meeting of the Voice Institute of the International Association of Laryngectomees, Dallas, TX.

Salmon, S. J. (1979). Methods of air intake for esophageal speech and their associated problems. In R. L. Keith and F. L. Darley, (Eds). *Laryngectomee Rehabilitation* (pp. 1–28). San Diego, CA: College-Hill Press.

Sanchez-Salazar, V., and Stark, A. (1972). The use of crisis intervention in the rehabilitation of laryngectomees. *J. Speech Hearing Dis., 37,* 323–328.

Shanks, J. C., and Duguay, M. J. (1974). Voice remediation and the teaching of alaryngeal speech. In S. Dickson, (Ed.), *Communication Disorders* (pp. 240–295). Glenview, IL: Scott Foresman.

Shedd, D., Bakamijian, V., Sako, K., Mann, M., Barba, S., and Schaaf, N. (1972). Reed fistula method of speech rehabilitation after laryngectomy. *Amer. J. Surg., 124,* 510–514.

Shedd, D., Schaaf, N., and Weinberg, B. (1976). Technical aspects of reed fistula speech following pharyngolaryngectomy. *J. Surg. Oncol., 8,* 305–310.

Shipp, T. (1967). Frequency, duration, and perceptual measures in relation to judgments of laryngeal speech acceptability. *J. Speech Hearing Res., 10,* 417–427.

Siegel, E., Konig, K., and Heidrich, R. (1969). Sociopsychiatric problems of laryngectomized patients. *Psychiatrie, Neurologie, und medizinische Psychologie, 21,* 330–336.

Simpson, I. C., Smith, J. C. S., and Gordon, M. T. (1972). Laryngectomy: The influence of muscle reconstruction on the mechanism of esophageal voice production. *J. Laryngol. Otol., 86,* 961–990.

Singer, M. I., and Blom, E. D. (1980). An endoscopic technique for restoration of voice after laryngectomy. *Ann. Otol. Rhinol. Laryngol., 89*(6), 529–533.

Singer, M. I., and Blom, E. D. (1981). A selective myotomy for voice rehabilitation after total laryngectomy. *Arch. Otolaryngol., 107,* 670–673.

Sisson, G. A., McConnel, F. M., Logemann, J. A., and Yeh, S. (1975). Voice rehabilitation after laryngectomy. *Arch. Otolaryngol., 101,* 178–181.

Sisty, N. L., and Weinberg, B. (1972). Formant frequency characteristics of esophageal speech. *J. Speech Hearing Res., 15,* 439–448.

Snidecor, J. (1969). *Speech rehabilitation of the laryngectomized* (2nd ed.). Springfield, IL: Charles C Thomas.

Snidecor, J. C. (1970). The family of the laryngectomee. In S. E. Gerber, (Ed.), *The family as supportive personnel in speech and hearing remediation* (pp. 12–30). Santa Barbara, CA: University of California Press.

Snidecor, J. C. (1971). *Laryngectomees and therapy* (videotape lecture). Presented at the eleventh annual meeting of the Voice Institute of the International Association of Laryngectomees, Kansas City, KS.

Snidecor, J. C. (1975). Some scientific foundations for voice restoration. *The Laryngoscope, 85,* 640–647.

Stetson, R. H. (1937). Esophageal speech for any laryngectomized patient. *Arch. Otolaryngol., 26,* 132–142.

Stoll, B. (1957). *An investigation into the relationships between certain communication factors and objective measures of the efficiency of the esopha-*

geal speech of laryngectomized patients. Final Report, Project 134, Office of Vocational Rehabilitation. *Amer. Otol. Rhinol. Laryngol., 67,* 550–557, 1958.

Stoll, B. (1958). Psychological factors determining the success or failure of the rehabilitation program of laryngectomized patients. *Ann. Otol. Rhinol. Laryngol., 67,* 550–557.

Tait, R. (1959). The oral vibrator. *Brit. Dent. J., 106,* 336–340.

Tait, R. (1960). The oral vibrator. *Brit. Dent. J., 109,* 506–507.

Tait, R. (1962). The oral vibrator. *Brit. Dent. J., 112,* 249–250.

Taylor, C. P. (1963). *Evaluation study report to the study committee of the IAL.* New York: American Cancer Society.

Tikofsky, R. S. (1965). A comparison of the intelligibility of esophageal and normal speakers. *Folia Phon., 17,* 19–32.

Vega, M. F. (1975). Larynx reconstructive surgery—A study of three year findings—A modified surgical technique. *The Laryngoscope, 85,* 866–881.

Waldrop, W. F., and Gould, M. A. (1956). *Your new voice.* Chicago: American Cancer Society, Illinois Division.

Wallen, V., and Webb, V. P. (1975). A survey of the background characteristics of 2000 laryngectomees: A preliminary report. *Mil. Med., 140,* 532–534.

Walsh, T. F. (1972). Sound the way for laryngectomees. *Patient Care, 6,* 58–89.

Weinberg, B., and Westerhouse, J. (1973). A study of pharyngeal speech. *J. Speech Hearing Dis., 38,* 111–118.

Winans, C. S., Reichback, E. J., and Waldrop, W. F. (1974). Esophageal determinants of alaryngeal speech. *Arch. Otolaryngol., 99,* 10–14.

Wolff, J. (1893). Üeber verbesserungen am künstlichen kehlkopf. *Arch. klinische Chirurgie, 45,* 237–257.

Zemlin, W. H. (1968). *Speech and hearing science.* New York: Prentice-Hall.

Zwitman, D., and Calcaterra, T. (1973). Phonation using the tracheoesophageal shunt. *J. Speech Hearing Dis., 38,* 369–373.

Chapter **3**

Methods of Air Intake for Esophageal Speech and Their Associated Problems

Shirley J. Salmon

This discussion will begin with an orientation to the anatomy and physiology associated with laryngectomy and esophageal speech since an understanding of it is basic to our topic. The information available about the associated anatomy and physiology has been obtained from surgeons who perform laryngectomies, analyses via fluoroscopy, still radiography, moving radiography, pharyngoesophageal manometry, electromyograms (EMGs), pneumography, and pneumotachography. A composite of information obtained from a number of such sources follows. It will lead to a clearer understanding of the structure of the esophageal speech mechanism and how air intake methods relate to its function during esophageal voice production.

ANATOMICAL CHANGES RESULTING FROM LARYNGECTOMY AND RADICAL NECK DISSECTION

"When total laryngectomy alone is carried out . . . the removed specimen typically consists of the hyoid bone, thyroid cartilage and contents, the strap muscles, epiglottis, cricoid cartilage and the upper two or three rings of the trachea" (Saunders, 1964, pp. 96–97). If cancer is present in the cervical lymph nodes, a radical neck dissection will likely be required on the right side, left side, or both sides of the neck. Then, according to Saunders, the following structures are routinely removed: the sternomastoid muscle, omohyoid muscle, internal jugular vein, spinal accessory nerve (XI), and submaxillary salivary gland. If there are specific indications, other structures that may be removed are the external carotid artery, a lobe of the thyroid, the strap muscles, cranial nerves X (vagus) and XII (hypoglossal), and the lingual branch of cranial nerve V (trigeminal) as well as a portion or all of the mandible.

As stated, total laryngectomy does not require removal of any cranial nerves. Radical neck dissection does require removal of the accessory nerve. Postoperatively this will result in a fairly significant shoulder drop on the operative side. Physical therapy may be advisable to help eliminate associated pain and stiffness. If more extensive neck surgery is required, cranial nerves X, XII, and the lingual branch of V may be involved. If so, associated impairments such as to oral-sensory function (touch, taste, and two-point discrimination) or lingual motor movements may be evident.

COMPARATIVE ANATOMY

A. *General Orientation of Structures Excised*
1. Following removal of the larynx, the trachea is sutured to the base of the neck to provide a permanent stoma for respiratory purposes.
2. The pharyngeal wall is then sutured together.
3. The inferior portion of the pharynx is joined to the upper esophageal area.
4. The superior portion of the pharynx is sutured to the base of the tongue.
5. If the suture lines do not heal well because of stitches either pulling through or breaking, a patient may develop
    a. *Fistula*—a tunnel from one opening to another that may result in the following:
        (1) The nasogastric tube must be used for a longer period of time.
        (2) A longer postoperative recovery period is necessitated.
        (3) The patient may be discharged to home with the nasogastric tube still in place.
        (4) Restriction of the use of neck-type artificial larynx unless cheek placement is utilized.
        (5) A delay in esophageal speech training.
        (6) The patient's depression may be intensified.

    b. *Diverticulum*—a pouch that is usually in the esophagus but could be in the pharynx that may result in the following:
- (1) A vulnerable structure for the collection of food or liquid.
- (2) The build-up of food may result in a bad taste or bad breath and may cause a feeling of something caught in the throat or a sensation of gagging.
- (3) The build-up of liquid or mucus may cause the esophageal voice quality to sound "gargly."

B. *The Hypopharynx*
1. The hypopharynx created by this suturing will vary in size and shape depending on the extent of surgery.
2. Tracings from lateral cinefluorographic films (Diedrich and Youngstrom, 1966) show that the hypopharynx is increased in size when comparisons are made between productions of sustained vowels by the same patient pre- and postlaryngectomy.
3. In general, the *length* of the hypopharynx postoperatively is shorter during vowel productions. However, the postoperative *width* of the hypopharynx is wider during most vowel productions.
4. Damsté (1958) and Diedrich and Youngstrom (1966) attempted to label and categorize the various shapes of the hypopharynx in esophageal speakers and then to relate the categories to good or poor esophageal speech skill. However, they were not successful in doing so since no significant correlations were obtained. Apparently, then, the shape or size of the configuration created by the hypopharynx, pharyngoesophageal (PE) segment, and upper esophagus has little to do with the acquisition or proficiency of esophageal speech.

C. *The Tongue*
1. Fibers from the base of the tongue are severed and joined with the pharyngeal suture line during surgery. They are no longer attached to the hyoid bone.
2. Some of the fibers of the tongue will be excised, perhaps causing shortening of the base of the tongue. If so, this effect, coupled with the shorter but wider hypopharynx postoperatively, may mean that the laryngectomee will need to develop compensatory articulatory movements. Since whispering is generally discouraged for fear that it may lead to development of buccal speech, early use of an artificial larynx seems the most logical way to help the newly laryngectomized acquire such compensatory movements.

D. *Comparison Between Speech Mechanisms: Normal and Esophageal*
1. Lauder (1978) has summarized the differences and similarities between the activator, vibrator, and articulators for normal speech production (lungs, vocal cords, articulators) and the esophagus, PE segment, and articulators used for esophageal speech production.
2. The esophagus is bounded superiorly by the hypopharynx and inferiorly by the stomach.
3. The esophagus is located immediately behind the trachea and lungs *and* it is within the thoracic cavity. Thus, the pressure within the esophagus can be influenced by intrathoracic pressure. This is an important fact to remember when considering the varying alterations in pressure that are associated with each method of air intake. The influence of intrathoracic pressure on esophageal pressure is highly stressed during any discussion of the "inhalation" method of air intake since more attempts are made to capitalize on it for this sort of intake procedure.
4. For both normal and esophageal speakers the esophagus is collapsed during a resting state. The intraesophageal air pressure at rest is negative and registers between -4 and -7 millimeters of mercury (mm Hg) below atmospheric pressure. This may decrease to -15 mm Hg on pulmonary inspiration.

E. *The Esophagus*
1. In his book *The Esophagus and Its Diseases,* Palmer (1952) reports that the length of the adult esophagus itself varies little according to sex or height. The average length is approximately 9 inches.
2. The diameter within the upper esophageal sphincter is a little over ½ inch, and the diameter at the inferior end just prior to its union with the stomach is less than one inch.
3. The distal or lower esophageal sphincter is often referred to as the cardiac sphincter. It is approximately 1 to 2 inches in length.
4. The sphincter at the PE junction is referred to by several names, the more common ones being upper esophageal sphincter and cricopharyngeal sphincter. It has been estimated to be approximately ½ inch long, which means that it is much shorter than its counterpart, the cardiac sphincter. Following laryngectomy the upper esophageal sphincter becomes the vibratory source for esophageal voice. Because the neoglottis is longer (⅘ inch to 1⅕ inches) than the upper esophageal sphincter (½ inch), it is referred to as the PE segment.
5. The various names used to label the PE sphincter probably result from confusion regarding how the sphincter operates. The

close proximity to (with fibers overlapping and even fusing) and the structural similarity between the cricopharyngeal muscle fibers and those belonging to the upper esophagus do not help clarify the situation. In addition, because knowledge of the innervation of the sphincter is less than adequate, it is difficult to differentiate structures involved in the sphincteric action. At the time of laryngectomy the fibers of the muscles within the PE area are severed and must be sutured back together. It seems reasonable to assume that both the number of fibers left to suture because of the extent of the lesions and the suturing procedure itself would influence the tightness or looseness of the sphincter observed clinically in patients. Some complain of difficulty in swallowing due to a feeling of tightness or of a "choking" sensation. Many of them talk about having to "wash" their food down. Also, when discussing their attempts to intake air, many of these same people describe a feeling of pressure in their throats that makes it difficult to move air downward owing to a "locking" sensation. The opposite extreme is represented by other patients who have no swallowing complaints and indicate little or no sensation of air passing into the esophagus during air intake. Patients of this type may not be able to achieve acceptable esophageal voice or volume level without some type of external pressure applied to their vibratory site.

F. *Tonicity of the PE Segment*

  1. Damsté (1958) has speculated that lack of tonicity within the cricopharyngeus muscle of esophageal speakers may make it difficult for the neoglottis to provide resistance to the expelled air from the esophagus during phonation. Since this resistance is considered necessary for good phonation, he believes that poor tonicity of the sphincter may prevent the acquisition of good esophageal voice. As mentioned previously, sometimes external pressure through styrofoam rubber, elastic bands, or digital pressure may be applied to increase tonicity of the muscle.

  2. The tonicity may be excessive. If the segment seems too tight, a bougie tube can be used for dilation. Another procedure described by Damsté might be tried if a physician is willing. It entails use of a syringe and a tube that has been inserted through the mouth and down into the esophagus. Activating the syringe forces air through the tube and into the esophagus. Reportedly, when the esophagus is sufficiently inflated, the PE segment will yield to the air pressure build-up below and esophageal voice will be produced. Damsté has suggested that repetition of this procedure provides the patient with sensory feedback so that eventually the capacity to open the PE

segment on a voluntary basis is achieved.

G.   *The Air Reservoir for Esophageal Speech*

1.   The capacity of the esophagus has been estimated by van den Berg and Moolenaar-Bijl (1959) to be approximately 80 cubic centimeters (cc) of air. This converts roughly to about 5 tablespoons.

2.   Most investigators seem to believe that only the upper one third of the esophagus is inflated during air intake by good or superior esophageal speakers.

3.   These observations appear to be supported by Snidecor and Isshiki (1965), who have also reported that the volume of air used by esophageal speakers *during continuous speech* is approximately 1 tablespoon. Incidentally, the study by Snidecor and Isshiki is one of several that negates the idea that the process for swallowing is similar to that for air injection. Care should be taken to avoid the word "swallow" in instructions for air intake.

The location of the air reservoir becomes an integral part of the definition of esophageal speech. According to Diedrich and Youngstrom (1966), "Esophageal speech is that in which the vicarious air chamber is located within the lumen of the esophagus and the neoglottis is located above the air chamber. The site of the neoglottis is located above the air chamber. The site of the neoglottis is the pharyngo-esophageal segment or junction and may contain fibers of the inferior constrictor, cricopharyngeus, and/or the superior esophageal sphincter which are predominately located at C5 and C6" (p. 108).

Thus, this discussion will exclude buccal speech, that resulting from air stored within the buccal area and squeezed in such a way that portions of the cheeks, tongue, or alveolar ridge become the vibrators. It also will exclude pharyngeal speech, that produced when air is stored in the pharynx and the tongue, soft palate, faucial pillars, or pharyngeal wall becomes the vibrator.

Thus, it is the PE constriction that is the vibratory site for esophageal speech. In order for esophageal phonation to occur, air must somehow pass down from the oral and pharyngeal cavities, through the segment, and into the esophagus. Then the air must be immediately redirected upward from the esophagus and pass through the PE segment in order to create sound.

In its natural or resting state, the PE segment is closed. Normally it opens only long enough to allow entry of liquids or food into the esophagus. It is typically in tonic contraction and normally prevents air from entering the esophagus and moving on down into the stomach. Thus, when a person desires to produce esophageal speech, he must learn some technique or techniques that enable him to transgress the normal resistance barrier of the PE segment and pass air in and out of it rapidly. It is this ability voluntarily to achieve rapid air intake and expulsion, into and out of the esophagus, that is basic to fluent esophageal speech.

In explaining the anatomy and physiology of the esophageal speech mechanism, Duguay (1977) likened the esophagus to a long, narrow collapsed balloon. At the top of the balloon is a rubber ring that, if closed tightly, would resemble the PE segment. To blow into the balloon a nonlaryngectomee, like an esophageal speaker, would have to build up enough oral-pharyngeal pressure to override the natural resistance of the rubber ring. If one is successful, the balloon will inflate. When the top ring of the balloon is pinched off to allow air to pass upward through the fingers, the natural elasticity of the balloon walls will help force the air upward. As it passes through the narrow opening at the top of the balloon, sound is produced. Such an analogy may clarify the idea that it is necessary to manipulate behaviors in three areas: (1) the oral-pharyngeal area, (2) the PE segment area, and (3) the esophagus. How can this be done?

It has been suggested by Damsté and others that for air intake purposes, the PE segment can either be voluntarily opened or forced open. If it can be opened voluntarily, then air that is circulating around in the mouth and pharynx might be drawn through the PE segment as with the inhalation method. On the other hand, if it must be forced open, then air in the mouth and pharynx must be compressed so that it exerts enough pressure above the PE segment to force it open, as is done, presumably, with the injection method.

In effect, the two primary methods of air intake are based on the two theories about how the PE segment opens for air intake and explusion.

Inhalation Method

With the inhalation method the tongue *never* occludes the oral cavity and there is little or no movement of the posterior tongue. The oral and nasal passages are open, and a completely patent airway is maintained between the lips or nose or both and the PE segment. The patient is instructed to close his mouth and to imagine breathing air in through his nose quickly. Sometimes, he is told to take a quick breath through his mouth and simultaneously inhale air into his lungs until they are about half full. Another technique utilized is to have the patient expel his breath via the stoma, then occlude his stoma with his fingers or handkerchief, open his mouth, and quickly suck air into his throat. These, then, are the frequently recommended instructions for teaching the inhalation method.

The purpose of these instructions is threefold. First, the act of quickly inhaling air through the stoma and into the lungs creates an instantaneous negative pressure within the thoracic cavity. This negative pressure is also reflected within the esophagus; consequently, the negative pressure within the esophagus during its *natural* state (-4 to -7 mm Hg) becomes *even more* negative (-10 to -20 mm Hg) with inspiration. This increased negativity within the esophagus makes it more likely that atmospheric air, registering positive pressure in the mouth and nose of the patient, will be drawn into the esophagus to equalize the pressure in both areas.

Second, instructions that encourage breathing air in through the nose or the mouth are designed to help the patient attain an open airway within the oral-pharyngeal area so that the positive pressure in the mouth can be drawn more readily through the PE segment by the negative pressure in the esophagus. The instructions, then, are designed to take advantage of the fact that positive pressure will move toward an area of negative pressure. Thus, if increased negativity can be created within the esophagus, it becomes even more of a vacuum and, it is hoped, the positive air available in the oral and pharyngeal cavities will be drawn or sucked through the PE segment.

Third, the instructions for breathing air through the nose or through the mouth are also given in the hope that there will be a reduction of tension throughout the entire oral, pharyngeal, and upper esophageal areas. The assumption is that the more patent the oral and pharyngeal airway, the more patent the PE segment. Theoretically, it should open more readily.

To elicit a quick inhalation and, consequently, a more rapid drop in esophageal pressure, Diedrich and Youngstrom (1966) have suggested the phrase "sniff air," which may help communicate better the "need for speed." The sniffing behavior may resemble that of a person with a head cold whose nose is so sore that he tries to "catch the drip" instead of using a handkerchief or tissue.

It is to be expected that the word "sniff" will conjure for the patient an image associated with preoperative behavior. Postoperatively, it is difficult or downright impossible for a patient to "sniff" through the nose but perhaps the imagery will cause him to inhale quickly *through the stoma.*

A sudden drop in negative pressure within the esophagus is only one part of the behavior attempted with the inhalation method of air intake. The other is an open airway within the oral cavity and hypopharynx so that air outside the mouth as well as air within the mouth (both of which are registering positive atmospheric pressure) can be drawn toward the negative pressure in the esophagus. To achieve such an open airway Diedrich and Youngstrom (1966) have suggested using the phrase "sucking air" through the mouth. In class lectures, Diedrich has also suggested that the laryngectomee might obtain a more open oral-pharyngeal airway if asked to imagine sucking in a mouthful of ground glass. Spriestersbach of the University of Iowa suggested the idea of sucking an apple down the throat. Patients can be encouraged to keep their throat open as they used to do when inhaling smoke from a cigarette or to try to replicate the open feeling in the back of their throat that occurs in the initial stage of a yawn. Recently, a patient reported that he could maintain a more open throat while attempting the inhalation method when he visualized a friend in college who, when competing in a chug-a-lug contest, seemed able to open his throat and pour down an entire bottle of beer without even swallowing!

Once the patient has demonstrated that he understands the concept of maintaining an open airway and has, simultaneously, inhaled air into his lungs until they are about half full, he is then instructed to expel his pulmonary air while he opens his mouth and attempts to say "ah." Sometimes the patient will be more effective when he is encouraged to feel the squeeze or contraction of his abdominal muscles as he releases the air from his lungs. The patient should be encouraged to expel his pulmonary air in a soft and easy manner. Otherwise the audible sound of air passing from the lungs and out the stoma will mask the esophageal sound he is attempting to produce through his mouth.

Maintaining a slow and steady expulsion of pulmonary air seems difficult for some patients, and many of them, unless discouraged early in therapy, will develop excessively loud wheezing noises through the tracheal stoma. Such wheezing noises are referred to as "stoma noise." Although it can be an associated problem with either method of air intake, it seems to be more of a problem for those who use the inhalation method of air intake.

To prevent stoma noise, some clinicians suggest to the patient that he try to hold his breath or "fix" the thoracic cage while attempting to produce esophageal voice, thereby reducing the chance for a distracting outflow of pulmonary air. Because of the direct link between the open stoma and the lungs it is, of course, impossible for the patient to inhibit all pulmonary airflow. However, the suggestion to "hold one's breath" will sometimes reduce both the amount and the speed of pulmonary air released through the stoma.

Laborwit (1970) proposes another means of inhibiting the extent of stoma noise. He suggests to the patient that the related anatomy resembles two sets of plumbing. The patient is encouraged to consider that one set of plumbing leads from the mouth, down his throat, through his esophagus, and into his stomach. The other set of plumbing is nearby but is totally separate; it leads from his stoma, through the tracheal area, and into his lungs.

At this point a discussion of anatomical drawings of the structures prior to surgery as compared to the postoperative anatomy may be useful. When a patient realizes that his voice is initiated and expelled from only one of the sets of plumbing, he may better understand that forcing air from his lungs in an attempt to achieve voice is pointless. In fact, it is detrimental because of its masking effect on the esophageal voice.

Other ways to approach the reduction of stoma noise entail use of the patients perceptual abilities. Often it is helpful to suggest that he alternate placing his fingers over the stoma and removing them from the stoma as he attempts to produce a series of esophageal sounds. When the patient literally feels the force of pulmonary air released from the stoma, he is sometimes able to decrease it. At the same time he can hear his esophageal voice with and without the masking effect of the stoma noise.

A useful gadget for increasing the patient's awareness of stoma noise is the "Talk-Back" device developed for helping children tune in better to their articulation errors. A microphone to a tape recorder can be placed strategically either to amplify or reduce the sound of stoma noise. Sometimes negative practice is helpful.

Shipp (1967) found that excessive stoma noise is a primary factor in determining whether judges find esophageal speech acceptable. His findings emphasize the importance of the speech clinician's consistent and conscientious efforts to prevent the patient from producing it, whenever possible.

Injection Method

For purposes of providing instructions to patients, it is easier to talk about two different types of injection.

The first type of injection method is injection via tongue pumping. Diedrich and Youngstrom (1966) refer to it as the glossopharyngeal closure type of injection. With this method the lips are usually sealed. The tip of the tongue *is* in contact with the alveolar ridge and the middle portion of the tongue is in contact with the hard and soft palate. When a pumpinglike motion of the tongue is initiated, the posterior portion makes a backward movement and thereby contacts the pharyngeal wall. During this pumping or rocking motion of the tongue, the velopharyngeal port is closed. Typically the patient is instructed to squeeze the tip of his tongue against the alveolar ridge, and as he uses the alveolar ridge as an anchor point, he is encouraged to perform rockinglike movements with the rest of his tongue. If the rocking motion is done correctly, it will often activate muscle movement in the upper region of the front of the neck or under the chin. Consequently, movement of the muscles in the region of the neck can be used as visible indicators of the patient's success at carrying out the instructions. To facilitate understanding these instructions, Diedrich and Youngstrom have suggested that the patient imagine taking a bubble of air and pushing it into the esophagus by wiping the roof of his mouth with the backward motion of the tongue and then squeezing or pumping the bubble into his esophagus. Lauder (1971) has suggested that the patient imagine his mouth is like a large paper sack full of air and that he use his tongue to push all of the air back and down into his throat.

Incidentally, intraoral pressure for injection can also be treated with tight lip closure and little or no tongue-tip involvement. In such instances, the air in the front of the mouth is squeezed backward with the cheeks as the middle portion of the tongue moves to come in contact with the hard and soft palate. So Lauder's suggestion about imagining that the mouth is like a large paper sack full of air can be adapted for the lip compression, with the cheeks pushing the air back instead of the tongue.

Another form of imagery used successfully is one whereby the patient is encouraged to squeeze air as far back into his throat as possible *without* swallowing. Compare this manipulation with the behavior of a small child when he is asked to take some medicine that he does not like, such as milk of magnesia. Occasionally it is helpful to use a gesture and, by placing the fingers of one hand into the palm of the other, demonstrate a side view of the pistonlike action that must be performed by the tongue.

Because teachers of esophageal speech used to believe that the motion of the tongue during this type of air injection resembled swallowing, this type of injection method was sometimes referred to as a "half-swallow," and in some of the outdated pamphlets laryngectomees are advised to "swallow air." To avoid confusion on the part of the patient, avoid making any comparison of air with swallowing. Instead, stress that with this air intake method, the laryngectomee must *not* swallow. One way of emphasizing the difference between the two behaviors is to have the patient who has achieved moderate success at injecting air on a voluntary basis alternate between the actual swallowing of coffee or water and his tongue-pumping attempts. This often helps him to develop some tactual discrimination and differentiate between the two behaviors, but not always.

In the early stages of learning this particular method of air intake, many patients will forget to replenish their air supply and in so doing alternate between voiced and nonvoiced productions. The need for systematic, follow-up injections should be underscored by suggesting to patients that obtaining voice is similar to obtaining money. They cannot cash a check (achieve voice) until they have first put money in the bank (injected air).

One problem commonly associated with injection via tongue pumping is what Diedrich and Youngstrom (1966) have called "klunking" and what others call "thumping." Snidecor (1968) states that it sounds like the words "punk" and "clump."

This klunking noise, which is audible during the intake of air and immediately prior to phonation, may be the result of too much air, injected too fast, and accompanied by too much tension within the pharyngeal or esophageal areas or both. Sometimes use of earphones with amplification, a stethoscope placed strategically, or playback of a speaker's voice from a tape recording will point out the klunking noise and encourage the laryngectomee to modify his behavior. Sometimes the simple suggestion that he speak more softly seems to help him reduce the amount of muscular tension exerted and in so doing decrease the audibility of the klunk.

The injection of too much air often results in its leakage from the esophagus into the stomach and frequently causes an accumulation of gas in the stomach and, occasionally, problems with distention. These problems often occur with the patient who produces a series of successive intakes prior to achieving any phonation or with the patient who has not developed smooth coordination between his efforts to achieve air intake and his efforts to expel air for esophageal voice. Too much air can sometimes be avoided by suggesting to the patient that he is behaving as if he were taking in several cupfuls of air, whereas only 3 to 4 tablespoons is all that is necessary to produce good esophageal voice. If the laryngectomee does accumulate a build-up of air within his stomach, he will often be really embarrassed by involuntary belching. Early in therapy it is a good practice to establish a permissive environment for such behavior and discourage any apologies. In attempts to play down our cultural disapproval of belching aloud, it is helpful to frequently tell the patient he is wasting good air that could be used for speech and point out that since it is free, he might as well *use* it by incorporating it into esophageal speech.

A second type of injection is what I will refer to as injection via consonant press. It is sometimes referred to as the plosive consonant method or plosive injection method. It is described most completely by Damsté (1958). With this method, air is compressed within the oral cavity via lip or tongue movements that accompany voiceless and, sometimes, voiced consonant productions. The velopharyngeal port is closed. Usually the patient is asked to produce a series of voiceless /p/, /t/, /k/, or /s/ sounds to determine which he is able to produce with the most plosion or frication. Occasionally a patient will demonstrate better frication with an /s/ blend. If so, he should be instructed to produce an /sp/, /st/, or /sk/. At other times, the patient may be able to achieve more frication with affricate productions. As the patient experiments with whichever of these sounds he produces most effectively, he should be encouraged to feel the compression of air within his mouth, and subsequently, the backward movement of some of the air as he produces the plosive consonants. Once a determination of which of the patient's sounds is more turbulent has been made, it can be explained to him that some of the air compressed in his mouth will be used to produce the forward movement of air, but some of it can also be forced backward into the throat and down into the esophagus. This "kick-back" of air into the throat and into the esophagus can be used for voicing when the consonant production is followed by a vowel. If the patient has difficulty compressing air out of his mouth with lip movements, it may be helpful to suggest the idea of spitting a grape seed from the edge of his lip or, as Snidecor (1971) recommends, to simulate the behavior of an old timer spitting tobacco juice. Gardner (1971) suggests that the popping of air against a piece of paper be used to demonstrate the type of tongue or lip action required to create the turbulence.

When the laryngectomee is not successful in compressing the air from his mouth and the hypopharynx down into the esophagus, it may be due to hypertension of the pharyngeal muscles as a result of his attempts to produce forceful consonants. Another reason may be that the PE segment is in such a state of excessive contraction that it prevents air passage to the esophagus and the result is a dilated hypopharynx. The air is trapped within the hypopharynx and cannot be maneuvered downward past the PE segment into the esophagus. When this occurs, the hypopharynx becomes the air chamber; as air is forced upward and outward from it, sound may be produced from the vibration of the tongue, hard or soft palate, faucial pillars, or the posterior pharyngeal wall. The patient will then, by definition, be producing pharyngeal voice. If this type of voice is reinforced by the clinician and established as an habitual pattern of behavior by the patient, it will be difficult for him to shift his sound source downward and to produce esophageal sound. Consequently, it is imperative that the clinician be alert to this kind of high-pitched, friction-like sound, which has a thinner, less-resonant quality. Its use must not be reinforced. Sometimes it is helpful to suggest that his voice sounds as if he is in the soprano or tenor range rather than the desired alto or bass range. Sometimes it helps to encourage him to push the air down lower and to provide models of esophageal voice.

It does not particularly matter which method of air intake is introduced first. Everyone develops a bias concerning one or the other that he or she prefers to teach. You may need to introduce all three methods and to jump back and forth among them, or some prefer to follow Diedrich's suggestion and have patients attempt the combined behaviors that result in use of all three methods.

Because your patient may not successfully carry out instructions for *one* method of air intake and you may need to change them or to switch to a different air intake procedure, it is imperative that you set the scene for lots of experimentation. Although you hope very much to help him achieve esophageal sound in the first session, it is better if he does not know this. It puts less pressure on him if you talk as if you do not expect any success for a while.

Before you begin trying to teach a patient to produce esophageal sound, be sure to find out if he already can. Ask if he knows how to belch or burp or if he has inadvertently made any esophageal sounds at home when air collected in his stomach while eating or when using an artificial larynx. If so, find out whether he can replicate such sounds volitionally. If he can, reinforce the behavior and begin shaping it for esophageal phonation.

This chapter has discussed the anatomy and physiology of the esophageal speech mechanism so that you might better understand how the different methods of air intake relate to its function and has suggested words or phrases that might be meaningful to your patients when you instruct them regarding each method of air intake. It is hoped the information is useful to you. Good luck!

QUESTIONS

1. What implications for speech could be associated with a patient who develops a fistula in the hypopharynx?
2. Differentiate between the shapes of the hypopharynx before and after surgery.
3. What factors could influence tightness (resistance) of the pharyngoesophageal (PE) segment?
4. Through what structures must air pass in order for a laryngectomee to successfully obtain an "air charge" using a pumping method? After listing these structures describe for each the pressure requirements that must be met in order for air to flow through the structure and those behaviors of the laryngectomee that are necessary to meet the requirement.
5. Write a topical outline you might follow in instructing a person to "inhale" air into the esophagus.

6. List some disadvantages to teaching a client to "swallow" air as a form of insufflation.
7. Behaviors associated with an audible "klunk" upon air charge include __________.
8. Why is it that some individuals can accomplish an air charge when attempting to produce a sibilant or plosive consonant?
9. List the various types of air charge and under each heading identify some of the reasons clients may fail to accomplish air charge by that method.
10. Hearing a patient belch provides what information that would reasonably let you assume the person's high probability of being able to produce sound using standard esophageal voice production methods?

REFERENCES

Berg, J., van den, and Moolenaar-Bijl, A. J. (1959). Crico-pharyngeal sphincter, pitch, intensity and fluency in oesophageal speech. *Practica Oto-Rhino-Laryngologica, 21,* 298–315.

Damsté, P. H. (1958). *Oesophageal speech.* Groningen: Gebr. Hoitsema.

Diedrich, W. M., and Youngstrom, K. A. (1966). *Alaryngeal speech.* Springfield, IL: Charles C Thomas.

Duguay, M. J. (1977). Esophageal speech. In M. Cooper and M. H. Cooper (Eds.), *Approaches to vocal rehabilitation.* Springfield, IL: Charles C Thomas.

Gardner, W. H. (1971). Twentieth Annual I.A.L. Convention, Kansas City, MO.

Laborwit, L. (1970). Fifteenth Postgraduate Course in Esophageal Speech. University of Miami School of Medicine, Miami, FL.

Lauder, E. (1971). Alaryngeal Voice Workshop. Lost Chord Club of Southern California, Los Angeles, CA.

Lauder, E. (1978). *Self-help for the laryngectomee.* 11115 Whisper Hollow, San Antonio, TX 78230.

Palmer, E. D. (1952). *The esophagus and its diseases.* New York: Paul B. Hoeber.

Saunders, W. H. (1964). *The larynx.* Summit, NJ: Ciba Pharmaceutical Company.

Shipp, T. (1967). Frequency, duration, and perceptual measures in relation to judgments of alaryngeal speech and acceptability. *J. Speech Hearing Res., 10,* 417–427.

Snidecor, J. C. (1971). Alaryngeal voice workshop. Lost Chord Club of Southern California. Los Angeles, CA.

Snidecor, J. C., (1968). *Speech Rehabilitation of the Laryngectomized.* Springfield, IL: Charles C Thomas.

Snidecor, J. C., and Isshiki, N. (1965). Air volume and air flow relationships of six male esophageal speakers. *J. Speech Hearing Dis., 30,* 205–216.

Chapter **4**

Developing Esophageal Communication

James C. Shanks

The topic of developing esophageal communication implies that one has been able to produce esophageal voice, along the lines outlined by Doctor Shirley Salmon. There appear to be five different parameters to the development of esophageal communication: (1) the nature of the communication, (2) an improvement in voice control, (3) the development of speech proficiency, (4) the acquisition of nonspeech attributes to assist communication rather than detract from it, and (5) a time frame under which the totality of communication proceeds.

The assessment of overall communication was an issue addressed in the Northwestern Otolaryngology Communication Profile. This scale was developed by Logemann, Fischer, and Becker in the late 1970s for head and neck surgery patients in the Otolaryngology Department at Northwestern University School of Medicine. However, it was first published in 1980 as an Appendix to a book on facilitation of speech (Shedd and Weinberg, 1980). Included in the scoring sheet for this chart (Fig. 4–1) is an assessment of (1) the amount, (2) the mode, and (3) the understandability of that communication. Each of these categories is assessed on a 60 point scale in five communication settings: at the place of residence, with friends, at work, on the telephone, and in other situations. Typically, there are some six questions regarding each setting. For example (Fig. 4–2), at the place where you live, if you really need someone's help, do you let him know? How do you do this? How well do you think people understand you? Other questions are: When you need something, do you ask for it? Do you answer questions of anyone where you live? Do you ask questions? If people are just talking where you live, do you

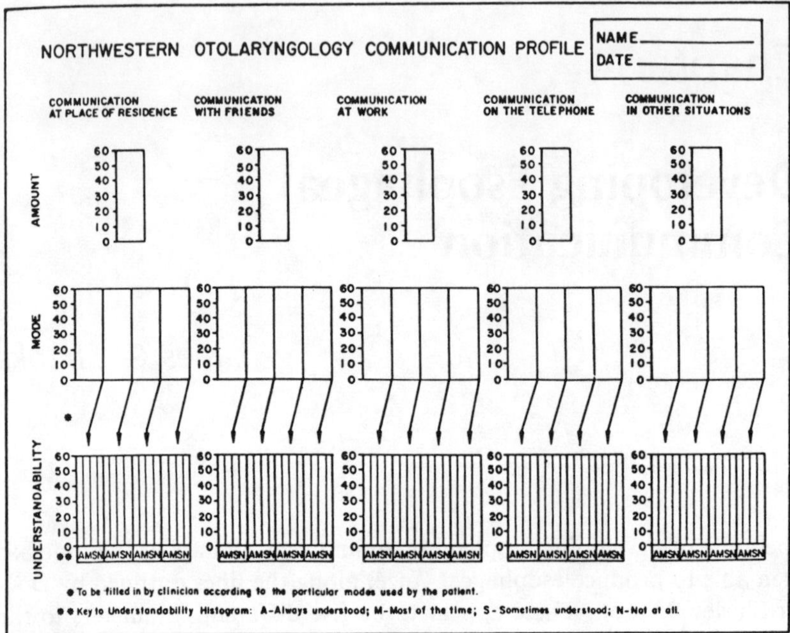

Figure 4–1. Scoring sheet for communication profile.

join in? If people are around, do you start talking to them? Through the use of such a scale, assessments may be made periodically to measure improvement in overall communication, not only concerning laryngectomy but for other disorders as well.

The overview of communication also was addressed in a study of cancer rehabilitation conducted under National Cancer Institute (NCI) auspices by Gonnella and co-workers (1978) at Emory University. Leaders throughout the country assume that speech should be intelligible by from 6 months (estimated by 10 per cent of the group) to 12 months (estimated by 85 per cent) after surgery (Figure 4–3). At the same time, effective communication was assumed by the respondents to exist from immediately after surgery to the 12 month termination point. How then is the development of esophageal communication quantified or scaled? Scales for this development have been in existence for more than a quarter of a century, beginning with the empiric notations made by Wepman, MacGahan, Rickard, and Shelton (1953). Subsequently, scales developed by Moore (1971), Robe, Moore, Andrews, and Hollinger (1956), and Barton and Hejna (1952) were similar to Wepman's. Irwin (1963) and

<u>COMMUNICATION AT THE PLACE WHERE YOU LIVE</u>

1. <u>If you really need someone's help, do you let him know?</u> Yes **No**

   a. How many times a day do you do this? (circle below)
      1   2   4   8   more than 8

   b. How do you do this? (circle below)
      Pointing &/or   Moving your mouth   Mechanical   Paper &
      gesturing   or whispering   larynx   pencil
           Laryngeal   Esophageal   Other:
           prosthesis   voice   __________

   c. How well do you think people understand you? (circle below)
      Always   Most of the time   Sometimes   Not at all

2. <u>When you need something do you ask for it?</u> Yes No

   a. How many times a day do you do this? (circle below)
      1   2   4   8   more than 8

   b. How do you do this? (circle below)
      Pointing &/or   Moving your mouth   Mechanical   Paper &
      gesturing   or whispering   larynx   pencil
           Laryngeal   Esophageal   Other:
           prosthesis   voice   __________

   c. How well do you think people understand you? (circle below)
      Always   Most of the time   Sometimes   Not at all

3. <u>Do you answer questions of anyone where you live?</u> Yes No

   a. How many times a day do you do this? (circle below)
      1   2   4   8   more than 8

   b. How do you do this? (circle below)
      Pointing &/or   Moving your mouth   Mechanical   Paper &
      gesturing   or whispering   larynx   pencil
           Laryngeal   Esophageal   Other:
           prosthesis   voice   __________

   c. How well do you think people understand you? (circle below)
      Always   Most of the time   Sometimes   Not at all

4. <u>Do you ask questions of anyone where you live?</u> Yes No

   a. How many times a day do you do this? (circle below)
      1   2   4   8   more than 8

   b. How do you do this? (circle below)
      Pointing &/or   Moving your mouth   Mechanical   Paper &
      gesturing   or whispering   larynx   pencil
           Laryngeal   Esophageal   Other:
           prosthesis   voice   __________

   c. How well do you think people understand you? (circle below)
      Always   Most of the time   Sometimes   Not at all

5. <u>If people are just talking where you live, do you join in?</u> Yes **No**

   a. How many times a day do you do this? (circle below)
      1   2   4   8   more than 8

   b. How do you do this? (circle below)
      Pointing &/or   Moving your mouth   Mechanical   Paper &
      gesturing   or whispering   larynx   pencil
           Laryngeal   Esophageal   Other:
           prosthesis   voice   __________

   c. How well do you think people understand you? (circle below)
      Always   Most of the time   Sometimes   Not at all

6. <u>If people are around where you live, do you start talking to them?</u>
   Yes No

   a. How many times a day do you do this? (circle below)
      1   2   4   8   more than 8

   b. How do you do this? (circle below)
      Pointing &/or   Moving your mouth   Mechanical   Paper &
      gesturing   or whispering   larynx   pencil
           Laryngeal   Esophageal   Other:
           prosthesis   voice   __________

   c. How well do you think people understand you? (circle below)
      Always   Most of the time   Sometimes   Not at all

Figure 4–2. Communication profile, where you live.

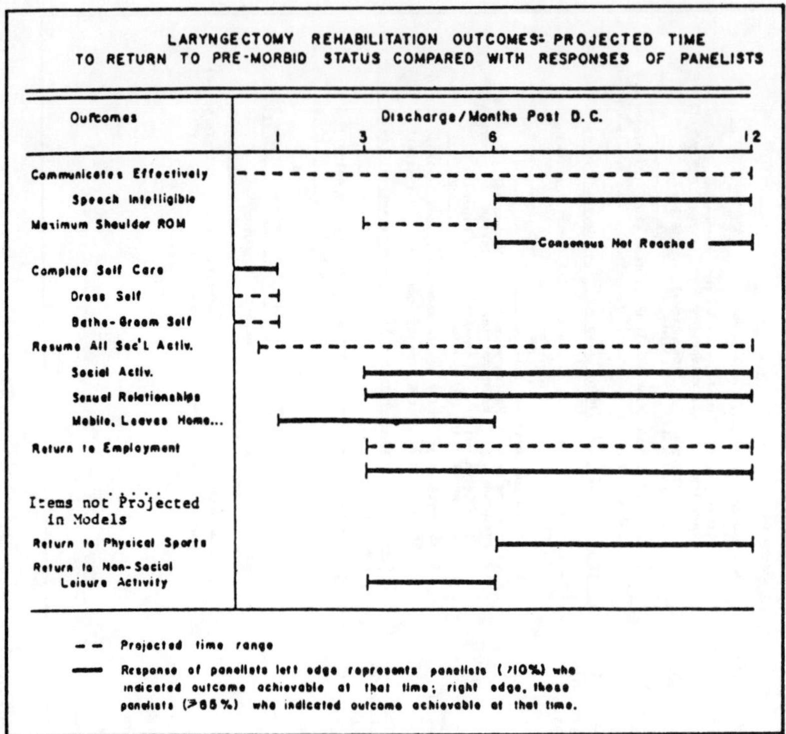

Figure 4–3. Projected laryngectomy rehabilitation.

most recently Gray (1973) have also developed scales. In general, these scales use the concept of rating dimensions of voice development as well as speech development.

In the assessment of voice improvement, it is helpful to go back to the basic parameters of sound: pitch, loudness, duration, and quality. To omit quality for the moment, the other attributes might be converted to frequency, intensity, and time. The acronym FIT is used to stand for *f*requency, *i*ntensity, and *t*ime. For esophageal as well as for laryngeal voice, the question remains: When is the voice "fit"?

The fundamental frequency of esophageal voice is lower than that of laryngeal voice, but can there be changes of frequency both in shift and during inflected speech? Esophageal speech need not be uttered at a monotone frequency level. The study of superior speakers by Snidecor

(1968) indicates that there can be a change of two or three tones in both inflection and shift. It should be noted that it is the superior speaker who achieves this change. The beginning speaker, for perhaps 6 to 12 months, should be content with whatever frequency he gets and should not concern himself with the modification of frequency in speech. Perhaps some inflection will emerge as the individual attempts in the first year of using esophageal voice to emphasize a word—to say "Oh!" or to say "I don't *want* to." A conscious effort in the second year after acquisition of voice to develop this pitch change to the maximum is more appropriate.

With respect to changes of intensity, it is recognized that the general intensity level of esophageal speech is lower than that of laryngeal speech, perhaps by 7 or 8 decibels (dB), with a restricted range of intensities available to the speaker. As in the case of frequency, it probably is well not to emphasize conscious expansion of the intensity range during the first few months or even the first year of speaking after laryngectomy. Despite this admonition, clinical practice suggests that most laryngectomees, all too aware of limitations of loudness, strive to speak more loudly. It is this clinician's sincere conviction that if the esophageal speaker is willing to try during the first year to speak as softly as he can with esophageal voice, the attempt must be made to help him learn to speak more loudly during the second year.

Clinically, the clinician might use a volume unit (VU) meter or a sound level meter to enable the laryngectomee to monitor the intensity level of his voice or speech utterance. Without equipment, the clinician might use the technique of determining how many feet away from the laryngectomee someone must be in order not to hear when esophageal voice is being produced in relative quiet.

The dimension of time in esophageal speech is fractionated by four component measures: (1) How long does it take to get air from the vocal tract into the esophagus? (2) How long does it take to reverse the direction of air flow so that sound is initiated? (3) How long can phonation be sustained? and (4) How much does the person voice within a given period of time such as a day? Over 20 years ago Berlin (1963) evolved some measures of esophageal speech that focused in great part on time. Consistency of phonation really refers to how many times a person produces voice on x number of trials. This is a quantitative measurement that may be made periodically.

The measure of time involved in charging the esophagus with air is subject to differing interpretations. In his description of this skill, Berlin (1963) noted a short latency between inflation of the esophagus and vocalization, apparently referring to the interval between inflation and the start of voice. However, he used a measure that began when the patient signaled that he was *beginning* to inflate his esophagus. Measured in this way, latency has to do both with the time needed to reverse the air flow and initiate phonation. Berlin's criterion of 0.4 seconds is reasonable for measures of pass-fail judgments. It may be noted that good speakers were able to achieve this intake of air in 0.2 of a second, a value in agreement with reports by Damsté (1958) and Diedrich and Youngstrom (1966).

Duration of phonation can likewise be measured in terms of seconds of sustained vowel production or repetition of an articulatory gesture with continuous phonation, such as repetition of the voiced syllable "da" as suggested by Berlin. As an activity the clinician might employ the rotation of the five vowel letters: a, e, i, o, u. This tool allows for a count of the number of discrete vowels uttered, even in the absence of a timer such as a watch. When the talker begins to sustain "a-e-i-o-u-a-e-i-o-u," it can be determined whether it is, in fact, 7, 10, 15, or even 25 separate vowels that have been uttered. Obviously such a clinical measure is influenced by the rapidity with which the individual shifts from one vowel to another. An application of Berlin's criteria in a clinical setting was made by Simpson and Martin (1975). Their data, like Berlin's, showed growth curves over time in the speaker's ability both to phonate consistently on demand and to sustain the isolated vowel /a/. Before concluding the discussion of these parameters of time, it should be noted that these tools not only provide test data by which progress can be measured but also supply a neat vehicle for practice in therapy that involves nonpropositional voicing.

Ideally, the talker should be able to get the air in quickly and the sound out in a prolonged fashion. It should be noted that some variability in each of these two skills may relate to the method of air intake used. It would be expected that the person who is an inhaler or a standard injector would be a bit longer in charging the esophagus but would have a longer duration. In contrast, the person relying primarily on consonant injection would be expected to get air in more quickly but to have a slightly shorter duration. A blend of both skills would be ideal to maximize time dimensions.

In measuring how much the individual voices during a given day, the clinician determines the amount of practice engaged in as well as the extent to which the laryngectomee uses his voice in communicative settings. To have all the skills and not to use them is indeed a tragedy. For example, one laryngectomee had opted for individual therapy, and as each Friday afternoon arrived, he would demonstrate skill in the production of voice as well as speech, but his wife would report that he had not spoken during the entire week since the previous clinical visit. This is sad. A pedometer exists to measure how many miles a person walks in a day; there ought to be a phonometer with a band around the neck to assess the total amount of voicing in a given day. This aspect, though difficult to measure, does relate back to the Northwestern scale and constitutes a desirable behavior to be aware of. Many laryngectomees who are proficient in speaking indicate that although it is not painful nor especially arduous, talking does take a certain amount of extra effort. Most laryngectomees indicate that they talk somewhat less with esophageal voice than they did with the preoperative laryngeal voice.

The fourth attribute of voice, quality, is difficult both to assess and to change. Although the dictum that quality is related to periodicity of phonation is acceptable, the question remains: How can you tell when voice is periodic when it emanates from the esophagus? One innovative clinical tool reported by Damsté (1958) involves the intentional playback at one-sixteenth the speed of a recorded utterance. Because the fundamental frequency of esophageal phonation hovers around 64 hertz (Hz), the one-sixteenth rate of playback is in the neighborhood of 4 cycles per second, yielding an auditory experience that is both perceptible and distinctive. Listen now to the voice of a person whose esophageal utterance appears to have suitable resonance and good quality. (Tape) Played back at one-half speed, the voice quality is still perceived as rather smooth, although speech begins to be reduced in intelligibility. (Tape) That same utterance at one-sixteenth of the original speech provides us with a listening experience somewhat analogous to waves washing in a cave on the ocean shore. (Tape) With this rhythmic "boom, boom, boom," one can confirm on a clinical level the basis for the apparent periodicity in connected utterance at standard speed playback.

How may the quality be faulty? The usual flow cited is that of a "wet" quality. All esophageal phonation involves the emergence of air bubbles through some degree of moisture in the hypopharynx, and this retention of fluid in the hypopharynx does not provide the penalty to pulmonary ventilation that would be the case for a laryngeal speaker. Thus it is not surprising that perception of a wet sound is made for some laryngectomees all of the time and for other larygectomees on occasion. Rather than suggest that the person insert a blotter into his hypopharynx, it probably is more appropriate to ask that the person swallow once, twice, or even three times before speaking. Another clinical tool to alter quality involves the alteration of tension at the PE itself. The application of a finger to the neck or a turn of the head may alter the mass and tension of the new glottis, thereby altering quality. Finally, the most practical suggestion to improve quality is to reduce the intensity of speech. Too often the speaker pays a price in quality when he attempts to produce loud speech.

In contrast to voice, the development of speech can be charted with a variety of measures, most of them quantified. The first area involves rate of connected speech. When it is recalled that young adults read aloud at a rate of 150 to 165 words per minute and when the difficulties attendant on the limited volume of air in the storage tank for esophageal voice are appreciated, it is not surprising that esophageal speech is slower than laryngeal speech. Snidecor (1968) observed good esophageal speech to involve utterance at the rate of 80 to 130 words per minute. Indeed, a rate of 100 to 110 words per minute, two-thirds the laryngeal rate, is an excellent standard to shoot for. At the beginning the rate of connected speech may be no more than 20 to 40 words per minute.

That the person may have his overall speech acceptability judged on the basis of rate should not be too surprising. Hoops and Noll (1969) found the rate measure of words per minute to be the measure most highly correlated with speech intelligibility and acceptability. This observation was true both when the listener was a speech pathologist familiar with esophageal speech and when listeners were unsophisticated, that is, were not familiar with esophageal speech. However, to say that a laryngectomee cannot speak at the rate of laryngeal utterance is not quite accurate. In the following tape sample, note how this particular laryngectomee was able, in a special situation, to speak at a rate of 260 words a minute, 100 more than the laryngeal standard. (Tape)

Another aspect of speech related to rate has to do with the grouping of words into suitable phrases. You may recall that Wepman's measures of speech proficiency really related to the capacity to string words together in sequence with word grouping and fluency being presumed. The adequacy of such word grouping, however, is not easy for the laryngectomee to master in esophageal speech. It is far better to use a slightly shorter phrase and not run out of air and voice within syllables or words than to keep driving the car until the tank runs dry between gas stations. It is better to say, "I work in (pause) Rochester," than to say, "I work in Ro (pause) chester." In attempting to expand voicing into phrases involving several syllables, laryngectomees might be well advised to practice groupings of numbers ("1-2-3" "4-5-6" "7-8-9") or letters ("a-b-c-d" "e-f-g-h"). Another clinical tool is the use of nursery rhymes that involve a meter conducive to the grouping of words by ideas (Gandour and Weinberg, 1982). It may be noted that the nonpropositionality of the nursery rhyme also reduces communicative pressure on the speaker.

Most speech clinicians would consider articulatory accuracy to be highly correlated with speech proficiency. It may be assumed that vowels as well as consonants will be produced and perceived accurately on standardized tests such as the vowel rhyme test or the consonant tests prepared by House, Williams, Hecker, and Kryter (1965) or the Multiple

Choice Discrimination Test (MCDT) lists of Schultz and Schubert (1969). These closed response sets enable the listener to select one of six potential utterances to determine agreement with the speaker's intent. In esophageal speech a voice signal is either present or absent, so theoretically voiceless consonants are not produced readily. Therefore, surd-sonant confusions may be expected in esophageal speech, as shown in a study involving a confusion matrix of various consonants (Sacco, Mann, and Schultz, 1967) (Fig. 4–4). When the sound /p/ was uttered or at least intended, it was perceived as /p/ 39 per cent of the time. As might be expected, a number of listeners perceived the sound as /b/, the voiced cognate of /p/. Indeed, the 22 perceptions of /b/ outnumbered all other "substitution" perceptions. However, when the consonant /b/ was uttered, 40 per cent of the time the listeners perceived it as /b/, while in 11 per cent of the listeners' judgments it was perceived as /p/. This seeming contradiction may stem from the fact that some esophageal voicing is achieved by inhalation or injection, which would lead to the perception of a voiceless sound as voiced, while speakers using consonant injection techniques for air charge are more likely to produce a voiced stop /b/ with sufficient pressure than one that is perceived as its voiceless cognate.

A study by Nichols (1974) also focused on perceptual confusion. The pattern was puzzling, however. The initial cluster /br-/ was perceived correctly 344 times, only 5 times as /pr-/, and 105 times as /r/ without the initial /p/. At the same time, initial /p/ was perceived correctly only 108 times, as /b/ 67 times, and as /bl-/ 247 times. Initial /t/ was perceived correctly 444 times, as /d/ 138 times. Initial /d/ was perceived correctly 483 times, as /t/ only 35 times. Initial /kr-/ was perceived correctly 214 times, as /gr-/ 221 times. Initial /g/ was perceived correctly 347 times, as /k/ 89 times. Initial /t/ was perceived correctly 414 times, as /dʒ/ 195 times. Initial /dʒ/ was perceived correctly 403 times, as /t/ 130 times.

Apart from voicing errors, there is considerable evidence that some classes of sounds cause more difficulty than others. Nasal sounds, for example, are reported by many investigators to pose serious problems. Perhaps, as noted by Diedrich and Youngstrom (1966), too many laryngectomees maintain velopharyngeal closure during nasal consonant utterance, reducing both the passage of sound through the nose and the perception of nasality. Just ask the laryngectomee to sustain an isolated hum or /m/. The muffled quality may contribute to an impression of reduced intensity even to the point of omission in the beginning speaker, whereas the better speaker should be able to sustain /m/ without reduced intensity or duration. After the laryngectomee has been speaking for some time, he may evolve his own technique for the production

Master confusion matrix for 256 syllables spoken by each of 19 subjects as judged by 10 listeners (converted to probabilities recorded as whole numbers).

RESPONSE

STIMULUS

	p	t	k	f	θ	s	ʃ	b	d	g	v	ð	z	ʒ	m	n
p	39	02	02	15	01			22	02	02	09	02			03	01
t	06	39	04	07	04			03	20	03	03	05		01	01	02
k	02	02	63	02	01			01	01	25	01	01		01		01
f	10	02	01	46	06	01		10	01	01	13	04	01		02	01
θ	07	10	03	14	14	01		07	10	03	06	18	02		01	05
s	01	04	01	03	04	35	12	01	02	01	01	03	23	09		01
ʃ	01	02	01	01	01	04	43		02	03	--	01	05	37		01
b	11	02	01	08	02			40	02	01	11	05			14	04
d	06	10	02	02	02			06	52	05	01	04		01	01	08
g	01	02	20	01	01		01	01	07	53	01	02	02	05		02
v	05	02	01	15	05	01		16	04	03	24	09	02	01	09	04
ð	06	07	03	13	13	01	01	04	09	03	06	22	04	01	02	05
z	01	04	01	02	04	09	05	01	07	03	02	07	43	10		02
ʒ	01	02	01	01	03	07	10		07	05	01	05	27	28		02
m	04		01	05	01			04	01	01	05	01			66	10
n	01	02	02	01	01			01	06	02	01	02			03	76

☐ = correct identifications

Figure 4–4. Perceived consonants in esophageal speech.

or approximation of /h/, the most difficult speech sound for the esophageal talker. The perception of this sound may be enhanced by a number
of clinical techniques: slightly longer duration, accompanying stoma

noise, or the insertion of an intrusive /k/. For a discussion of techniques to enhance the perception of /h/ and other consonants, see Shanks and Duguay (1984). Now I would like to play an audio tape of the only esophageal speaker I am aware of who can produce an isolated /h/. (Tape)

With the realization that articulation, phrasing, and rate are not ends in themselves but means to the end of intelligible, acceptable speech comes the recognition that one hazard to intelligible speech in everyday situations is noise competing with the signal. A study by Horii and Weinberg (1975) is relevant. It shows that vowel sounds uttered by esophageal talkers are subject to the same reduced intelligibility in noise as are those of laryngeal speakers. However, there is greater penalty to the intelligibility of consonants spoken by esophageal speakers in noise. Moreover, not all consonants are penalized equally, with liquid glides and nasals suffering in comparison to laryngeal voice more than the stops and fricatives. Clinically, this simply means that the esophageal speaker should try both to avoid speaking in the presence of loud noise and to work on his consonant articulation to the end that his speech be judged as both intelligible and acceptable.

A number of behaviors that are not phonemic and are not truly speech elements influence esophageal communication. One category of behaviors should be absent; namely, bad habits or distractors that may be seen or heard. Included in the visual category are facial grimace, poor eye contact, eye closure, untoward head movement, and head flexion or extension during air intake. Auditory behaviors that should be minimized or eliminated include the stoma blast while speaking, that is, an undue gush of air through the stoma, and the klunk or thump accompanying an injection of air, whether that thump be produced singly or doubly. These behaviors are inappropriate in that they draw the attention of the listener-viewer and interfere with intelligibility of communication.

Another category of behavior should be present. It is appropriate to develop the time-filling "uh" that characterizes laryngeal speech. An audible laugh should also be developed, in addition to the body shake and thigh slapping reminiscent of Kruschev's outbursts. Laughter may be facilitated by stomal exhalation concomitant with esophageal phonation as developed by Texan Ken Kellam. (Tape)

Finally, the totality of esophageal communication will develop over time. This requisite ingredient, time, may be on the order of 6 months, but it is more likely to involve a year or more. Notice how this esophageal talker progressed over time, as shown by periodic recordings. (Tape)

The individual who cares enough about his own speech to record it periodically and to analyze it for errors that may then be worked on exemplifies laryngectomees who are serious in their efforts to develop esophageal communication. Although they may do these chores on their own, it is assumed that a qualified teacher will expedite the development of esophageal communication.

QUESTIONS

1. Surveys would suggest that intelligible speech using esophageal voice might be developed within what time span after laryngectomy?
2. When would be an appropriate time to consider training pitch and intensity changes?
3. What time frame should characterize an air charge?
4. What are some ways a clinician might estimate a client's duration of phonation and what "target" would you recommend?
5. Duration of phonation might vary as a function of the air charge method. List the methods of air charge according to the expected duration.
6. Describe Damsté's method of evaluating quality of voice (periodicity).
7. Explain why application of digital pressure to the anterior part of the neck might improve voice quality.
8. How fast do you think a laryngectomized speaker should talk?
9. Shanks recommends several procedures to aid "phrasing." What guideline would you provide your client regarding stopping to take in more air?
10. What is meant by "surd-sonant confusions"?

REFERENCES

Barton, J., and Hejna, R. (1952). *A study of certain factors relating to success or non-success in the acquisition of esophageal speech.* Unpublished seminar report, Northwestern University.

Berlin, C. I. (1963). Clinical measurement of esophageal speech. I. Methodology and curves of skill acquisition. *J. Speech Hearing Dis., 22,* 42–51.

Damsté, P. H. (1958). *Oesophageal speech after laryngectomy.* Groningen: Hoistema.

Diedrich, W., and Youngstrom, K. A. (1966). *Alaryngeal speech.* Springfield, IL: Charles C Thomas.

Gandour, J., and Weinberg, B. (1982). Perception of contrastive stress in alaryngeal speech. *J. Phonetics, 10,* 347–349.

Gonella, C., Parker, D., Hollender, J., Lowell, G., Petterson, P., and Miller, S. (1978). *Normative Criteria for Cancer Rehabilitation. Rehab. Res.* Monograph Series No. 1, Atlanta: Emory University.

Gray, E. T. (1973). *Esophageal Voice and Speech Development: A Workbook.* Melbourne, FL: Brevard Graphics (1973).

Hoops, H. R., and Noll, J. D. (1969). Relationship of selected acoustic variables to judgments of esophageal speech. *J. Commun. Dis., 2,* 1–13.

Horii, Y., and Weinberg, B. (1975). Intelligibility characteristics of superior esophageal speech presented under various levels of masking noise. *J. Speech Hearing Dis., 18,* 413–419.

House, A. S., Williams, C. E., Hecker, M. H., and Kryter, K. D. (1965). Articulation testing methods: consonantal differentiation with a closed-response set. *J. Acoust. Soc. Am., 37,* 158–166.

Irwin, J. A. (1963). Teaching beginning esophageal speech. Indianapolis, IN: Third I.A.L. Voice Institute.

Moore, G. P. (1971). Voice disorders organically based. In L. E. Travis (Ed.), *Handbook of speech pathology and audiology* (Chapter 21). New York: Appleton-Century-Crofts.

Nichols, A. (1974). Confusions in recognizing phonemes spoken by esophageal speakers: I. Initial consonants and clusters. *J. Commun. Dis., 9,* 27–41.

Robe, E. Y., Moore, P., Andrews, A. H., and Holinger, P. H. (1956). A study of the role of certain factors in the development of speech after laryngectomy: I. Type of operation. *Laryngoscope, 66,* 173–186.

Sacco, P. R., Mann, M. B., and Schultz, M. C. (1967). Perceptual confusions among selected phonemes in esophageal speech. *Ind. Speech Hearing J., 26,* 19–33.

Schultz, M. C., and Schubert, E. D. (1969). A multiple choice discrimination test. *Laryngoscope, 79,* 382–399.

Shanks, J. C., and Duguay, M. (1984). Voice remediation and the teaching of alaryngeal speech. In S. Dickson (Ed.), *Communication disorders: Remedial principles and practices* (2nd ed.) (Chap. 5). Glenview, IL: Scott Foresman.

Shedd, D., and Weinberg, B. (1980). *Surgical and Surgical Prosthetic Approaches to Speech Rehabilitation,* Boston, MA: G. K. Hall.

Simpson, M. L., and Martin, D. E. (1975). The use of an electronic apparatus to develop early esophageal voice skills. *J. Mich. Speech Hearing Assn., 11,* 210–214.

Snidecor, J. C. (1968). *Speech rehabilitation of the laryngectomized* (2nd ed.). Springfield, IL: Charles C Thomas (1968).

Wepman, J. M., MacGahan, J., Rickard, J. C., and Shelton, N. W. (1953). The objective measurement of progressive esophageal speech development. *J. Speech Hearing Dis., 18,* 247–251.

Chapter **5**

Some Obstacles in Learning Esophageal Speech

P. Helbert Damsté

PHARYNGEAL VOICE

The attempts of a patient to produce the new voice by small aircharges that do not reach the esophagus, bringing into vibration pharyngeal mucosa instead of the esophagus-pharynx transition is called pharyngeal voice. The sound is different from that of esophageal voice, but some speech pathologists find it hard to recognize the difference. Witness that they continue to practice and reward this mode of phonation instead of discontinuing the exercises and switching to methods that will elicit esophageal sound.

It may be that recognizing the difference requires a musical sense of hearing with good discriminatory ability for timbre. A pharyngeal voice can have a higher fundamental frequency than the mean frequency of 65 hertz (Hz) of esophageal voices, but esophageal voices, even excellent ones, can also be of high fundamental pitch. A pharyngeal voice is always of short duration (0.25 second), but so are many esophageal voices in their early stages. No, the only discriminative, audible sign of pharyngeal voice is its peculiar timbre. The vowel formants are higher than would be expected from a person of the patient's size and stature, because the resonant cavity, the oropharynx, is of relatively small size. That in turn is due to the high position of the sound generator (Figure 5–1).

Pharyngeal voice is usually caused by the ill-directed practice of the plosive consonant method: air is not injected into the esophagus but is trapped in the hypopharynx and returned through a pseudoglottis at the level of the base of the tongue. In this way the patient acquires a persist-

    P. Helbert Damsté

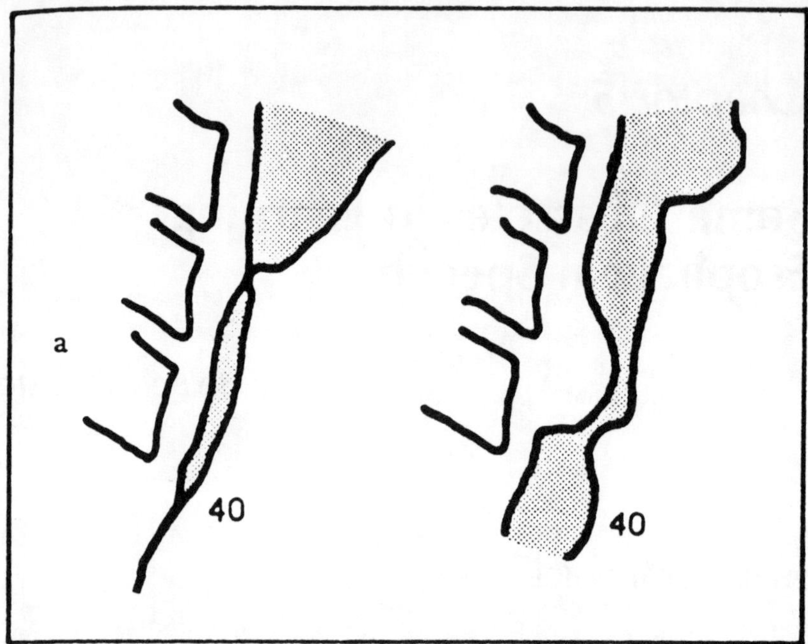

Figure 5–1. Tracings of lateral radiograph of the neck of a laryngectomized person during attempts to speak. Left, Pharyngeal voice. The air is brought into vibration at a narrowing of the pharynx at the level of the fifth cervical vertebra. There is a very small air chamber underneath. The esophagus does not contain any air. Right, 6 weeks later. The narrowing where the vibrations are generated is at the level of the sixth cervical vertebra. The esophagus is filled with air.

ent habit of contracting the inferior constrictor muscles of the pharynx and the entrance of the esophagus. This results in a strong involuntary constriction of the structures that in esophageal voice serve as the new vibrator. In a few cases a light or moderate stenosis of the entrance to the esophagus has predisposed such a dysfunction to develop. Whether this has been the case is easy to find out by questioning the patient if he regularly has difficulty in swallowing solid food. Must he chew his meat very carefully in order to be able to swallow it? In any case of unexplained problems in learning esophageal speech it is advisable to do a radiological examination to exclude possible fistulas or diverticula.

As it has hardly ever been possible to guide the patient out of his dead alley of pharyngeal voice back to the correct road to esophageal voice without special manipulations, the following procedure is recommended.

The patient is informed in detail about the differences between pharyngeal and esophageal phonation; a tape recording of a previously retrained patient can be used as illustration. This encourages the patient to consent to and cooperate with the first part of the treatment, which, at least for the first time, is an unpleasant experience. It consists of swallowing a flexible esophageal dilator, a bougie approximately 14 millimeters (mm) in diameter. When an organic narrowing is suspected or likely, a bougie of smaller diameter is used. If the pharynx has been anesthetized, the bougie is usually well tolerated. On following days the anesthetic can be diminished and finally omitted altogether when the patient has become accustomed to swallowing the bougie. It is left in place for 5 or 10 minutes.

After the bougie has been removed, the air will pass more easily through the pharyngoesophageal barrier if certain precautions are taken:

1. The patient should not be reminded in any way of his former attempts to speak. The only voice sound that is asked is a deep burp, gradually modified into vowel-like sound such as *ow* or *aow*. This is to prevent any association with articulatory movements, which would immediately trigger the pharynx constriction.

2. The surest way to elicit esophageal sounds is by inserting a catheter through the nose into the uppermost part of the esophagus and injecting air by squeezing a rubber balloon that is attached to the catheter. This is combined with exercises for general and local relaxation: relaxing the shoulders, the neck, and the jaw; chewing; yawning; and anything else that may relax the patient, such as humor.

3. When the passive injection of air produces constant results of immediate phonation when a sufficient volume of air is pumped in, inhalation through the catheter can be tried. The balloon is removed. The patient is allowed to take air into the esophagus by inhalation; as long as the catheter is in place, it will admit air without much resistance. During expiration, when the patient attempts to phonate, the orifice of the catheter is closed off with the fingers so that the air can leave only by way of the esophagus and pharynx.

4. Inhaling air followed by phonation is then practiced without a catheter. This is again combined with measures directed at relaxation and suggestions for a wide pharynx: pretending to gulp beer, stretching the neck, and putting the jaw forward. The pressure in the esophagus can be lowered by nearly closing off the tracheostoma near the end of an inspiration.

5. It is important that, as soon as air is heard to enter the esophagus, this fact is brought to the patient's attention and rewarded. As a next step, this signal should immediately be followed by reversing

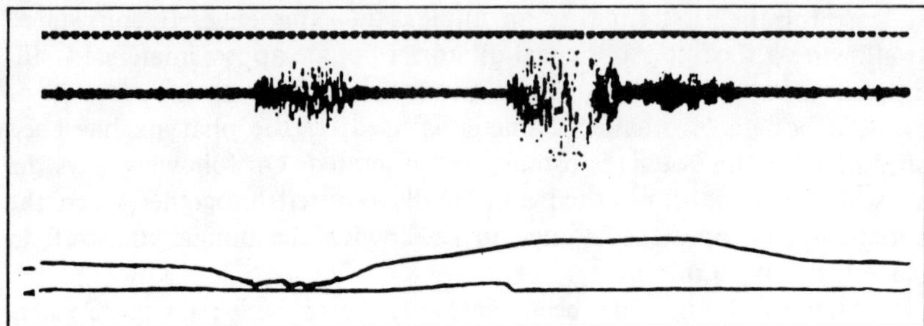

Figure 5–2. From top to bottom, time signal indicating 0.02 sec., sound track, pressure in the esophagus, pressure in the pharynx. This is a recording of "two-way speech": the patient emits sound on inhaling air (lowering of the esophageal pressure) and again when he lets the air out (rising of the pressure in the esophagus). There is no change in the pharyngeal air pressure except for the small rise and fall for the pronunciation of the occlusive before the second vowel sound was emitted. The syllable spoken was "pa."

the airstream, thus producing the sound of air leaving the esophagus. If the patient has control over this air in–air out, he has reached the stage of two-way speech (Fig. 5–2). From there he can go on by learning to take air in silently and eventually progress to the discovery of air-injection (Fig. 5–3).

THE SHAPE OF THE PSEUDOGLOTTIS

The extent of the surgery and the postoperative course, especially with regard to healing of the wound, determine for a large part the end result of voice rehabilitation. There are differences in the amount of muscle tissue at the pharyngoesophageal (PE) junction and its structural relationship to the connective tissue that surrounds the lumen of the new

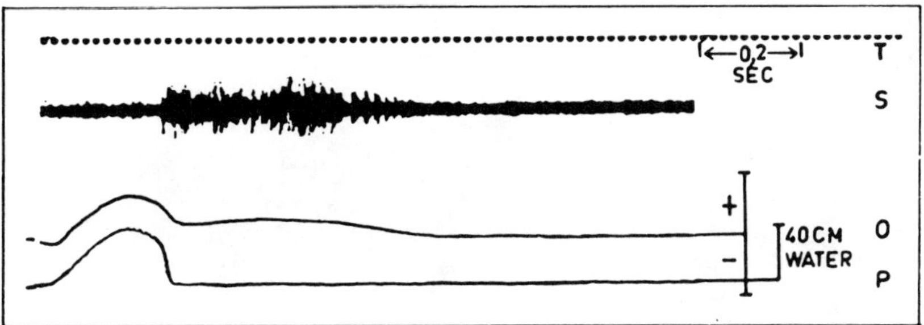

Figure 5–3. Here the same syllable "pa" spoken by the same patient as in Figure 5-2 a few weeks later. A large rise of pressure in the pharynx immediately followed by a rise in the esophagus precedes the vowel sound. The elevation coincides with the pressure rise for the plosive but is much larger: The air injection for filling the esophagus coincides with the hold before the plosive.

upper digestive and vocal tract. Thus the form of the PE segment can vary from wide to narrow, from long to short, and its shape can be flat, round, and prominent (Fig. 5-4).

Considerations to examine in some detail include (1) the features that, as a consequence of surgery and wound healing, are permanent and unchangeable and (2) the features that can be changed by goal-directed practice. The configuration of the pharyngeal voice (see Fig. 5-1) is an example of the second sort, although an organic stricture or stenosis may have predisposed to its development. The configurations of Fig. 5-4 were originally considered to be features of the organic kind. It was later found that this is not always so. The oppositions flat-round and flat-prominent are seen to occur in one individual when he phonates soft and loud. Some persons who establish a flat type of PE segment can train themselves to develop a pseudoglottis that has a more prominent shape. This does not exclude the possibility that in other persons who

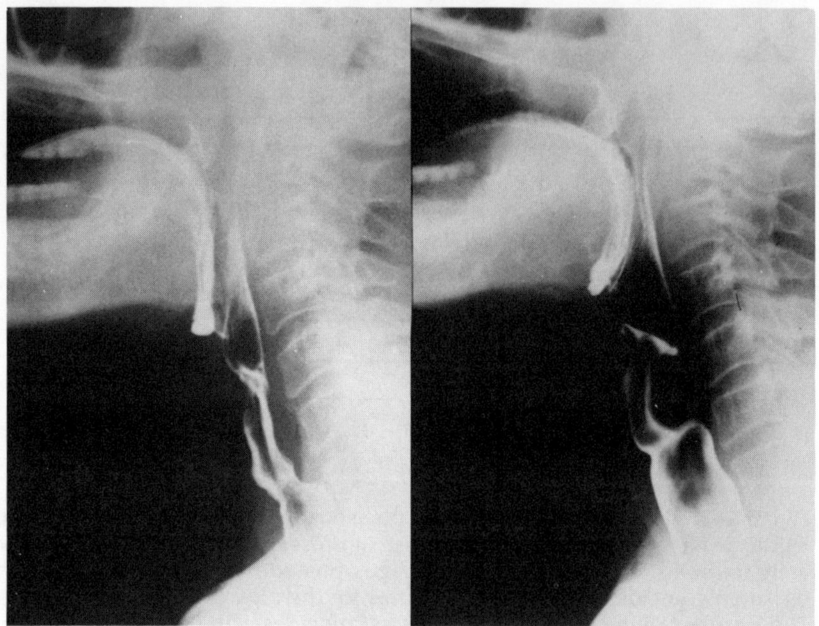

Figure 5–4. Different configurations of the pseudoglottis in one speaker during soft (left) and loud (right) phonation.

are deprived of sphincter musculature or of its innervation the flat shape is an unchangeable characteristic that cannot be improved on by practicing. These persons will keep a small voice volume, and some are suitable candidates for a spandex ribbon or another external pressure device.

Important and not infrequent organic feature are pouches and diverticula in the PE segment. They have an adverse influence on the voice when they are situated in the cranial part of the "siphon" (Fig. 5–5). There they form niches that contain stagnating secretions. As a result, the voice pulses are irregular and the audible impression is one of a wet, gurgling sound. In one patient the origin of a shallow diverticulum in the anterior wall of the PE segment could be traced back to a fistula, where the suture had broken down. This patient, when he appeared to be unable to produce voice, was examined by means of a lateral x-ray after he swallowed a contrast medium. When a deep, blind-ending fistula was found, therapy was discontinued and the fistula was allowed to heal. All that remained of the accident with the suture was a small irregularity in the anterior lining of the PE segment. In other cases, however, wound-healing complications may affect the form of the PE segment and cause its shape

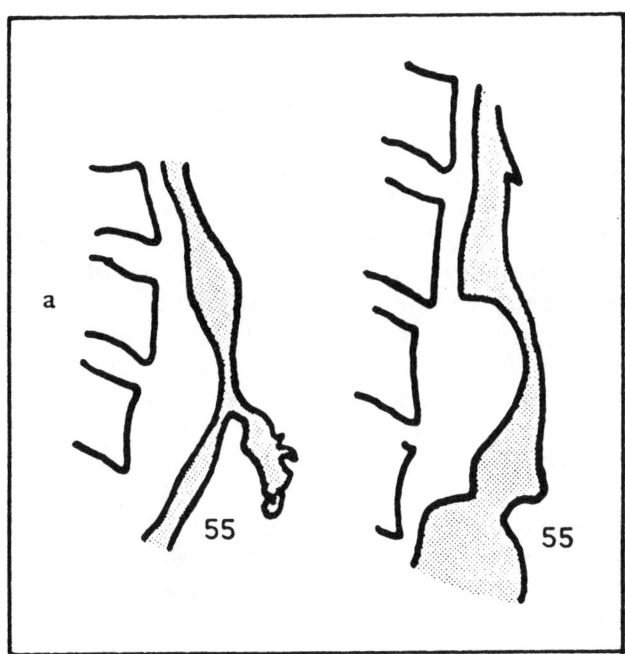

Figure 5–5. Pouch or diverticulum (right) that has remained as a consequence of broken down suture of the pharyngeal wall (left).

to be too irregular to allow clear phonation. It is important for future
voice rehabilitation that the pharyngeal wall be stitched with the utmost
care, saving as much muscle tissue as possible.

The next adverse factor to be discussed is the extensive type of surgery with plastic reconstruction of the pharynx. This operation is performed by few surgeons and aims at removal of postcricoid carcinoma
situated in the hypopharynx, just above the entrance of the esophagus.
A tumor in this location causes severe dysphagia and, if not removed,
eventually necessitates a gastrostomy. It occurs typically in women and is
often preceded by a chronic hypopharyngitis; swallowing complaints can
therefore have existed for a long time. The problem with the removal of
this kind of tumor is that not only must the entire larynx be removed but
a large part of the pharyngeal mucosa and a part of the upper esophagus
must be taken as well. There is too little tissue left for the reconstruction of that part of the digestive tract, and extra tissue will have to be
mobilized from elsewhere. Several surgical techniques are used. One is
the insertion of a piece of colon in the void between the pharynx and the
esophagus. Other surgeons let both ends meet by pulling the stomach up

from its usual site under the diaphragm into the thoracic cavity. In both groups of patients fair postlaryngectomy voices have been reported. In a third type of reconstruction a large skin flap is obtained from the area of the chest and shoulder on one side; it is formed into a tube and moved into the area of the operation in two stages. There it is sutured between the esophagus and what is left of the pharynx. This author had a chance to see six patients treated with a deltopectoral flap operation by Doctor Stell at Liverpool. They had some swallowing difficulties that could be overcome, but regaining a voice appeared to be very difficult. They had had intensive speech therapy for prolonged periods of time, and the best some of them could produce was a form of pseudo–whispered speech. One or two had a pharyngeal voice that was somewhat more satisfactory, and only two had developed what could be called an esophageal voice. Two years had already elapsed since the operation. A possible explanation for the delay in voice development is that the skin tube needs such a long time before its tissues have completely adapted to the new surroundings. The adaptation that takes place can be a rearrangement of the collagen fibers that would make the PE segment more supple. The lateral radiograph of one of these patients shows an esophagus with a narrow lumen that is not filled with air. Even though the pharynx did not seem to be extremely narrow, none of these patients had succeeded in using an electronic larynx, most probably because the thick pharyngeal lining (skin flap) absorbs too much of the sound energy.

QUESTIONS

1. Contrast the site of the neoglottis for esophageal voice and pharyngeal voice. How can a clinician help the patient recognize differences between these two types of voice?
2. Differences in the shape of the PE segment would most likely influence what perceptual aspect of voice—pitch, loudness, or quality—and why?
3. How might wide-field excision of a cancer within and outside the larynx affect subsequent voice production?

REFERENCES

Damsté, P. H., and Lerman, J. W. (1969). Configuration of the neoglottis: an x-ray study. *Folia Phoniat.*, 21, 347–358.

Chapter 6

The Artificial Larynx: Types and Modifications

Eric D. Blom and Shirley J. Salmon

This chapter provides a review of currently available artificial larynxes. In some instances homemade modifications are provided that, based on subjective clinical evaluation, might improve the design and versatility of a number of the instruments described. Pneumatic instruments are discussed first; then mouth-type electronic larynxes. Speech pathologists who intend to offer comprehensive alaryngeal speech therapy should be completely familiar with these instruments, be able to demonstrate their use either personally or with videotaped samples, and have available as many of them as possible for trial purposes.

The major portion of this chapter has been adapted from Blom's chapter, ''The Artificial Larynx: Past and Present,'' which appears in *The Artificial Larynx Handbook* edited by Shirley J. Salmon and Lewis Goldstein in 1978. The authors are indebted to Grune & Stratton, Inc., for their permission to reproduce this material.

PNEUMATIC ARTIFICIAL LARYNXES

Tokyo Artificial Larynx

The Tokyo device is an inexpensive Japanese-made instrument consisting of either a steel or a soft rubber cover that fits over the stoma, a steel pipe leading to and away from a cylindrical chamber that houses a stretched rubber membrane held in position by a rubber band, and a plastic or rubber mouth-tube (Figs. 6–1 and 6–2). The frequency can be changed by adjusting the width and tension of the vibrating membrane

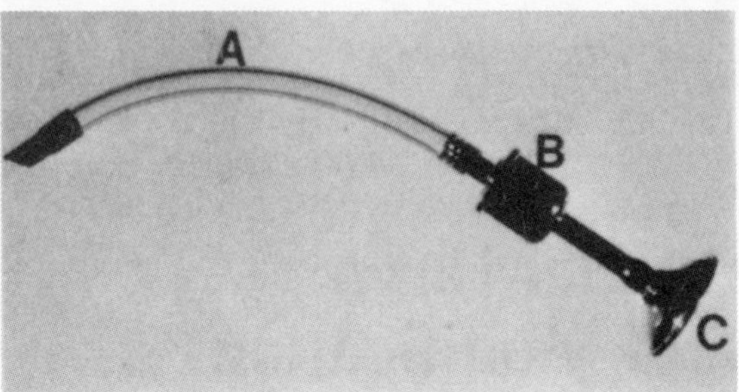

Figure 6–1. Tokyo artificial larynx. A, Mouth tube. B, Vibrator chamber. C, Steel stoma cover.

or by varying breath pressure during use. Varying breath pressure also results in a significant variation in intensity. Speech with the Tokyo device has been described by Weinberg and Riekena (1973).

Simple modifications to "the Tokyo" make it more functional. To negate the necessity of moving the Tokyo from the stoma on each inhalation, a ⅜ inch hole drilled in the cylindrical body of the instrument provides a convenient finger-controlled breathing port (see Fig. 6–3). A soft-flanged fistula tube serves nicely in cases in which the standard steel or rubber tracheostoma cover does not adequately fit over the stoma.

Another effective modification with the Tokyo as well as with other mouth-type devices consists of using a dental saliva-ejector tube to replace the more conventional tygon mouth tubing (Fig.6–3). This kind of tube offers the following advantages: (1) a wire running through the tubing gives firmness and at the same time makes it possible to bend the tubing into permanent shape; (2) greater thickness decreases sound radi-

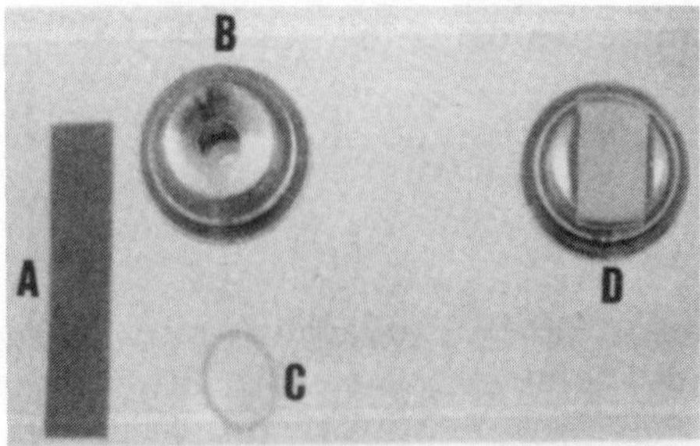

Figure 6–2. Tokyo artificial larynx vibrator assembly. A, Rubber membrane. B, Top view of chamber interior. C, Orthodontic rubber band. D, Assembled vibrator.

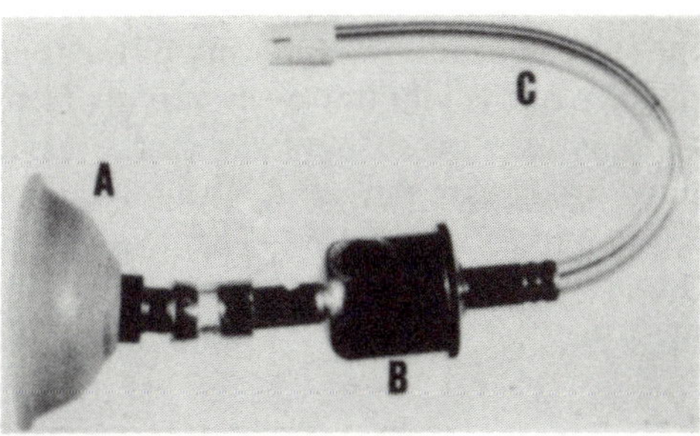

Figure 6–3. Modified Tokyo artificial larynx. A, Rubber stoma cover. B, Finger-controlled breathing port. C, Dental saliva-ejector tube.

ation through the tubing wall; and (3) a small, slitted cap over the end of the tube decreases intake of saliva and skin tissue into the tube orifice when the tube is in the mouth.

The Tokyo is available from Mr. Red Woodward, 3132 Waits Avenue, Fort Worth, TX 76109, at an approximate cost of $26.

In 1975 Nelson, Parkin, and Potter (1975) described two modifications of the Tokyo. Rigidity and curvature of the mouth tube are achieved by constructing the tube out of prebent stainless steel and by capping the portion that actually goes into the mouth with a short piece of plastic tubing. To overcome the difficulties presented by an irregularly angled stoma, a swivel-joint connector is incorporated on the proximal end of the device between the steel connecting tube and the tracheostoma cover. Cost of the modified device is reported to be in excess of $140.

Osaka Artificial Larynx

The Osaka artificial larynx (Fig. 6–4) is another Japanese-manufactured instrument basically similar to the Tokyo. The tracheostoma cover and

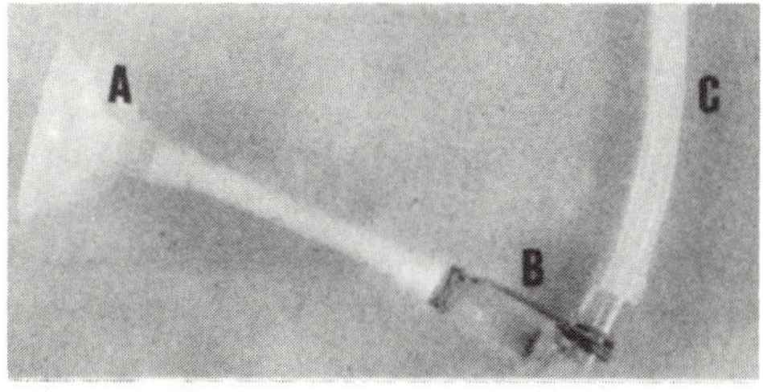

Figure 6–4. Osaka (Yamamura) artificial larynx. A, Stoma cover. B, Vibratory mechanism. C, Mouth tube.

housing for the rubber vibrator are made of lightweight plastic. It is possible to change the frequency and intensity of the tone by altering the physical characteristics of the vibrator or by varying breath pressure during use. The Osaka is referred to by some as the Yamamura and was formerly distributed by the late Reverend Yoshimi Yamamura (R. Woodward, personal communication, 1976). The Osaka can be purchased from Mr. Red Woodward, 3132 Waits Avenue, Fort Worth, TX 76109, for approximately $30.

Van Humen Artificial Larynx ("Dutch" DSP8)

The Van Humen artificial larynx has a plastic mouth-tube, a nylon vibrator housing, an adjustable rubber membrane, and an air-filled cover that fits over the stoma (Fig. 6–5). The design permits the user to breathe normally and also to speak without removing the device from the stoma. This Dutch-made instrument is infrequently seen in the United States, but is available from Memacon, Pres. Kennedy Laan 263, P.O. Box 56, Velp 6200, Netherlands, at a cost of approximately $80.

ELECTRONIC MOUTH-TYPE ARTIFICIAL LARYNXES

Cooper-Rand Electronic Speech Aid

Probably the most widely known mouth-type electronic larynx is the Cooper-Rand. This instrument basically consists of a battery-powered pulse generator connected by a wire to a handheld tone generator (Fig.

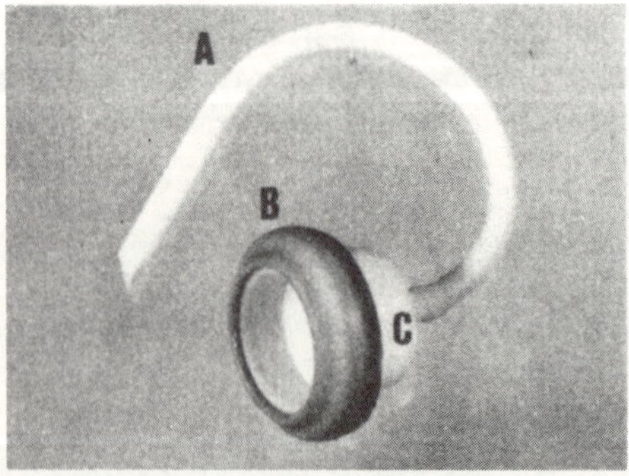

Figure 6–5. Van Humen (DSP8) artificial larynx. A, Mouth tube. B, Vibratory mechanism. C, Air-filled stoma cover.

6–6). Sound is directed into the mouth by a short piece of plastic tubing. Switches incorporated on the battery case permit variation in both frequency and intensity. Recently the manufacturer of the Cooper-Rand made several needed improvements. The cords supplied with the instruments are now of a heavier gauge and are thus less likely to break. Both the conventional plastic mouth-tubes and the saliva-ejector tubes described previously are included with the instrument. The manufacturer now advises the user that the two-pronged cord can be plugged into the handheld transducer in only one direction. Plugging in the cord in reverse results in an impedance mismatch and a noticeable reduction in intensity. The Cooper-Rand, with two Eveready 411 batteries, filter holder and filters, is available from Luminaud, P.O. Box 257, 7670 Acacia Avenue, Mentor, OH 44060, at an approximate cost of $204.

MODIFICATIONS OF THE WESTERN ELECTRIC NO. 5 ELECTRONIC LARYNX

Creech (H. B. Creech, personal communication, 1976) recently described a simple and inexpensive modification of a standard Western Electric No. 5 neck-type electronic larynx into a mouth-type instrument (see Fig. 6–7). The tapered tip of a 2 ounce plastic irrigating syringe is cemented with epoxy over the screw-on cap of a Western Electric No. 5, thereby enclosing the sound transducer. Dental acrylic is then applied around the circumference of the cap to secure the syringe tip further and to enhance the appearance of the instrument. This modified electronic

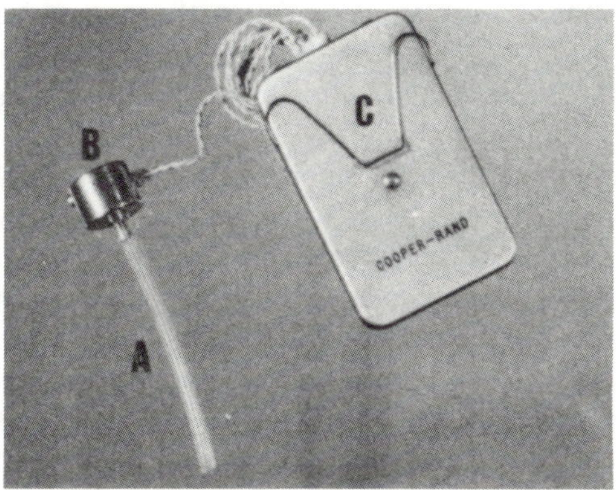

Figure 6–6. Cooper-Rand electronic larynx. A, Mouth tube. B, Handheld tone generator. C, Pulse generator and battery case.

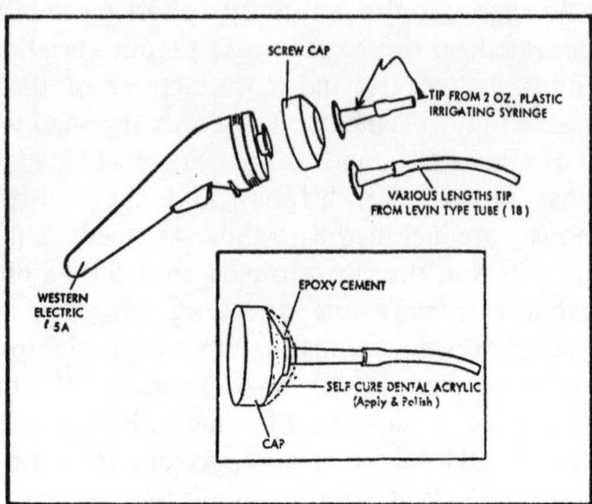

Figure 6–7. Mouth-type Western Electric No. 5 electronic larynx modification by Creech.

larynx, either with or without a short piece of plastic tubing attached to the end of the syringe tip, is used in a manner similar to that of any other mouth-type artificial larynx. With the purchase of extra screw-on caps from the Bell Telephone Company (approximately $4.00 each), the modified instrument can easily be switched back to a neck-type instrument by simply replacing the modified cap with a standard cap.

Williams and Ostroy (W. G. Williams, personal communication, 1976) have developed a unique mouth-type electronic larynx using a Western Electric No. 5 as the basic unit. Their modification consists of replacing the standard transducer with a conventional hearing aid receiver (Fig. 6–8). An aluminum coverplate is used to stabilize the plastic mouth-tube that fits over the nub of the hearing aid receiver. This modified instrument produces a tone almost totally devoid of extraneous noise radiating from the head of the unit. Another important feature of this modification is that battery drain is decreased significantly (0.2 watts drain versus 1.5 watts). If the original transducer is saved, the instrument can be changed back into a neck-type electronic larynx when desired.

According to Williams, the modification consists of removing the complete vibrating diaphragm unit and replacing it with a standard body hearing aid receiver. The receiver acts as a transducer or a speaker. The hearing aid receiver is glued securely in place within the space originally occupied by the vibrating diaphragm. The two wires from the Western Electric No. 5 circuit and the two short (unbraided) wires from the hearing aid receiver cord are soldered together, using the basic unit that sup-

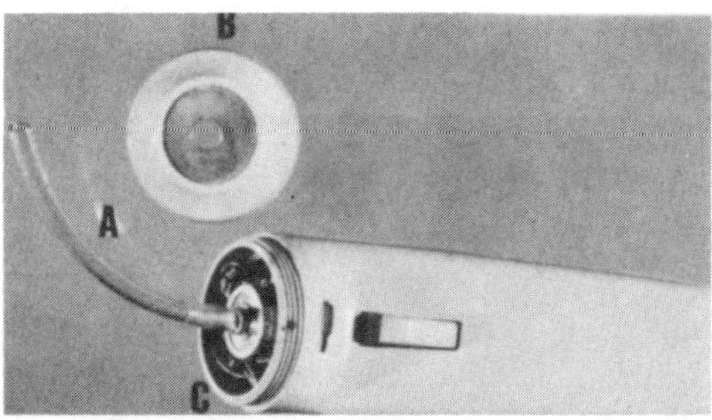

Figure 6–8. Mouth-type Western Electric No. 5 electronic larynx modification by Williams and Ostroy. A, Mouth tube. B, Screw-on cap with aluminum coverplate. C, Body-type hearing aid receiver.

plies the energy to activate the hearing aid receiver. The electrical circuit of the Western Electric No. 5 is retained unless a small optional modification is desired. A 10K resistor can be connected in series with the variable tone control and 910K resistors in order to eliminate cut-off of the tone oscillator at its highest frequency. A 3 inch piece of tygon tubing is fitted over the nub of the hearing aid receiver. An aluminum coverplate is cut and fitted into the opening of the screw-on cap that previously accommodated the head of the vibrating diaphragm assembly. A hole large enough to allow the tygon tubing to slip freely through is drilled in the center of the aluminum coverplate. The completed cover is then screwed down snugly to the body of the Western Electric No. 5. The final product is well finished and attractive. It should be noted that this modification nullifies the manufacturer's warranty.

Zwitman and Disinger (1975) reported a modification that consists of inserting a bypass plug into the circuitry of a Western Electric No. 5 electronic larynx to convert it into a mouth-type instrument. The modified device consists basically of a standard neck-type transducer, a bypass plug, a cord leading to a handheld body-type hearing aid receiver, and a plastic mouth-tube (see Fig. 6–9). The instrument permits the user to select either mouth-type or neck-type use.

Knox (A. Knox, personal communication, 1977) explained how to make the modification. The Zwitman modification is possible by a theoretically simple but technically exasperating addition of a shorting jack to the main frame of the device, which shunts the power from the output transducer to a hearing aid transducer when the alternate output plug is inserted in the jack.

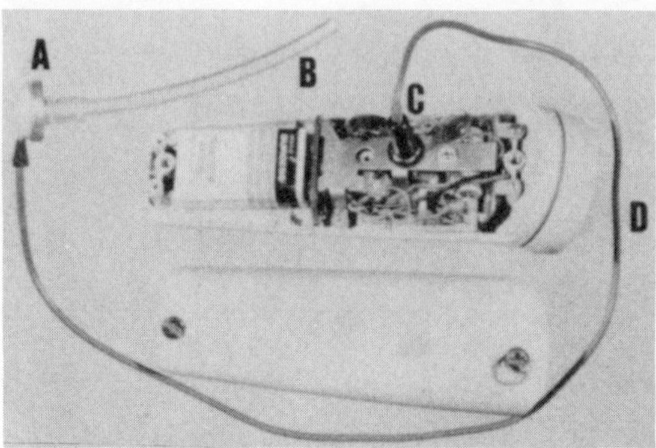

Figure 6–9.   Mouth-type Western Electric No. 5 electronic larynx modification by Zwitman and Disinger. A, Body-type hearing aid receiver. B, Mouth tube. C, Shorting jack and plug. D, Cord.

As shown in Fig. 6–9 the jack is located directly opposite the control knob, where according to Knox it does not interfere with the user's grip. It can be fastened on the main frame, and therefore wiring between the main frame and the removable back is not necessary. A hole is cut into the removable back to receive the plug from the mouth-type transducer. The miniature shorting jack is typical of those used for personal speakers on transistor radios. The main frame is drilled and reamed out carefully to receive the threaded sleeve of the jack encased from both sides of the chassis by extruded fiber washers for electrical isolation. The red lead is then cut and wired both to the sleeve of the jack and to its power source. The normally closed terminal of the jack is wired to the green lead of the conventional Western Electric No. 5 transducer. The connection between them is opened when the plug is inserted, and output is routed to the hearing aid transducer. The conventional output transducer as measured on an impedance bridge has 20 ohms' impedance at 1 kilohertz (KHz). A 15 ohm Telex RTR-04 hearing aid receiver is used because of the closeness of the impedance and the heavy-duty cord. A miniature plug is put on the cord, replacing the ¼ inch standard plug.

This plastic mouth-tube can be any soft plastic tube with an adaptor to a ¼ inch interior dimension. In a demonstration instrument, a tube from a disposable plastic nasal cannula (Hudson No. 1102) was used by cutting off part of the slip-on adaptor for the oxygen tank. The thick, soft plastic wall worked very well. When the plug was inserted in the jack, the instrument reverted to a neck-type artificial larynx. This modification nullifies the manufacturer's warranty.

AUREX NEOVOX M-550 INTRAORAL CONVERSION

Intraoral Adaptors

Recently several manufacturers of neck-type electronic artificial larynxes have made intraoral adaptors available. These adaptors permit easy conversion of the neck-type electronic devices into mouth-type ones. Although the adaptors are uniquely constructed so they are not interchangeable, the adaptor in Figure 6–10 is generally representative of their design. They consist of a rubber cap and a plastic mouth-tube for collecting sound and conveying it into the mouth. The conversion results in an instrument that is satisfactorily devoid of extraneous noise. The prices of intraoral adaptors range from $16. to $20. and can be ordered from the manufacturers of the Aurex Neovox, Rehaton, Romet, and Servox devices. Addresses for these companies are listed in the section pertaining to electronic neck-type artificial larynxes.

Interdental Speech Aids

An artificial larynx that can be placed on a dental plate in the mouth and concealed within the oral cavity has been envisioned by several. The first prototype, the Oral Vibrator, was invented in England by Tait and Tait in 1959 but is not commercially available. The most recent, the Speech Master, was manufactured by the Xomed Corporation and was sold between 1982 and 1984. Recently, however, it has been withdrawn from the market.

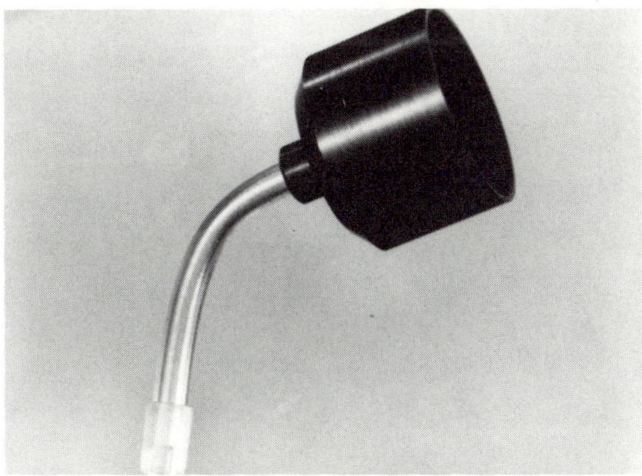

Figure 6–10.   Illustration of a typical intraoral adaptor.

Research with an interdental device is ongoing in Natroma Heights, Pennsylvania, by Joseph A. Resnick, but the Resnick Emitter has not yet been marketed (Joseph A. Resnick, personal communication, 1984).

ELECTRONIC NECK-TYPE ARTIFICIAL LARYNXES

Western Electric 5A and 5B Electronic Larynxes

The most popular neck-type electronic larynx is probably the Western Electric 5A (low pitch for male) and 5B (high pitch for female). This instrument is a handheld, battery-powered transducer that transmits sound into the resonance tract when correctly placed against the neck (Fig. 6–11). Correct placement varies among users and must be determined by experimentation. It may be the midline junction between the neck and the floor of the mouth, the anterolateral aspect of the neck, or even the side of the face in instances when no suitable spot can be found on the neck and a mouth-type instrument is not available. For users who at first find it difficult to find the appropriate spot on the neck consistently, a piece of tape on the predetermined spot may held considerably.

The Western Electric No. 5 has an external variable frequency control incorporated in the on-off tone activation switch. The internal preset frequency range of the instrument can be adjusted to meet individual preference by loosening a set screw with an Allen wrench (Fig. 6–12) and slowly adjusting a nearby screw while operating the instrument (Fig. 6–13). Caution must be exercised when retightening the set screw to assure that the

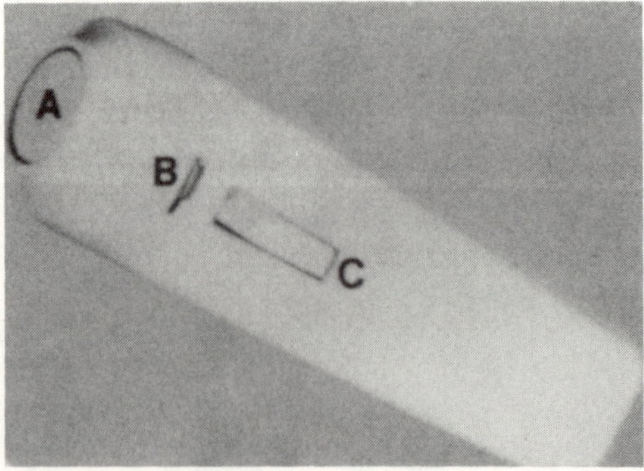

Figure 6–11. Western Electric No. 5 electronic larynx. A, Electromagnetic transducer. B, Power switch. C, Frequency control and on-off tone activation switch.

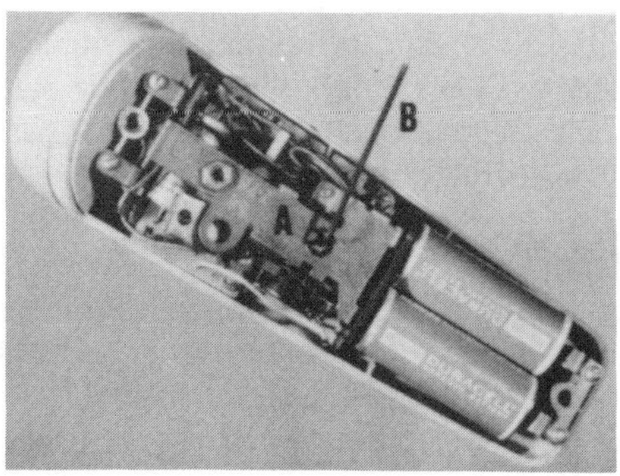

Figure 6–12. Preparing to adjust frequency range on the Western Electric No. 5 by loosening set screw (A) with Allen wrench (B).

tone activation switch (variable pitch button), which is kept centered in its slot by the set screw, is centrally positioned before tightening. There is no provision for intensity variation. Extraneous noise radiating from the head of the instrument can be reduced by unscrewing the cap and packing a sound-absorbing material in the space around the transducer. Decreasing the degree to which the cap is screwed on (by about one and one-half turns) also seems to reduce extraneous vibratory noise in exceedingly loud instruments.

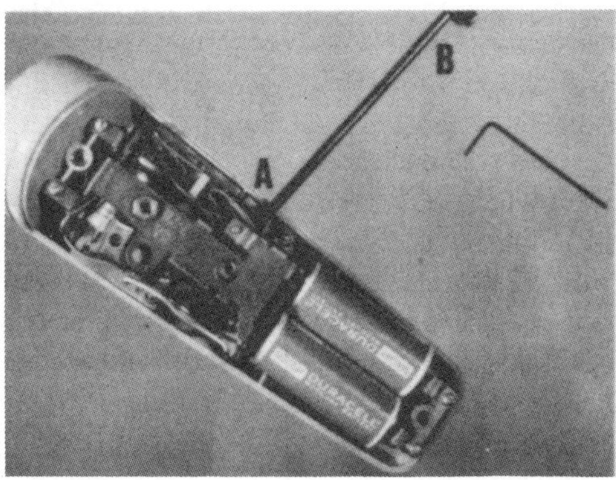

Figure 6–13. Adjusting Western Electric No. 5 frequency adjustment screw (A) with a screw driver (B).

Although AT&T is phasing out this device with replacement of a 5C, the 5A and 5B instruments are expected to be seen for a long time owing to previous popularity. When they become inoperable, arrangements for their repair or trade-in on a 5C device can be made by contacting American Telephone and Telegraph Company (AT&T), Special Needs Center, Parsippany, New Jersey 07054; call toll-free 1–800–233–1222. The complete exchange of an inoperable 5A or 5B device for another repaired 5A or 5B artificial larynx is also possible. Send the device (modified or not) with a check for $64.50 to AT&T Consumer Products, Special Needs, 32000 Aurora Road, Solon, OH 44139, or call (216) 248-4410. The Western Electric 5A and 5B devices operate on two batteries (Eveready 164, Mallory TR164, Burgess H164, or RCA 164) that have a retail cost of approximately $7.50 each.

A little-known and relatively simple modification of the battery compartment of the Western Electric No. 5 electrolarynx can significantly alleviate battery cost and unavailability (Blom, 1978). The modification consists of slightly altering the battery compartment so that it will accept one standard 9 volt battery (Fig. 6–14). Figure 14 shows the instrument unmodified (A). By unscrewing the metal clip and cutting off the two centered points of plastic in the floor of the case (B), the empty battery compartment (C) will accept a standard 9 volt battery (D). The battery should be carefully inserted (to avoid damage to contacts) so that the positive and negative terminals of the battery make good contact with corresponding electrical contacts in the battery case. It might be necessary to carefully pry these metal contacts slightly forward to insure firm contact with the terminals of the battery. If necessary, a small piece of foam rubber or tissue paper can be packed in the battery compartment to eliminate battery movement. This modification nullifies the manufacturer's warranty.

With normal use a 9 volt battery will last 8 to 10 days. Although this is only one third as long as the two standard 5.6 volt batteries, three replacements of the 9 volt battery per month cost only $2.75 ($0.75 each). Even the better grade of alkaline 9 volt batteries retail for only $1.25 each for a total of $3.75 for three replacements each month. Monthly replacement of the two standard 5.6 volt batteries can cost from $5.50 to $10.00. Equally significant is that 9 volt batteries are readily available at any drugstore or supermarket, while the standard 5.6 volt batteries are frequently difficult to procure.

Popular brandname 9 volt batteries and their respective model number are: Mallory MN 1604 (alkaline), Eveready 522 (alkaline), Mallory M1604, Burgess 2U6, Eveready 216, and Ray-O-Vac 1604. Assessment of battery-life characteristics has revealed that the alkaline 9 volt batteries (Mallory MN 1604, Eveready 522) last longer than the carbon zinc batter-

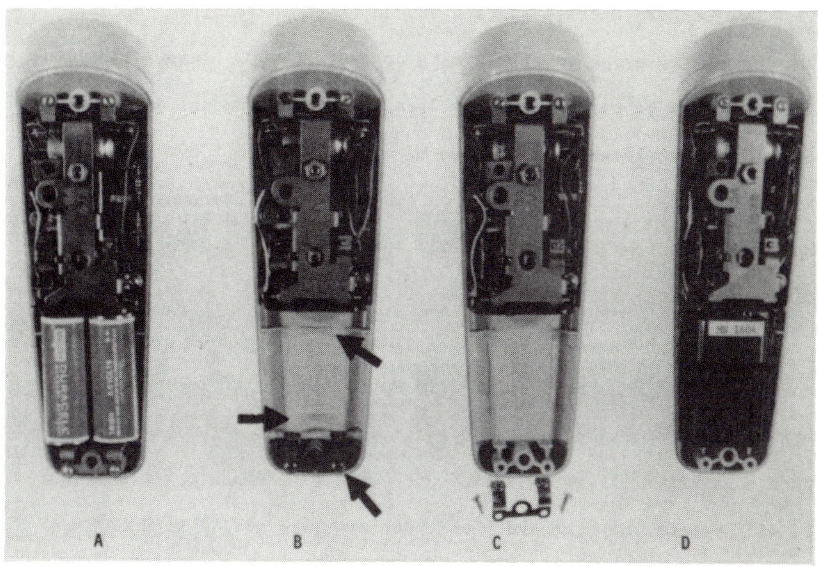

Figure 6–14. Conversion of the Western Electric No. 5 electronic larynx to a 9 volt power supply. A, Artificial larynx with two standard batteries. B, Remove metal clip and two centered points of plastic. C, Metal clip and two centered points of plastic removed. D, Artificial larynx with single 9 volt battery.

ies. Cheap nonbrandname 9 volt batteries should be avoided, since they frequently have a short battery life. Recently introduced rechargeable nickel-cadmium 9 volt batteries cannot be used in the Western Electric No. 5 electrolarynx without considerable compartment modification to accommodate their slightly larger size.

Western Electric 5C Electronic Artificial Larynx

The Western Electric 5A and 5B Electronic Larynxes recently have been redesigned, resulting in the production of a new Western Electric 5C (Fig. 6–15). According to the manufacturer, the 5C was developed to eliminate major difficulties that were resulting in frequent repairs and consumer inconvenience.

The transducer or vibrator head has been more securely fastened. The variable pitch control has been replaced with a single on-off switch. Frequency can be preset by turning a small screw inside the instrument, thus eliminating the need for two separate male and female pitch units. Intensity can be reduced by unscrewing the collar around the vibrating head

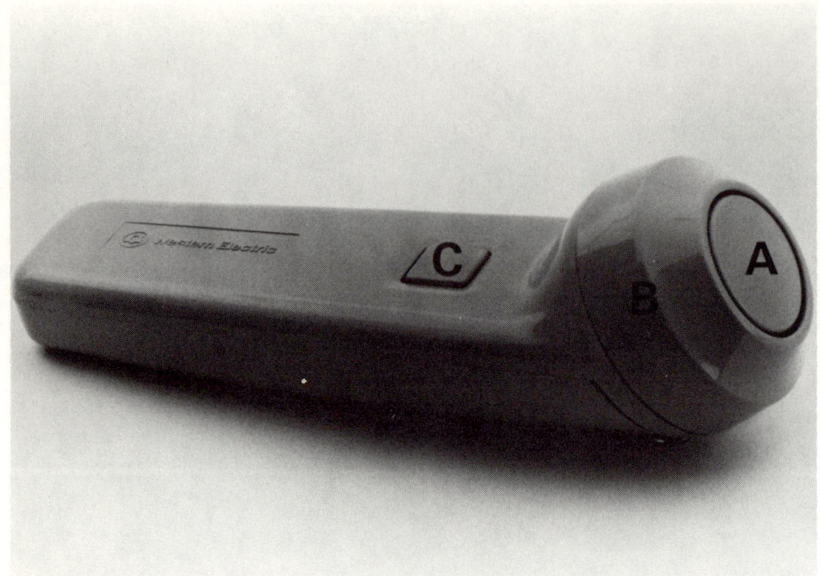

Figure 6–15.   Western Electric No. 5C electronic artificial larynx. A, Vibrator head. B, Collar. C, On-off control.

approximately one and one-half turns. The 5C employs a new circuitry that uses a regular 9 volt alkaline battery. A rechargeable 9 volt battery may also be used. The Western Electric 5C replaced the 5A and 5B units in 1985. Information about purchase of the 5C is available from American Telephone and Telegraph Company (AT&T) Special Needs Center, New Jersey; call toll-free 1–800–233–1222. The price of the 5C is $92.00 and includes the device and a 9 volt alkaline battery.

Park MKII Artificial Larynx

Another neck-type device available in the United States is the Park MKII Artificial Larynx Vibrator (Fig. 6–16). This instrument basically consists of a small, battery-powered motor that drives a spring-loaded piston against a diaphragm and thus produces sound. The mechanism is housed in a lightweight cylindrical case with an angled vibrator head. The intensity of the instrument is fixed, but frequency can be preset by adjusting a locking ring around the head of the vibrator. The Park MKII, with a standard 1.5 volt battery, is available from Park Surgical Company, Inc., 5001 New Utrecht Avenue, Brooklyn, NY 11219, at an approximate cost of $195.

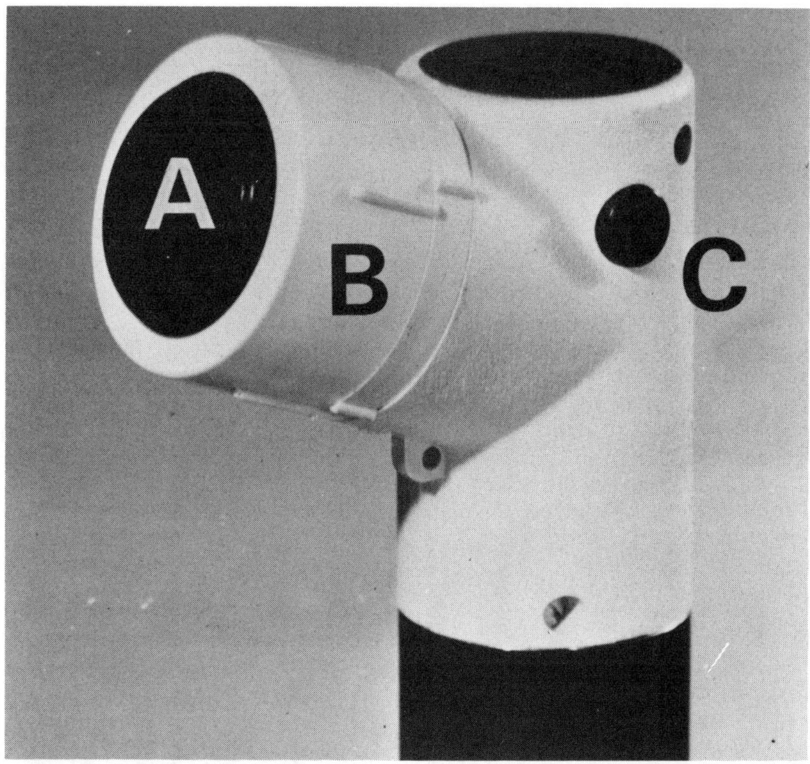

Figure 6–16. Park MKII electronic larynx. A, Vibrator head. B, Locking ring. C, On-off tone button.

Park Electronic Artificial Larynx JM 011

The Park JM 011 (Fig. 6–17) is one of the newest neck-type electronic larynxes to be introduced in the United States. Although it was not made available to us for comparison with other devices, it is reported to be similar to the Rehaton, discussed later in this chapter. It is one of the smaller lightweight devices available. Sound is produced by means of a piston striking a diaphragm. Tone and volume can be adjusted by turning the appropriate controls on either side of the instrument. The price of $400.00 includes the device with battery charger, two rechargeable batteries, an oral adaptor, and a carrying case. It is available from Park Surgical Co., Inc., 5001 New Utrecht Avenue, Brooklyn, NY 11219.

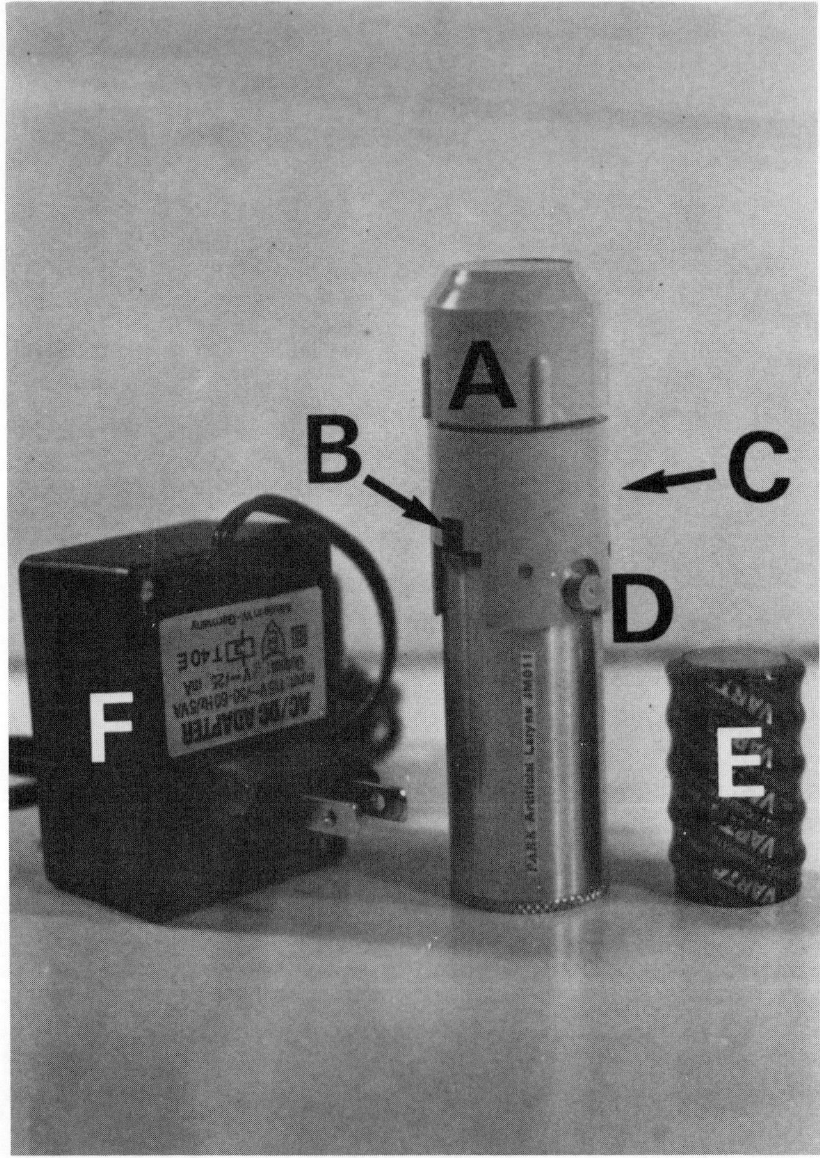

Figure 6–17. Park JM 011 electronic larynx. A, Collar around vibrator. B, Volume control. C, Tone control. D, On-off button. E, Rechargeable battery. F, Battery charger.

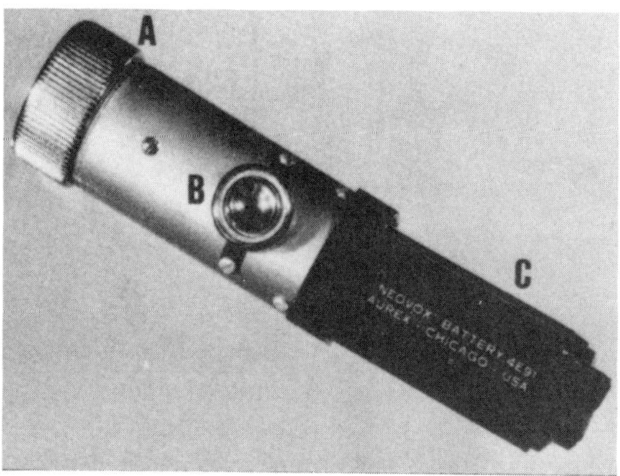

Figure 6–18. Aurex "Neovox" M-520T electronic larynx. A, Chrome collar around vibrator mechanism. B, On-off tone activation switch. C, Battery.

Aurex "Neovox" Electronic Larynx

The Aurex "Neovox" M-520T is a battery-powered instrument that produces sound by means of a piston striking a diaphragm (Fig. 6–18). The Aurex has an on-off tone activation switch with a ring around it that can be rotated to adjust intensity to a desired level. Although the manufacturer advises against altering the chrome collar located around the vibrating head of the instrument, minor alterations (less than one turn) do result in noticeable frequency variation. Under no circumstances should the cap be removed. The Aurex "Neovox" can be purchased from the Aurex Corporation, 844 West Adams Street, Chicago, IL 60607, for approximately $356.50. This price includes a rechargeable battery and battery charger. Replacement batteries are priced at $20. each.

Servox Electronic Larynx

The Siemens Servox is a high-quality German instrument (Fig. 6–19). Sound is produced when a piston strikes a fixed diaphragm at a high velocity. The best quality of sound can be achieved by rotating the screw cap in which the diaphragm is mounted until the piston barely strikes this diaphragm at its farthest point of contact. Frequency and intensity may be adjusted by rotating individual-function switches. Additionally, minimal frequency variation (5 to 20 Hz) can be achieved while talking

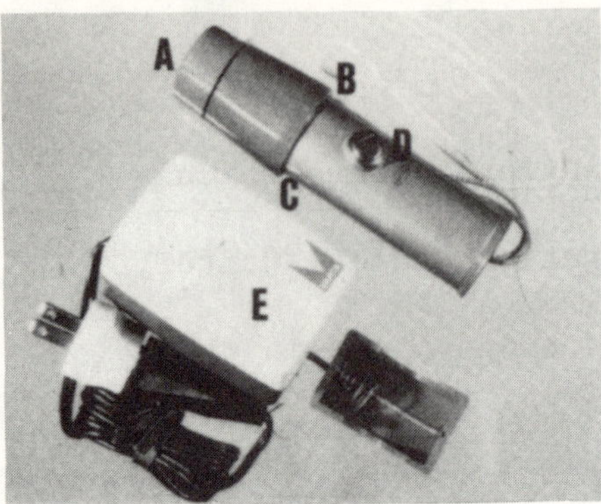

Figure 6–19. Siemens Servox electronic larynx. A, Vibrator mechanism. B, Frequency control switch. C, Intensity control switch. D, On-off tone activation switch. E, Battery charger.

by applying increased pressure to the tone activation switch. The Servox can be purchased from the Siemens Corporation, 685 Liberty Avenue, Union, NJ 07083, for $450. This price includes a rechargeable battery, a charger, and a carrying case.

Rehaton Electronic Larynx

The Rehaton Speech Aid (Fig. 6–20) is another German-made instrument, smaller and lighter in weight than the Servox. Sound is produced by means of a piston striking a diaphragm. Quality of sound can sometimes

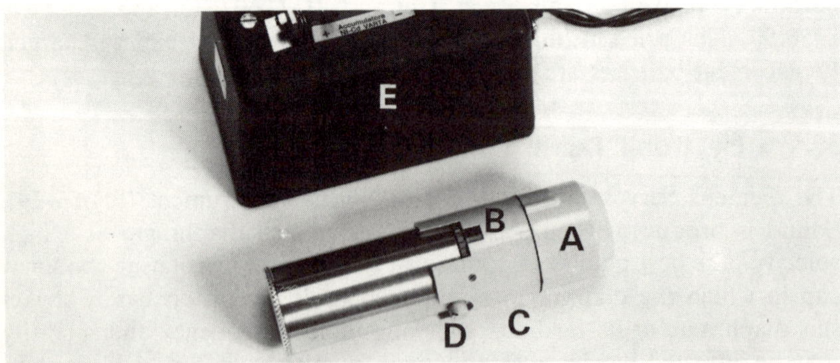

Figure 6–20. Rehaton Speech Aid. A, Screw cap around vibrating mechanism. B, Intensity control wheel. C, Frequency control wheel. D, On-off tone button. E, Battery charger.

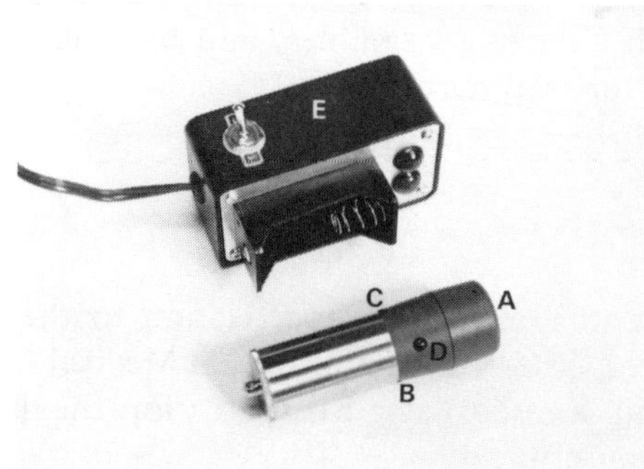

Figure 6–21. ROMET Speech Aid. A, Rigid vibrator. B, Frequency control disc. C, Intensity control disc. D, On-off tone button. E, Battery charger.

be improved by rotating the screw cap of the vibrator membrane. Intensity and frequency can be adjusted by turning the appropriate red-rimmed wheel on either side of the device. The Rehaton can be ordered directly from the Bavarian Laryngectomee Club, VEREIN-KEHLKOPFLOSEN, Schmellerstr. 20 Rgb., D-8000 Munchen 2, Federal Republic of Germany, or from the U.S. distributor: Dean Rosecrans, Post Office Box 710, Nampa, ID 83651. The price of $290. includes the device, two rechargeable batteries, a battery charger, and a carrying case. An oral adaptor can be purchased for an additional $20.

ROMET Speech-Aid Electronic Larynx

The ROMET is the smallest electronic neck-type speech aid available (Fig. 6–21). It is approximately 3¾ inches long, 1 inch in diameter, and weighs only 5 ounces. Sound is produced when a piston strikes a rigid diaphragm. When ordering, the customer selects volume (low, moderate, high); sound (soft or sharp), and pitch (low, medium, high). In this way the manufacturer adjusts each instrument to meet individual needs. In addition, the owner may alter frequency and intensity by rotating appropriate disc controls. The device is powered by a 1.5 volt rechargeable battery. It can be purchased for $295. from ROMET, Inc., P.O. Box 132, Westerly, Rhode Island 02891. Price includes the speech aid, two rechargeable batteries, and a charging unit.

The preceding presentation, although not intended to be an exhaustive review, has provided a description of commercial artificial larynxes currently available to speech pathologists and laryngectomees in the United States. Speech pathologists who desire to be well equipped to offer comprehensive alaryngeal speech therapy should be completely familiar with these instruments, be able to demonstrate their use either personally or with videotaped samples, and have as many of them as possible available for trial purposes.

ACKNOWLEDGMENT

The authors wish to extend their appreciation to the Medical Media Production Services, Veterans Administration Medical Center, Indianapolis, Indiana, and Kansas City, Missouri, for the illustrations that appear in this manuscript.

QUESTIONS

1. Under what two major classifications can most types of artificial larynxes be placed?
2. Under what conditions presented by a patient might you consider recommending an electric intraoral device?
3. When would it be appropriate to recommend a pneumatic artificial larynx rather than an electric neck-type?
4. How could a person without a tracheal stoma demonstrate the use of a pneumatic type of device?

REFERENCES

Blom, E. D. (1978). A practical change to an artificial larynx. *I.A.L. News, 23,* 5.

Nelson, I. W., Parkin, J. L., and Potter, J. E. (1975). The modified Tokyo larynx. *Arch. Otolaryngol., 101,* 107–108.

Tait, V., and Tait, R. V. (1959). Speech rehabilitation with the oral vibrator. *Speech Pathol. Ther., 2,* 64–69.

Weinberg, B., and Riekena, A. (1973). Speech produced with the Tokyo artificial larynx. *J. Speech Hearing Dis., 38,* 383–389.

Zwitman, D. H., and Disinger, J. L. (1975). Experimental modification of the Western Electric No. 5 electrolarynx to a mouth-type instrument. *J. Speech Hearing Dis., 40,* 35–39.

Chapter 7

Acoustical Properties of Esophageal and Tracheoesophageal Speech*

Bernd Weinberg

Human speech production is a diverse and fascinating endeavor. The diversity of this endeavor is highlighted by the capacity for human communication by speech to be examined from several levels: physiological, acoustical, psychophysical, linguistic, and psycholinguistic levels underlying both production and perception of speech. These underlying levels or processes are interrelated parts of a uniquely human endeavor. Moreover, major questions, issues, and clinical and investigative activities in speech pathology ultimately force clinicians to deal with the interrelationships among physiological, acoustical, psychological, and linguistic levels of speech performance.

In this chapter various acoustical properties of two major types of alaryngeal speech, esophageal and tracheoesophageal speech, are described. An exploration of this topic is undertaken for several reasons. First, knowledge about acoustical properties of alaryngeal speech represents an important body of information and a significant area of theoretical and applied study. Second, knowledge about acoustical properties of alaryngeal speech can be interpreted in such a manner as to enlarge understanding of speech production following larynx removal. Increased understanding is accomplished by uncovering relationships among

*Preparation of this chapter was supported, in part, by the National Institute of Neurological, Communicative Disorders and Stroke research grant #NS15371–06.

acoustical properties and physiological, psychological, and linguistic aspects of alaryngeal speech production. This chapter has been prepared in such a manner as to make some of these relationships explicit.

ESOPHAGEAL AND TRACHEOESOPHAGEAL SPEECH: AN INTRODUCTION

Normal speech production is accomplished by generating source sounds in the larynx or at various sites in the vocal tract and differentially modifying these sounds by acoustic filtering. Contemporary descriptions of speech production embrace what is known as source-filter theory of speech production. Normal speech production is executed by exhaling pulmonary air to provide energy to generate source sounds within the vocal tract or by interrupting exhaled air with the vocal folds to produce a quasiperiodic sound source or voicing. In either circumstance, pulmonary air is used to energize a source, and these sound sources are differentially modified by resonant properties of the vocal tract.

There are circumstances in which people must produce speech using a radically altered mechanical system. Patients who have undergone total laryngectomy are in such a situation. As indicated elsewhere in this text, surgical removal of the larynx is a form of laryngeal cancer treatment. Total laryngectomy necessitates removal of the entire larynx. All structures between, and often including, the hyoid bone and the upper tracheal rings are resected. As part of this surgical procedure, the trachea is rotated forward and sutured to the base of the neck to create a permanent respiratory stoma on the neck wall.

Contemporary approaches to speech restoration following total larynx removal include (1) assisting patients to learn to produce esophageal speech, (2) developing speech that is mediated, in part, on a surgical-prosthetic basis, and (3) assisting laryngectomized patients to produce speech powered by some type of prosthetic artificial larynx. In this chapter only esophageal and tracheoesophageal speech is discussed. This topical limitation is occasioned, in part, by a need to limit the scope and length of presentation. In addition, comprehensive information about acoustical properties of speech produced by laryngectomized patients using artificial larynges is not provided because of a paucity of information on this topic. Finally, the diversity in acoustic outputs directly attributable to the nature of the excitation sources used in commercially available devices occasions wide variation in acoustical properties. This broad range of acoustical properties is too extensive to review in a chapter of this scope.

Instead, two forms of alaryngeal speech are considered: esophageal and tracheoesophageal speech. The former is a time-honored form of alaryngeal speech used by thousands of laryngectomized patients. The latter is a more recent form of alaryngeal speech mediated, in part, on a surgical-prosthetic basis. Among contemporary surgical-prosthetic methods, tracheoesophageal puncture is the most widely used. In addition, esophageal and tracheoesophageal speech share some common features. For example, esophageal and tracheoesophageal speech rely on surgically reconstructed upper esophageal segments as voicing sources. Esophageal speech is energized by air initially insufflated into the esophagus from the mouth or the nose and pharynx or both, whereas tracheoesophageal speech is energized by pulmonary air.

ACOUSTICAL PROPERTIES OF ESOPHAGEAL SPEECH

Phonatory Characteristics

Total laryngectomy always results in a sacrifice of tissue essential to normal vocal function. As indicated earlier, esophageal and tracheoesophageal speakers rely on surgically reconstructed tissue for a voicing source. Both kinds of speakers also use altered respiratory inputs to drive and modulate their voicing source and phonatory apparatus. A large number of investigations have been undertaken to define acoustical properties emerging from the esophageal phonatory process (see Weinberg, 1980, 1982, and references therein for detailed reference citations). Published information dealing with acoustical properties of tracheoesophageal voices is beginning to emerge, but it remains somewhat limited and largely unreplicated (Robbins, 1984; Robbins, Fisher, Blom, and Singer, 1984a, 1984b).

One consistent finding emerging from these works is that both esophageal and tracheoesophageal speakers exhibit extensive variation in average voice fundamental frequency (F_0) (Hoops and Noll, 1969; Robbins et al., 1984a, 1984b; Shipp, 1967; Snidecor and Curry, 1959, 1960). In view of the extensive intersubject variation in average F_0 that exists among speakers in both of these groups, serious questions might be raised about the usefulness of average F_0 data for either of these groups of alaryngeal speakers. Average F_0 for male esophageal speakers is reported to be about 65 hertz (Hz). Average F_0 of esophageal voice also has been reported to vary as a function of speaker sex (Weinberg and Bennett, 1972), although this observation has not been independently verified. The average F_0 for 15 male tracheoesophageal speakers has recently been noted to be about 100 Hz (Robbins et al., 1984b). Robbins and colleagues attributed this increase (100 Hz for tracheoesophageal versus 65 Hz for esophageal) in average F_0 to differences in the nature of respiratory influences between esophageal and tracheoesophageal voice production. The recent work of Moon (1985) suggests that neither group nor individual tracheoesophageal speaker average F_0 can be predicted on the basis of any single influence or combination of respiratory influences. Although data from the Moon (1985) project show that aerodynamic influences do mediate tracheoesophageal voice production, the impact of these influences on average F_0 is probably not as straightforward as Robbins and co-workers have suggested. Hence, specification of factors that influence or mediate average oscillatory rates of the [tracheo]esophageal voicing sources represents a highly promising area of future research. Clearly one important defining property of esophageal and tracheoesophageal voices is the large intersubject variation in average F_0. The range in average F_0 for speakers in both groups extends from about 30 to over 200 Hz.

Existing published data (see references cited previously) also reveal that esophageal and tracheoesophageal speakers phonate over a wide range of fundamental frequencies. On the average, esophageal speakers exhibit F_0 standard deviations of 2 to 4 semitones and 90 per cent ranges of 13 to 14 semitones, or slightly over one octave. Tracheoesophageal speakers have average F_0 standard deviation of about 6 semitones (Robbins et al., 1984a).

A second important defining characteristic of esophageal and tracheoesophageal voices is large intersubject variation in vocal quality characteristics. No esophageal or tracheoesophageal speaker has been documented to have normal voice quality. In view of the nature of the voicing sources used to support [tracheo]esophageal voice, normality in vocal quality should not be expected. Vocal qualities noted among esophageal and tracheoesophageal speakers include rough-hoarse, strain-tense, and wet-bubbly vocal qualities (Smith, Weinberg, Feth, and Horii, 1978; Weinberg, 1981, 1982). Recently a number of clinicians, including this writer, have noted breathiness consistently present during voice production by some tracheoesophageal speakers. Finally, note should be made that some esophageal and tracheoesophageal speakers also produce a variety of extraneous (e.g., stomal noise, air intake noises, and air leakage around and through prostheses) sounds that both detract from overall perceived acceptability and signal deviancy or abnormality.

Speech Characteristics

Total laryngectomy also occasions substantial changes in nonphonatory aspects of alaryngeal speech production. For example, esophageal speakers consistently deliver speech at a rate that is significantly reduced in comparison with normal. Snidecor and Curry (1959, 1960) have shown that speech rate of superior esophageal speakers ranged from 85 to 129 words per minute, with a group average of 113 words per minute. The reduction in esophageal speech rate is due, in part, to an increase in the amount of time these speakers spend in silence. The increase in silence time is occasioned by the esophageal speaker's limited ability to sustain voicing. For example, esophageal speakers produce fewer words per breath group than normal (e.g., about 5.0 versus 12.4 words, on the average). Recent data (Robbins et al., 1984a, 1984b) suggest that tracheoesophageal speakers deliver speech at a more rapid rate: the average was about 125 words per minute for 15 male tracheoesophageal speakers. The increased rate of delivery of tracheoesophageal speech can be attributed to the use of pulmonary rather than insufflated air and the absence of the need to pause frequently for esophageal air filling.

Comprehensive data about articulatory changes occasioned by larynx removal is lacking. Larynx removal must alter articulatory behavior (see Weinberg, 1980, for details). This is true because total laryngectomy disrupts muscular support for the tongue, occasions major changes in articulatory aerodynamics, and produced alteration in vocal tract morphology. In addition, the intrusion of gestures essential to esophageal air filling must exert disruptions in dynamic articulatory behaviors of esophageal speakers.

The results of numerous studies (Creech, 1966; Hyman, 1955; McCroskey and Mulligan, 1963; Sacco, Mann, and Schultz, 1967: Tikofsky, 1965; Weinberg, 1980) show that esophageal speech is characterized by a reduction in speech intelligibility. Although it is now clear that, on the average, esophageal speakers exhibit reduced intelligibility, the nature of articulatory performances of this group is not well understood. In view of the importance of articulation to communication efficacy, this area merits serious investigation.

Information about acoustical properties of articulatory by-products in alaryngeal speech is scarce. Sisty and Weinberg (1972) have shown that formant frequency characteristics of vowels produced by esophageal speakers are elevated, a finding interpreted to show that laryngectomized patients have shorter than normal vocal tracts. Christensen and Weinberg (1976) have shown that the spoken vowels of esophageal speakers are consistently longer than those spoken by normal speakers, a finding supportive of the view that articulatory behavior is altered.

Additional acoustic properties of speech influenced by total laryngectomy are speech intensity characteristics. Smith and co-workers (1980) have shown that esophageal speech is characterized by an increased prevalence of lower-level speech output in comparison with normal speech; on the average, the median intensity levels of esophageal speech are about 6 to 10 decibels (dB) less than normal speech. Recent observations of Robbins and colleagues (1984b) suggest that median intensity of tracheoesophageal speech is about 10 dB more intense than normal, a finding that should be substantiated before widespread conclusions or interpretations are offered.

Acoustic manifestations of prosody in alaryngeal speech are now reviewed. Prosodic aspects of speech contribute to speech understanding, naturalness, proficiency, and normality. Acoustical and perceptual investigations of intonation (e.g., Bev loves Bób versus Bev loves Bób?), contrastive stress (e.g., Bév loves Bob versus Bev loves Bób), lexical stress (e.g., óbject versus objéct), and syntactical stress (e.g., bláckboard versus black bóard) have been completed only recently (Gandour and Weinberg, 1982, 1983, 1985; Gandour, Weinberg, and Garzione, 1983; Gandour, Weinberg, and Kosowsky, 1982; Weinberg and Gandour, 1985).

Some findings of these studies are summarized here. Esophageal and tracheoesophageal speakers are able to signal intonation contrast successfully (Gandour and Weinberg, 1983). The physical properties of the intonation patterns produced by normal, esophageal, and tracheoesophageal speakers have also been examined (see Gandour and Weinberg, 1985, for details). For example, the F_0 contours of all sentences spoken by a normal speaker are displayed in Figure 7–1. Examination of these contours reveals that questions were signaled consistently with a terminal rise in F_0, statements with a terminal fall in F_0. In the pair in which Bev is stressed, F_0 falls slightly in Bob in declarative tokens and rises sharply on Bob in interrogative tokens. In the pair in which Bob is stressed, F_0 rises and falls on Bob in declarative tokens and rises sharply on Bob in interrogative tokens. The F_0 contours for other normal speakers were similar to those illustrated in Figure 7–1.

The F_0 contours of all sentences spoken by one esophageal speaker are displayed in Figure 7–2. Three aspects of these contours merit discussion. First, this speaker's F_0 contours are noisy approximations of those produced by normal speakers. This speaker was nonetheless able to signal intonation in a manner indistinguishable from that of normal speakers. Readily observable frequency perturbations and interruptions in voicing are evident in this speaker's F_0 contours. Such characteristics reflect that the voicing characteristics of esophageal speakers are considerably more aperiodic and less reliable than those of normal speakers (Smith et al. 1978). Second, the mean *absolute* F_0 during sentences produced by this speaker is approximately one octave below that of sentences produced by normal speakers. This finding conforms with the results of numerous earlier studies of esophageal phonation (Weinberg, 1980, and references therein). Third, systematic differences in the shape of F_0 contours, rate of changes in F_0, peak F_0, and endpoint F_0 are evident in

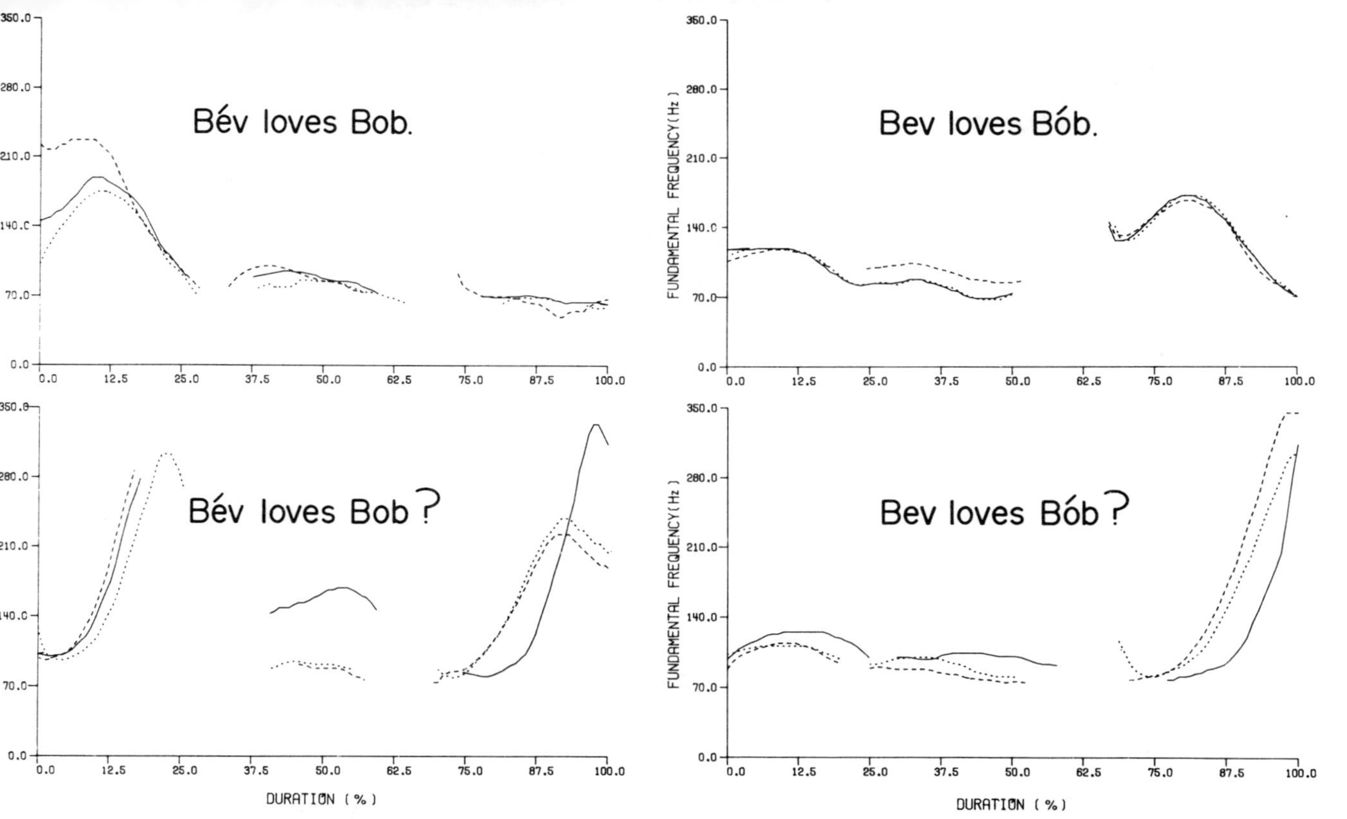

Figure 7–1. F_0 contours of 12 sentences spoken by one normal speaker. Individual sentences are indicated by solid (token #1), dotted (token #2), and dashed (token #3) lines. Words assigned contrastive stress are indicated by superscript acute accent signs. Duration is normalized for speaking rate.

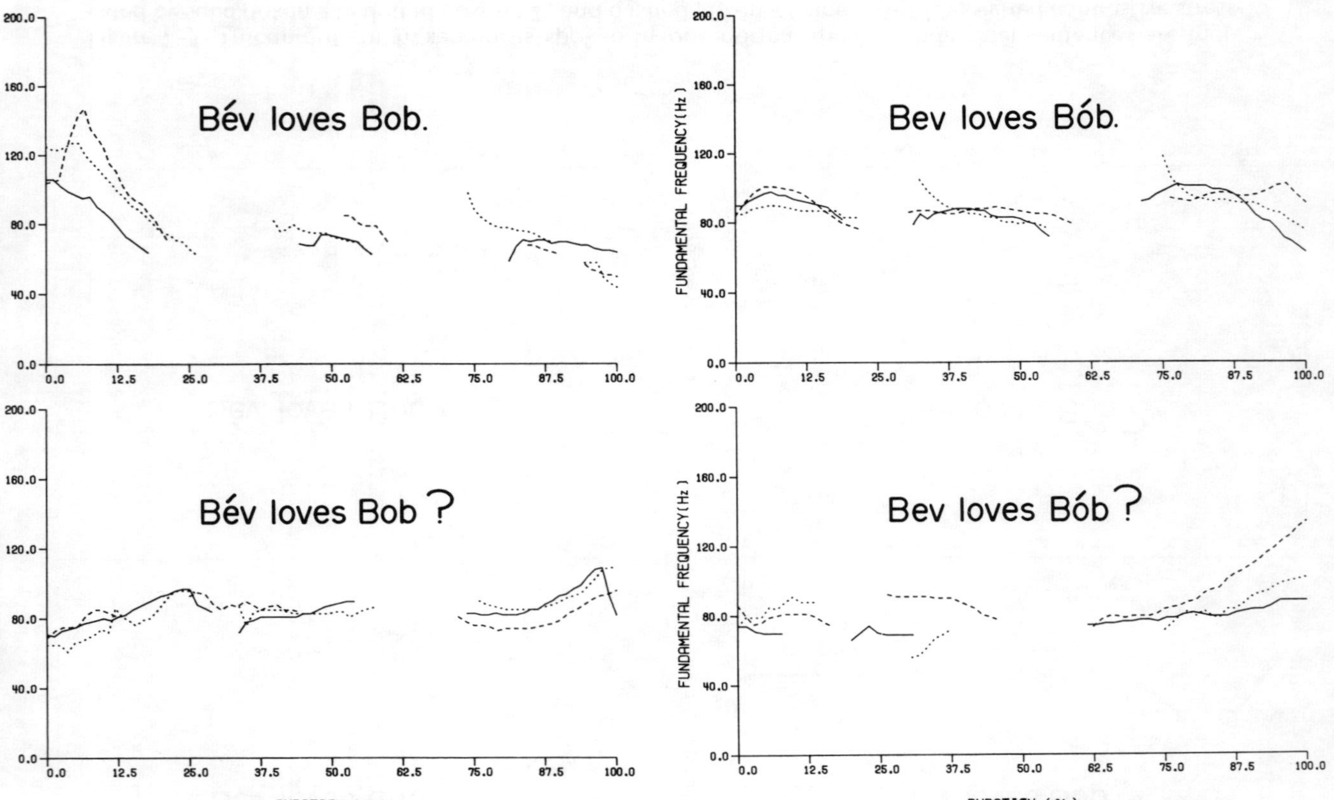

Figure 7–2. F_0 contours of 12 sentences spoken by one esophageal speaker. See also legend for Figure 7–1.

these contours, depending on whether the sentence spoken is a statement or a question. Thus, this speaker, as well as other esophageal speakers studied, was able to control *relative* differences in F_0 to distinguish statements from questions.

F_0 contours of all sentences spoken by a tracheoesophageal speaker are displayed in Figure 7–3. His contours are also noisy approximations of those produced by normal speakers, yet they exhibit systematic, relative differences in F_0 variation as a function of statement versus question production. Since the voices of other tracheoesophageal speakers were largely aperiodic, reliable F_0 measurements for them were unobtainable. That these tracheoesophageal speakers were able to signal intonational contrasts with largely aperiodic excitation emphasizes again the reality that perceptual judgments of pitch attributes of alaryngeal voices may not "be related in a one-to-one fashion to F_0" (Angermeier and Weinberg, 1981, p. 89).

Taken together, these findings suggest that surgically reconstructed pharyngoesophageal segments of some laryngectomized patients, powered either by air insufflated into the esophagus or by diverted pulmonary air, provide an adequate, nonconventional phonatory apparatus that enables some laryngectomized speakers to control and modulate F_0 for the purpose of signaling intonation patterns.

In addition, it has been shown that esophageal and tracheoesophageal speakers are also able to signal contrastive stress in a highly effective manner (see Gandour and Weinberg, 1982, for details). The physical properties underlying stress patterns produced by normal, esophageal, and tracheoesophageal speakers have also been examined in detail. Three aspects of these stress patterns are highlighted. First, all normal speakers and most of the esophageal and tracheoesophageal speakers studied produced systematic differences in peak F_0 as a function of stress position (see Figure 7–4). Second, all normal speakers and half of the esophageal and tracheoesophageal speakers studied produced systematic differences in peak intensity between stressed and unstressed syllables (see Figure 7–5). Third, all the speakers who signaled contrastive stress successfully, normal and alaryngeal alike, produced systematic differences in varying degrees in the duration of both syllables and contiguous pauses between stressed and unstressed syllables (see Gandour and Weinberg, 1985, for details).

Among normal, esophageal, and tracheoesophageal speaker groups, there was a nonsignificant group effect for the differences in relative magnitude of peak F_0, peak intensity, syllable duration, and pause duration between stressed and unstressed syllables (cf. McHenry, Reich, and Minifie, 1982). There was, however, considerable variation in the relative

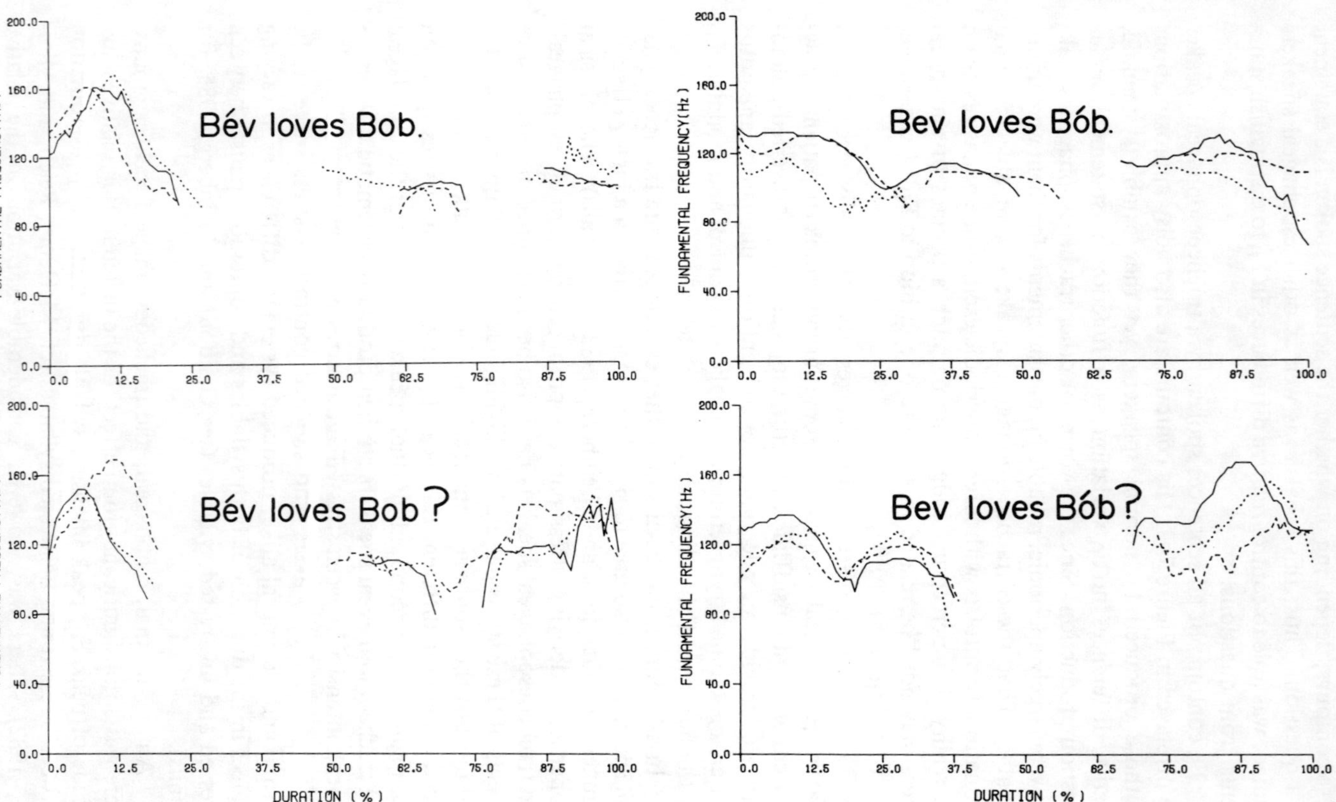

Figure 7–3.   F$_0$ contours of 12 sentences spoken by one tracheoesophageal speaker. See also legend for Figure 7–1.

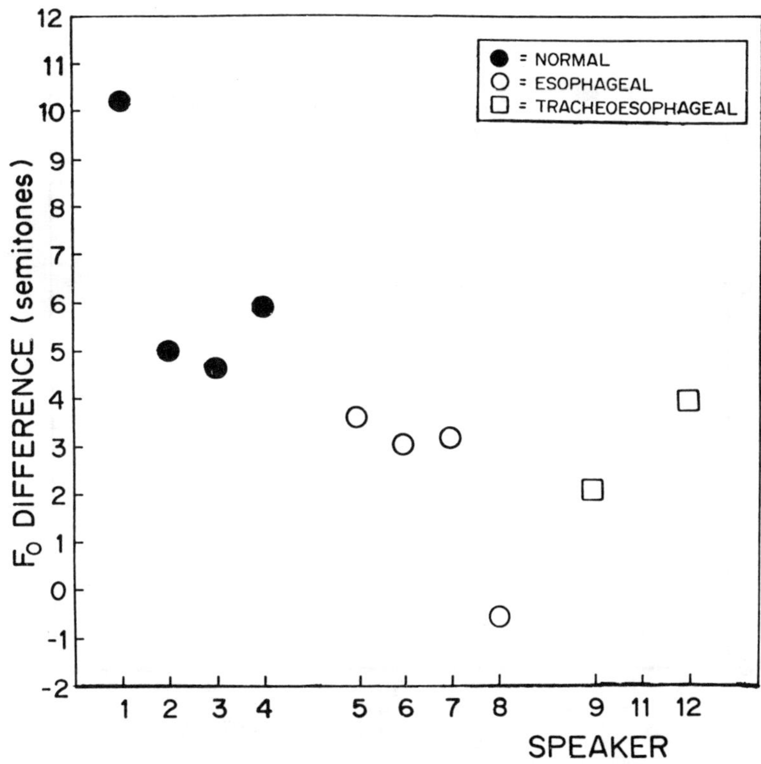

Figure 7–4. Average differences in peak F_0 between stressed and unstressed syllables for normal, tracheoesophageal, and esophageal speakers.

weighting of these four acoustical properties on the perception of contrastive stress among individual speakers within each of these three groups (see Weinberg and Gandour, 1985, for details).

These findings support the view that listeners rely on a variety of acoustical properties to perceive stress. It appears that esophageal and tracheoesophageal speakers use the same properties as normal speakers to mark stress. In view of the fact that the vibratory source is the same in these two groups of alaryngeal speakers, albeit driven by different airstream mechanisms, the F_0 findings emphasize that some esophageal and tracheoesophageal speakers are physiologically capable of controlling F_0 to signal contrastive stress.

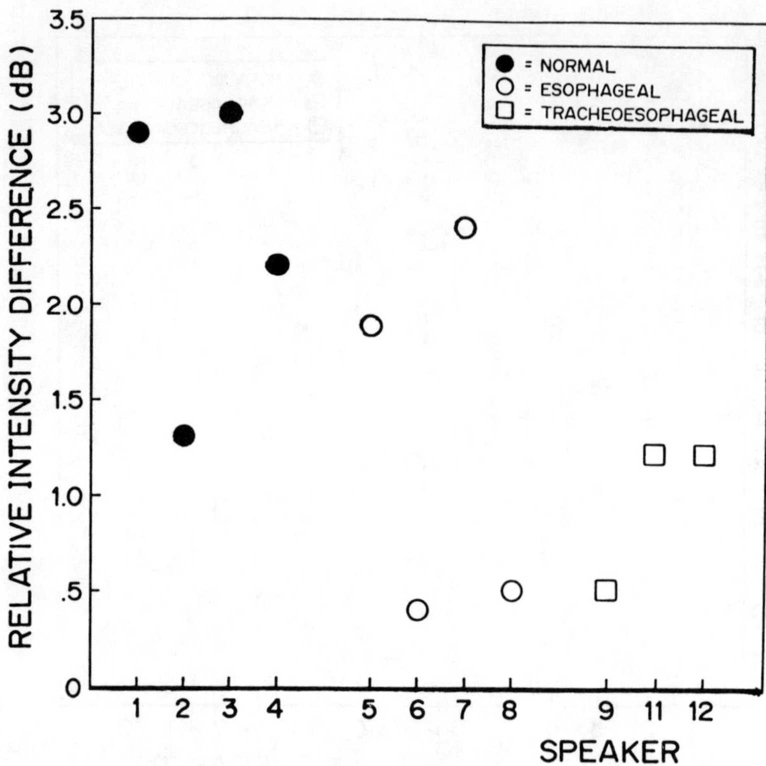

Figure 7–5.   Average differences in peak relative intensity between stressed and unstressed syllables for normal, esophageal, and tracheoesophageal speakers.

Esophageal and tracheoesophageal speakers are also able to achieve lexical and syntactical stress contrasts at high levels of proficiency (see Gandour et al., 1983; Gandour, et al., 1982, for details). The acoustical properties underlying productions of these periodic contrasts in alaryngeal speech will be described elsewhere.

The results of studies dealing with prosodic characteristics of speech after laryngectomy reveal several factors that influence the control of prosody in alaryngeal speech. First, the particular form of alaryngeal speech used by laryngectomized patients may play a critical role in the realization of certain linquistic contrasts within the same language. Second, for a single speaker, a given form of alaryngeal speech may not be used equally well to achieve different prosodic contrasts within the same language. Third, for a given prosodic contrast, the same form of alaryngeal speech may not be used equally effectively by different speakers of the same language.

A fundamental assumption underlying the conduct of this work has been that surgical removal of the larynx eliminates the normal mechanism of phonation and substantially alters the mechanics of speech production. The assumption has been made that surgical removal of the larynx does not impair or disturb the linguistic form of the laryngectomized speaker's message. Thus, the extent to which prosodic contrasts may be realized in given forms of alaryngeal speech depends partially on the specific physical properties on which a given contrast is based and partially on the constraints of the altered speech production apparatus used by laryngectomized patients.

As noted in earlier sections of this chapter, acoustical investigation of esophageal and tracheoesophageal speech has, until recently, provided mostly descriptive information about long-time F_0, intensity, and duration characteristics of major forms of alaryngeal speech. Although major differences in long-term physical properties between alaryngeal and normal speech have been documented, the results of our recent studies indicate that such differences are largely irrelevant from a linguistic perspective. For example, findings indicate that some esophageal and tracheoesophageal speakers are able to vary physical properties (F_0, intensity, and duration) of speech to mediate successfully the perception of intonation and contrastive stress. These findings emphasize that some of these speakers produce appropriate *relative* differences in acoustical patterns critical to the realization of linguistic contrasts, while significant *absolute* differences in F_0, intensity, and duration characteristics between alaryngeal and normal speech serve largely to signal nonlinguistic sources of variation.

The results of our research indicate that some laryngectomized patients are able to produce highly acceptable prosodic patterns. This observation suggests that many laryngectomized patients have the capacity to produce speech characterized by prosodic patterns and proficiency levels that exceed those typically sought by professional workers in the field of speech pathology. Speech pathologists should (1) evaluate how well laryngectomized patients are able to realize prosodic contrasts and (2) provide direct therapy to enhance production of appropriate prosodic patterns in patients who exhibit deficits in their fundamental aspects of speech production (Weinberg and Gandour, 1986).

QUESTIONS

1. Identify the average F_0 for speakers using standard esophageal voice in terms of Hz and of notes on a piano. Do the same for speakers using tracheoesophageal speech.
2. What is incorrect with the concept that laryngectomees speak in a monotone?
3. Compare (in words per minute) the rate of speaking a laryngectomee using standard esophageal voice production probably would employ with that of your own rate and then explain why the laryngectomee would most likely be slower.
4. Weinberg cites two ways in which a laryngectomee's vowel sounds are different than normal. What are they?
5. If a laryngeal talker spoke at a level of 70 dB, how intense would you expect a laryngectomee's voice to be?
6. Explain the vocal differences between "Bev *loves* Bob" and "Bev loves Bob?" and then speculate as to how alaryngeal speakers might accomplish such differences.

REFERENCES

Angermeier, C., and Weinberg, B. (1981). Some aspects of fundamental frequency control in esophageal speech. *J. Speech Hearing Res., 24,* 85–91.

Christensen, J., and Weinberg, B. (1976). Vowel duration characteristics of esophageal speech. *J. Speech Hearing Res., 19,* 678–689.

Creech, H. B., (1966). Evaluating esophageal speech. *J. Speech Hearing Assn. of Virginia, 7,* 13–19.

Gandour, J., and Weinberg, B. (1982). Perception of contrastive stress in alaryngeal speech. *J. Phonetics, 10,* 347–350.

Gandour, J., and Weinberg, B. (1983). Perception of intonation contrasts in alaryngeal speech. *J. Speech Hearing Res., 26,* 142–148.

Gandour, J., and Weinberg, B. (1985). Production of intonation and contrastive stress in esophageal and tracheoesophageal speech. *J. Phonetics, 13,* 83–95.

Gandour, J., Weinberg, B., and Garzione, B. (1983). Perception of lexical stress in alaryngeal speech. *J. Speech Hearing Res., 26,* 418–424.

Gandour, J., Weinberg, B., and Kosowsky, A. (1982). Perception of syntactic stress in alaryngeal speech. *Lang. Speech, 25,* 299–304.

Hoops, H. R., and Noll, J. D. (1969). Relationships of selected acoustic variables to judgments of speech proficiency. *J. Comm. Dis., 2,* 1–13.

Hyman, M. (1955). An experimental study of artificial larynx and esophageal speech. *J. Speech Hearing Dis., 20,* 291–299.

McCroskey, R. L., and Mulligan, M. (1963). The relative intelligibility of esophageal speech and artificial larynx speech. *J. Speech Hearing Dis., 28,* 37–41.

McHenry, M., Reich, A., and Minifie, F. (1982). Acoustical characteristics of intended syllabic stress in excellent esophageal speakers. *J. Speech Hearing Res., 25,* 564–573.

Moon, J. (1985). *Aero-dynamic and myoelastic contributions to tracheoesophageal voice production.* Unpublished doctoral dissertation, Purdue University, West Lafayette, IN.

Robbins, J. (1984). *Acoustic differentiation of laryngeal, esophageal and tracheoesophageal speech. J. Speech Hearing Res., 27,* 577–585.

Robbins, J., Fisher, H. B., Blom, E. C., and Singer, M. I. (1984a). A comparative study of normal, esophageal and tracheoesophageal speech production. *J. Speech Hearing Dis., 49,* 202–210.

Robbins, J., Fisher, H. B., Blom, E. C., and Singer, M. I. (1984b). Selected acoustic features of tracheoesophageal and laryngeal speech. *Arch. Otolaryngol., 110,* 670–672.

Sacco, P. R., Mann, M. B., and Schultz, M. C. (1967). Perceptual confusions among selected phonemes in esophageal speech. *J. Indiana Speech Hearing Assn., 26,* 19–33.

Shipp, T. (1967). Frequency, duration and perceptual measures in relation to judgments of alaryngeal speech acceptability. *J. Speech Hearing Res., 10,* 417–427.

Sisty, N., and Weinberg, B. (1972). Vowel formant frequency characteristics of esophageal speech. *J. Speech Hearing Res., 15,* 439–448.

Smith, B. E., Weinberg, B., Feth, L., and Horii, Y. (1978). Vocal roughness and jitter characteristics of vowels produced by esophageal speakers. *J. Speech Hearing Res., 21,* 140–249.

Snidecor, J. C., and Curry, E. T. (1959). Temporal and pitch aspects of superior esophageal speech. *Ann. Otol. Rhinol. Laryngol., 68,* 1–14.

Snidecor, J. C., and Curry, E. T. (1960). How effectively can the laryngectomee expect to speak? *Laryngoscope, 70,* 62–67.

Tikofsky, R. S., (1965). A comparison of the intelligibility of esophageal and normal speakers. *Folia Phon., 17,* 19–32.

Weinberg, B. (1980). *Readings in speech following total laryngectomy.* Baltimore: University Park Press.

Weinberg, B. (1981). Speech alternatives following total laryngectomy. In J. Darby (Ed.), *Speech evaluation in medicine.* New York: Grune & Stratton.

Weinberg, B. (1982). Speech after laryngectomy: An overview and review of acoustic and temporal characteristics of esophageal speech. In A. Sekey and R. Hanson (Eds.), *Electroacoustic analysis and enhancement of alaryngeal speech.* Springfield: Charles C Thomas.

Weinberg, B., and Bennett, S. (1972). Selected acoustic characteristics of esophageal speech produced by female laryngectomees. *J. Speech Hearing Res., 15,* 211–216.

Weinberg, B., and Gandour, J. (1986). Prosody in alaryngeal speech. In W. Perkins (Ed.), *Seminars in speech and language.* New York: Thieme-Stratton.

Chapter **8**

The Role of the Rehabilitation Team in Counseling the Family and Friends of the Laryngectomee

Paula A. Square

We, as speech pathologists, almost unanimously agree that counseling of the laryngectomee, his family, and his friends is vital to the total rehabilitation process. Varied and divergent opinions, however, were presented as to what counseling should include and when, how, and by whom such counseling should be delivered.

Doctor Hartman stated that primary consideration of a counseling program should be directed not only to the laryngectomee but also to his spouse and children, employer and work colleagues, relatives, and neighbors, a fact seemingly agreed upon by all panel members. In addition, all seemed to agree that counseling should begin following the initial diagnosis of laryngeal cancer and the recommendation for laryngectomy and that it should be continued well beyond the postoperative discharge period.

Doctor Salmon viewed the counseling process as affecting three discrete stages of the rehabilitation process in which the needs of the laryngectomee, his family, and friends focus on different concerns. The first stage occurs during the preoperative period when all are thinking about surgery in terms of survival and its most obvious after-effects. Salmon was of the opinion that at this time, the laryngectomee and his family and friends need to interact closely with only a small nucleus of profes-

---

Panel Participants: David E. Hartman, R. Wayne Holland, Shirley J. Salmon, James C. Shanks.

sionals, including the surgeon, nurses, and anesthesiologist; a counselor; a speech pathologist; and, often, a religious representative of their choice. Doctor Hartman concurred with this concept as he listed the pertinent issues to be discussed preoperatively: (1) what is "wrong" and the necessity for surgery to maintain life, (2) what the surgery basically involves, (3) the definite anatomical and physiological changes and the probable psychosocial alterations resulting from surgery, (4) changes in lifestyle necessitated by surgery, and (5) changes in speech and the necessity for using alternate forms of communication. Doctor Shanks pointed out that the findings of research completed by Gonnella and co-workers (1978) show that it is during this stage that counseling focuses on the imparting of information rather than instruction, treatment, or evaluation. During this information-imparting stage of counseling, the physician appears to be the central figure as judged by the rehabilitation professionals surveyed by Gonnella.

The second stage for patient and family occurs immediately postoperatively. According to Salmon, the patient's and family's attention is initially focused on recovery but gradually shifts to thoughts about discharge from the hospital to the home. Concerns include having enough knowledge to assure adequate medical care in the home, acquisition of alaryngeal speech, payment of hospital and surgical bills, and initial adjustments that each family member may be responsible for or may feel responsible to make. Because the kinds of problems become broader in scope, the number of professionals with whom the patient and family might logically interact increases. According to Salmon, the individuals who might assume major involvement during this stage are the nurses, a speech pathologist, an alaryngeal speaker and spouse, an American Cancer Society representative, a physical therapist, a counselor, and someone who can interpret insurance and disability benefits. According to Shanks's synopsis of the Gonnella study, the scope of the counseling program now increases to include not only the imparting of information but also some aspects of instruction. The survey by Gonnella and colleagues (1978) of rehabilitation specialists indicated that many such specialists must become involved in the counseling process at this time and that throughout all, the family should be involved.

Salmon suggested that the third stage of the process, the postdischarge stage, centers around the long-term effects of laryngectomy. According to a survey of spouses of laryngectomees completed by Salmon, aspects of daily life become paramount, including communication; employment; social, psychological, sexual, financial, marital, and familial matters; and alcoholism. Salmon was also of the opinion that it is during this period that the laryngectomee and his family experience real feelings of abandonment because most members of the rehabilitation team are no longer involved when discharge from the hospital takes place. Comprehensive services are rarely resumed on a routine basis, except on request. It appears that all too often the rehabilitation team is nothing more than a hospital discharge team.

Agreed upon by all panel participants was the idea that one person must be willing to suggest to the patient and family the names of professionals or referral sources to contact when problems arise during the postoperative period. The identity of the person who should assume this role, however, was not agreed upon. Shanks was of the conviction that any professional with a good knowledge of laryngectomy and resulting psychosocial-familial problems may act as the counselor or resource-referral agent. He stated that speech pathologists should feel a professional obligation beyond that of dealing solely with communication deficits. If a speech pathologist possesses the knowledge and the time and is confronted with the opportunity to counsel, he or she should provide this service. Salmon, on the other hand, felt that speech pathologists may not be as proficient in the area of counseling skills as they are led to believe during their graduate training. She was of the opinion that because speech pathologists may be ill-equipped to counsel patients about problems of daily living, they do nothing to resolve the global problems of the laryngectomee and his family and friends. Instead, they may antagonize them and frustrate themselves even to the point of sacrificing valuable therapy time.

Both Salmon and Holland outlined practical approaches to the dilemma of counseling the laryngectomee and his friends and family. At the Veterans Administration Medical Center in Kansas City, Missouri, Salmon actively engaged the interest and cooperation of a social worker on staff to implement a counseling program. All prospective laryngectomees and their families are referred to this trained therapist preoperatively and are seen by her during their postoperative recovery period on a daily basis before discharge. Later, as outpatients, all laryngectomees and close family members meet for hourly group sessions weekly. In addition, the laryngectomee and the spouse, family, or both meet individually with this therapist when necessary. Because this program embraces the preoperative, postoperative, and long-range discharge periods, this therapist is responsible for making referrals to appropriate members of the "rehabilitation team" at the appropriate times. Problems of daily living after discharge are discussed in a group setting, thereby affording the laryngectomized persons and their families support from others undergoing similar problems.

As Coordinator of Speech Pathology Services at the Michigan Cancer Foundation in Detroit, Holland has devised a biannual team-counseling program for laryngectomees and their families and friends.

The program consists of a 5 hour educational seminar for the family and friends of laryngectomees, with a concurrent seminar for the laryngectomees themselves. Lectures are delivered by each member of the rehabilitation team, including a surgeon, a speech pathologist, a social worker trained in head and neck rehabilitation, a rehabilitation nurse, a vocational rehabilitation counselor, and a laryngectomized speaker. Both lectures and rap sessions are included in the seminar program. Holland stated that as a result of completing this seminar, the family and friends have obtained a foundation of information that allows them to have a more positive influence in the rehabilitation efforts of their laryngectomee. Counseling efforts, however, are not concluded following the all-day "Teach-In." At the completion of the "Teach-In" the participants are enrolled in psychosocial group therapy sessions. These sessions are held in 8 week blocks with groups separated into male, female, family, and friends. These group meetings are designed to assist the participants in all adjustment areas associated with the laryngectomee experience. The rehabilitation team, in addition, holds additional weekly meetings to discuss events that transpire in the psychosocial groups. Each team member can then alter his or her plans of treatment in order to benefit optimally his or her group's participants and thus aid the rehabilitation prognosis of each laryngectomee involved in the program. Furthermore, support to the laryngectomee and family and friends is not considered complete following the 8 week group sessions; 6 week follow-up contacts are arranged with the patient and his family until the patient ceases his rehabilitation program. Thereafter, contact with the patient and family continues on a biannual to annual basis.

The pragmatic approaches to counseling outlined by Salmon and Holland help to resolve the conflict that speech pathologists may feel concerning their obligations to the laryngectomee and his or her family. Thanks to such programs, the time spent with the speech pathologist can be devoted solely to the development of communication skills. Nevertheless, it should be mentioned that the speech pathologist may be the only professional from the rehabilitation team with a broad-enough knowledge to arrange, organize, and administer such counseling programs and seminars. According to Shanks, speech pathologists fully realize the scope of the problems of the laryngectomee and understand the principles involved and to whom to refer patients. Their knowledge is therefore of great value in instituting such programs. Furthermore, many rural geographical areas do not offer the resources available in metropolitan areas. In such instances, Shanks felt that the speech pathologist is professionally obligated to institute Lost Chord or New Voice Clubs even if the enrollment is as few as two members. Laryngectomees must be urged to become functioning members of society. This goal is often not realized without the assistance of support groups that help the laryngectomee and his family adjust to their problems of daily life by offering knowledge and emotional support through this difficult period.

QUESTIONS

1. To what extent do you agree with Dr. Hartman's proposed "targets" of counseling?
2. In Salmon's first stage of counseling, what topics listed by Hartman should you be concerned with most? List issues you would raise in an information-sharing capacity.
3. In the second stage of counseling, from the postoperative period to discharge from the hospital, what should be the involvement of a speech pathologist or laryngectomized speech instructor in terms of appropriate concerns to discuss?
4. Recognizing that few of us have the capability to tap a rehabilitation team as described by Holland, what do you advocate beyond issues of speech development as topics for discussion with your clients?

REFERENCES

Gonnella, C., Parker, D., Hollender, J., Lowell, G., Pettersen, P., and Miller, S. (1978). *Normative criteria for cancer rehabilitation. Rehab. Res. Monagr. Series, No. 1.* Atlanta: Emory University.

Chapter **9**

The Intermediate Stage of Teaching Alaryngeal Speech*

Melvin Hyman

In this chapter, methods for teaching the laryngectomee multisyllable vocal units as well as word and phrase production will be discussed. The patient, having progressed through the initial stage of esophageal speech training, should have satisfactorily developed a technique for air intake and usage and be capable of producing tone on demand. Specific techniques and practice materials to help the patient through the intermediate stage will be described.

THE INTERMEDIATE STAGE OF TRAINING

Syllable Drill

The purpose of this procedure is to encourage the patient to produce more than one syllable per air intake. This drill is used after the patient has satisfactorily completed the initial stage, as demonstrated by his ability to produce a monosyllabic unit (consonant-vowel) following air intake. Plosive and sibilant sounds are used in this drill in order to take advantage of the injection possibilities associated with the production of these sounds.

---

*This paper is based in part on Hyman, M. (1971). Primary stage of teaching alaryngeal speech. In S. Rigrodsky and J. Lerman (Eds.). Therapy for the laryngectomized patient (pp. 29–41). New York: Columbia University Teachers College Press.

Several authors, including Doehler (1956), Hyman and Keller (1960), Nelson (1949), and Gardner (1971), advocate similar techniques in learning to produce two or more syllables per air intake. Various combinations of consonant and vowel sounds can be created that may be used by the clinician for practice with the laryngectomee.

At first the patient is asked to produce a single consonant-vowel syllable, prolonging the vowel. This can be practiced until the patient is capable of maintaining the phonation for approximately 2 seconds. These same nonsense monosyllables can be used for the production of from two to approximately five syllables per air intake. Care should be taken to permit the patient to achieve success and not to tax his abilities beyond what he is capable of producing. It is suggested that the units be grouped by twos and then built gradually into longer units until five syllables are achieved.

As part of this procedure, it is recommended that the patient be instructed to vary the duration, intonation, and loudness of the syllables produced. For example, equal duration, intonation, and loudness can be given to all the syllables produced; then the patient can be told to increase the duration of the first syllable and to shorten those that follow; then increase loudness on the second syllable; alternate intonation every other syllable, and so forth.

Word Drill

If the patient is successfully producing consonant-vowel syllables containing plosive and sibilant sounds, the clinician may introduce single-syllable words in which these sounds occur in the initial position, the final position, or both, while varying the vowels used. Examples of such words appear in Table 9-1. The procedures described in the previous section on syllable drill can be used for the word drill.

The use of one-syllable words that do not begin or end with plosives and sibilants can then be introduced, for example, *yes, no,* and *fine* as well as *hi, bye* (it will be said as /a/ but the listener will hear /ha/), and counting from one to ten. Although these are usually more difficult to produce, they add utilitarian value to this stage of communication. These five words will enable the patient to communicate to some degree with his family and friends. The patient is able to greet people (''hi''), indicate agreement (''yes'') or disagreement (''no''), answer the usual question that is asked when one has been hospitalized: ''How are you?'' (''fine''—if the patient has a positive attitude—or ''lousy'' if it better suits the patient's temperament), and bid a person goodbye (''bye'').

Table 9–1. Word Drill

/t/	/p/	/s/	/st/	/sp/	/ʃ/	/t/	/k/
tap	pat	sat	stack	spat	shack	chat	cat
tack	pap	sap	stop	spot	shot	chap	cap
tot	pass	sass	start	spark	shop	chop	cash
top	patch	sack	stock	space	shock	chart	cast
tart	past	sop	stark	spade	shark	chock	cot
tape	pack	sock	state	spoof	shape	chase	cop
taste	pot	sake	steak	speck	shake	chaste	cart
take	pop	say	stay	speech	shoot	chew	carp
toot	part	suit	stoop	speak	shoe	Chet	Kate
two	park	soup	stew	spit	sheet	check	cape
tooth	pace	Sue	step	spurt	sheep	cheat	case
test	paste	set	steep	sport	sheik	cheap	cake
teach	pay	said	stitch	spore	ship	cheek	Kay
teak	pooch	seat	stick	spite	show	chip	kept
tip	pet	seep	stow	spy	shirt	chick	keep
tick	pep	cease	store	spike	shirk	church	kit
tote	pest	seek	stalk	spout	short	chore	kiss
toast	peck	sit	sty		shore	chalk	kick
toe	peat	sip	stout		shy		coat
terse	peep	sick			shout		cope
turk	peace	soap			shook		coast
taught	peach	sew					coach
tore	peek	search					Coke
torch	pit	sought					curt
toss	pop	sore					curse
talk	pitch	source					Kirk
tight	pick	salt					caught
type	pope	sight					course
tie	post	side					cork
tike	poach	soot					kite
took	pert						couch
	purse						cook
	perch						
	perk						
	pour						
	porch						
	pork						
	pipe						
	pie						
	pike						
	pout						
	pouch						
	put						

Producing Two- and Three-Syllable Words and Phrases

When the patient demonstrates that he is capable of producing three to
five monosyllabic words per air intake, it is useful to introduce multisyllabic words and phrases beginning with plosives and silibants and extend
the practice to include all vowels and consonants. It is at this point that
the patient is coming closer to maximum speech communication.

Table 9–2. Multiple Syllable and Phrase Drill

pass/ the/ salt	pass the salt
ba/ na/ na	banana
pe/ pper/ pot	pepper pot
di/ nner/ time	dinner time
ta/ king/ it	taking it
grand/ fa/ ther	grandfather
buy/ some/ bread	buy some bread
don't/ for/ get	don't forget
pre/ tty/ soon	pretty soon
te/ le/ phone	telephone
pump/ kin/ pie	pumpkin pie
cut/ some/ cake	cut some cake
kick/ the/ stick	kick the stick
cook/ the/ stew	cook the stew
cut/ the/ grass	cut the grass
stop/ and/ see	stop and see
suit/ and/ tie	suit and tie
stitch/ in/ time	stitch in time
six/ ty/ six	sixty six
che/ rry/ tree	cherry tree
jum/ ping/ Jack	jumping Jack
shoe/ shine/ brush	shoeshine brush
sho/ vel/ snow	shovel snow
check/ and/ see	check and see
they/ are/ there	they are there
Thanks/ gi/ ving	Thanksgiving
three/ do/ llars	three dollars
fa/ vor/ ite	favorite
va/ len/ tine	valentine
mea/ sure/ ment	measurement
mail/ them/ now	mail them now
my/ daugh/ ter	my daughter
rea/ lly/ did	really did
li/ bra/ ry	library
li/ ttle/ dog	little dog
red/ or/ blue	red or blue
went/ to/ church	went to church
he's/ at/ school	he's at school
a/ nice/ day	a nice day
our/ back door	our back door
a/ large/ piece	a large piece
at/ the/ store	at the store
in/ our/ car	in our car

The words and phrases in Table 9-2 are examples for combining monosyllables and short words into multisyllabic words and phrases. The words are separated into syllables according to the *oral* production of each word and not in the manner found in most standard dictionaries. The patient should produce each syllable, as divided by the slant lines, separately and then combine two syllables and then three. The same should be done for each word in the phrase. Practice in varying the duration, intonation, loudness, and pause time between words is a critical component of this exercise.

In this way multisyllabic words and phrases are first broken down into smaller units and then gradually built back up to form the original word or phrase. The patient may combine numbers, words, or phrases to form two- and three-syllable drills. Blending exercises will help to increase the number of syllables produced with each intake of air since some phonation time is eliminated. As an example, in the words *good time*, the /d/ phoneme is imploded but not exploded. Another example of blending is in the words *Bob will*. A slight explosion of the /b/ phoneme may be produced as one goes quickly on to produce the /w/ phoneme; many speakers may use only the imploded phrase of the /b/ and glide quickly to the /w/ sound. Thus a series of isolated sounds is avoided, and speech may be produced that is fluent and rhythmical rather than pedantic.

ARTICULATION SHARPENING

Snidecor (1968) states that "given reasonable loudness and quality, intelligibility or understandability is almost entirely a result of effective articulation" (p. 185). Thus it is important that there be precision in articulation. Care, however, must be taken that the articulation not be overprecise, for such exaggeration will lead to unnatural or affected speech and may cause difficulty in fluency.

Sounds That May Need Special Attention

The Nasals.   The nasal sounds should be prolonged sufficiently to ensure good nasal resonance. Nonsense syllable practice will help attain this quality. Some examples are:

/ma/, /mo/, /mi/, /mei/, /mu/
/na/, /no/, /ni/, /ner/, /nu/
/mana/, /mano/, /mani/, /manu/
/nama/, /namo/, /nami/, /namu/
/aŋ/, /iŋ/, /ʌŋ/, /ieŋ/, /uŋ/
/aŋuŋ/, /iŋaŋ/, /eŋʌŋ/, /uŋiŋ/

Words and phrases containing various combinations of nasal sounds should then be used for the purpose of producing good nasal resonance. Humming and having the patient feel the vibrations coming from his nose also help to attain this quality.

The Fricatives.   The fricatives, particularly the /s/, may tend to be weak or missing, especially in the initial position of a word. The speaker may not be giving enough time to the sound or the tongue may be in a position in which air cannot escape between the teeth (tongue tip against the back of the incisor teeth). Practice of this sound in isolation, nonsense syllables, and words may be necessary. For example:

> Produce each /s/ in isolation: s - s - s - s
> Produce the following nonsense syllables: /sa/, /so/, /si/, /sei/, /su/.
> Produce the following words: sat, soap, seed, sake, soup, bus, toss, ice, icy, bossy.

Consonant Clusters.   Some patients may have difficulty in combining two consonants or a consonant and a vowel sound. This has been noticed, not infrequently, when the patient is producing the linguavelar sounds /k/ and /g/ in combination with another sound in the initial position. Exercises using the /k/ and /g/ in isolation and then in nonsense syllables will help to coordinate the production of the velar sounds and those that follow them. A few examples are:

k - l	p - l	c - r	p - r
kl	pl	cr	pr
klick	play	crowd	proud
g - l	b - l	g - r	b - r
gl	bl	gr	br
glad	blade	great	broom

The /h/ Sound.   It is well known that the esophageal speaker has difficulty in producing the /h/ sound owing to the lack of a continuing air supply. Most speakers simply omit this sound from their speech, and the listener conveniently "hears" the missing sound through the context of the sentence. In the sentences *I am going 'ome* or *This is my 'ouse,* the listener fills in the /h/ sound without much trouble or loss of intelligibility for the speaker. Gestures as well as the immediate previous conversation will be of assistance; for example, *It is very late. I am going 'ome.* When it is advisable for the patient to be able to produce a fairly intelligible /h/ phoneme, the clinician may wish to employ a method that appears to work satisfactorily. Hodson and Oswald (1958) teach the /h/ sound by having the patient produce the /k/ sound at first. The patient is then asked to lower the tongue slightly at the back, allowing breath to escape. This produces the German *ich*. The tongue is then lowered still further, so that a very small space between the back of the tongue and the soft palate exists. The outgoing air emanating through this space should produce a good /h/ sound.

Producing Final Consonants

The esophageal speaker's intelligibility may be further increased if final consonants are accurately heard by the listener, particularly at the ends of phrases and sentences. This does not mean that the articulation should be overprecise but should be precise enough to avoid confusion between words that are similar except for the final consonants. Drills stressing final consonant production and discrimination for individual words and phrases should be used with patients who consistently omit final consonants or unvoice the final phoneme.

Each member of the following pairs of words contains the same initial consonant and vowel but differs in the final consonant, which is a voiceless or voiced cognate:

bat—bad	not—nod
pot—pad	seat—seed
mat—mad	bus—buz
tack—tag	nap—nab
Dick—dig	tap—tab
let—led	lap—lab
fat—fad	breath—breathe

LOUDNESS FLEXIBILITY

One of the problems esophageal speakers encounter is inability to vary the loudness of the voice. With the small amount of air from the esophagus that can be used in phonation, it is difficult for them to increase their loudness level. However, there are certain exercises and techniques that may be used to help them develop loudness flexibility.

1. Instruct the patient to use a larger mouth opening.
2. Exercises from soft voice to loud voice can be employed to help esophageal speakers develop a greater range of loudness. The following exercises are suggested. Words in italics are to be produced with greater loudness. This will aid not only in giving variety to the esophageal voice but also in giving meaning to the sentences.

Turn it on.	*Sit* over there.
Turn *it* on.	Sit *over* there.
Turn it *on*.	Sit over *there*.
Her name is Jane.	*I* want some coffee.
Her *name* is Jane.	I *want* some coffee.
Her name *is* Jane.	I want some *coffee*.
Her name is *Jane*.	

Other exercises may be made up stressing various words to give change in loudness and meaning.

3. The following technique used by some clinicians is recommended for use with caution, following consultation with the patient's physician. When the musculature is lacking in tonus, an elastic band (garter) with snappers may be used around the speaker's neck to increase tonus and produce a louder voice. Care should be taken that the band is not too tight. The same effect may be produced by having the speaker place his hand on the side of his neck, so that slight pressure is applied to the cricopharyngeal area.

PITCH FLEXIBILITY

Since the fundamental pitch of alaryngeal speakers is usually quite low (60 to 90 hertz [Hz]), the voice may sound monotonous. Alaryngeal speakers may be able to attain two octaves in pitch range, but few use much of this range. At low fundamental pitches, the listener may not perceive many of the pitch variations.

1. Step approach: The speaker intones the vowel /a/ at discrete pitches from his lowest to his highest pitch. Through practice, the range may be increased.

                                      /a/

                     /a/

      /a/

2. Glide method: In this exercise, the /a/ is produced (a) from low to high in a continuous glide, (b) from high to low in a continuous glide, and (c) in a combination of both.

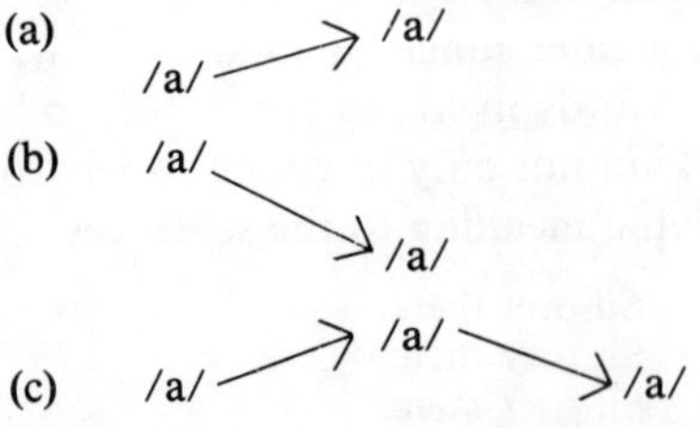

3. Practice may also be given in trying to raise the pitch at the end of sentences containing questions.

How are you?
How do you feel?
Are you hungry?

4. In speakers with vocal cords, increasing loudness tends to raise the pitch. This phenomenon is also true for the alaryngeal speaker.
5. Limericks, poetry, nursery rhymes, and songs may also be employed to increase variety in pitch.

CAUTIONS FOR THE CLINICIAN AND PATIENT

In his or efforts to produce speech, the patient may use various movements and techniques that make his speech unintelligible and esthetically unacceptable to the listener. These extraneous movements and noises should be eliminated or modified from the onset so that they do not become habitual.

Physiological Aspects

Loud Gulping or Klunking.   The loud klunking that is heard in some patients is usually due to excessive strain and tension. The patient may be taking in too much air or using several injections of air before attempting the production of the word. Reduction of tension through relaxation exercises, lessening the amount of pressure exerted by the tongue, and a relaxed atmosphere in the clinical situation will all help to eliminate these extraneous noises.

Grimaces and Head Movements.   In attempting to produce the sound, the patient may use facial grimaces and head movements. He often believes he needs these for speech. Practice before a mirror in a relaxed situation will convince the patient that he can speak without them.

Excessive Air from the Stoma.   This condition may occur when the patient attempts to speak with increased loudness. The excessive air from the stoma masks his speech and shortens the length of his phrase. Rapid contraction of the abdominal muscles may result in a rapid expulsion of air out of the trachea (Diedrich, 1971). Practice in breathing easily through the stoma several times and then saying the word with the same easy and almost effortless contraction of muscles will eliminate the masking. Thus, the patient should be taught to exhale through the stoma with less force during speaking.

Concomitant Organic Impairments.   Structures other than the larynx may have been partially or totally removed during the original operation, which may have a direct bearing on the individual's ability to produce speech. Since laryngectomies occur primarily in the 40 to 65 year old age group, concomitant factors such as hearing loss may also affect the patient's speech. Amplification and visual, tactile, and kinesthetic methods may be of assistance in teaching such patients.

Psychological Aspects

It is not unusual for these patients to have periods of depression. The operation may have a disturbing effect on the sense of belonging and the self-concept of the patient. Barton (1965) stated that the psychological trauma experienced by some patients appears not to be a result of the loss of the sense of smell and taste or of the need to become a "neck breather" but of the realization that they have become dependent on others. It may, therefore, be necessary to refer such patients for psychological counseling.

The depression may become even more evident when the patient reaches a plateau in learning speech. It is the clinician's responsibility throughout this period of learning to reinforce the patient's efforts and to work to maintain a high level of motivation, so that the patient can successfully cope with the moments when he apparently is making little progress in his speech rehabilitation.

Counseling the spouse and other members of the family is essential. For instance, they may expect too much too quickly. It is usually helpful to tell the family what the patient is expected to practice for the next therapy session. They should be informed of ways in which they may help the patient, such as waiting patiently for the patient to say a word (not unlike the therapy for a stutterer) or conducting short conversations with the patient that require him to use words that he can produce or that he is practicing. Often it is necessary for the clinician to tell the family that the patient is expected to practice in a room by himself to assure that he will be more relaxed in his practice sessions.

Speaking to the family will also give the clinician the opportunity to discuss any questions or problems that they may have in relation to the patient. The allaying of fears and doubts on the part of the family will help give the patient the optimum environment in which to learn esophageal speech successfully.

The clinician must get to know his or her patient in order to determine ways to motivate him and to learn what can be expected of him in terms of his frustration tolerance. Periodic interviews with the family as well as a good clinician-patient relationship within the therapy session will aid the clinician in dealing with the patient. For a more detailed account of the adjustment problems of the female laryngectomized patient, the reader is referred to Gardner (1966).

SUMMARY

Methods for teaching the laryngectomee multisyllabic vocal units, words, and phrase productions were discussed. Exercises for articulation sharpening, variety in pitch and loudness, elimination of concomitant distractions were described. The clinician should keep in mind the following:

1. *Good posture.* Just as good posture is important for good speech in laryngeal speakers, it is equally if not more important for the esophageal speaker.
2. *Relaxation.* A relaxed atmosphere, in which the patient has optimal use of muscles directly or indirectly involved in speech production, is necessary for learning esophageal speech.
3. *The meaning of percentages.* Keep the statistics in mind, but they may not mean much for you. Statistics of 70 or 80 per cent do not mean anything if your patient is in the other 30 or 20 per cent category. Know what he does and how he does it and what he does not know how to do; work from there.
4. *Practice makes permanent.* Only if the patient practices in the correct manner is he able to approach perfection.

QUESTIONS

1. Judging from Hyman's opening paragraph, what do you envision as the content of a "preliminary stage" of esophageal speech instruction?
2. How long should a client sustain a sound before you should consider moving him into bisyllable productions?
3. Since laryngectomized individuals cannot use pulmonary air for consonant productions, how can they be expected to produce these sounds? (What is the physiology of consonant production for laryngectomees?)
4. How does Hyman advocate that laryngectomees produce /h/ by compensation?
5. Hyman discusses the importance of the final consonant. Do you think he really is addressing the issue of final consonants or of avoiding voice-voiceless confusions?
6. When does Hyman recommend attention be placed to the elimination of "distractors" from speech? What are the more common liabilities associated with producing speech with esophageal voice?
7. What is the significance of the statement "Practice makes permanent"?

REFERENCES

Barton, R. T. (1965). Life after laryngectomy. *Laryngoscope, 75,* 1408–1415.

Diedrich, W. M. (1971). Primary stage of teaching alaryngeal speech. In S. Rigrodsky and J. Lerman (Eds.), *Therapy for the laryngectomized patient.* New York: Teachers College Press.

Doehler, M. (1956). *Esophageal speech: A manual for teachers.* Boston: American Cancer Society.

Gardner, W. H. (1966). Adjustment problems of laryngectomized women. *Arch. Otolaryn., 83,* 31–42.

Gardner, W. H. (1971). *Laryngectomee Speech and Rehabilitation.* Springfield, IL: Charles C Thomas.

Hodson, C. J., and Oswald, M. V. O. (1958). *Speech recovery after total laryngectomy.* London: E. and S. Livingstone.

Hyman, M., and Keller, M. (1960). *How to speak again.* Bowling Green, OH: Bowling Green State University.

Nelson, C. (1949). *You can speak again. A manual for laryngectomized patients.* New York: Funk and Wagnalls.

Snidecor, J. C. (1968). *Speech rehabilitation of the laryngectomized, 2nd ed.* Springfield, IL: Charles C Thomas.

Chapter **10**

Evaluating Esophageal Speech Development and Proficiency

Daniel E. Martin

INTRODUCTORY COMMENTS

Skill in evaluating esophageal speech proficiency is based, in part, on a thorough understanding of the nature of esophageal speech. Clinicians who want to expand their services to the rehabilitation of laryngectomees should have a good grasp of the available literature on laryngectomee rehabilitation. Familiarity with the literature will assist them in gaining a more comprehensive understanding of the area from several perspectives, including anatomical and physiological aspects, acoustical features, rehabilitative techniques and procedures, and evaluation tools.

In order to judge esophageal voice and speech progress effectively, as well as global speech skills at the conclusion of a therapy program, the clinician should internalize a grasp of the range of voice and speech attributes of esophageal speakers. How good is a really good esophageal speaker? Good in what frame of reference? What pitch levels and melodic intonation characteristics best exemplify esophageal speech? How loud is average esophageal voice in relation to laryngeal voice? Is esophageal voice quality a constant, or are there noticeable differences among speakers? If you were an experienced esophageal speech instructor who had taught many laryngectomees to use esophageal speech effectively, would you have instant recognition of different patients who telephoned you just by their voice and speech characteristics? These are examples of some of the questions that speech clinicians should ask themselves and that this chapter will address.

A critical, educated ear is one of the most important tools a clinician must possess in order to judge effectively the voice and speech characteristics of laryngectomized clients. Developing a critical and educated ear and developing good listening abilities are based to a large extent on exposure to and experience in listening to a variety of esophageal speakers. Perhaps speech pathologists, upon completion of a seminar like this, would benefit from listening to tape recordings containing large numbers of esophageal speakers at varying levels of development and with different voice and speech characteristics.

Speech clinicians may find it useful to view each patient's speech development on two levels, a macroscopic level and a microscopic level. Macroscopic viewing means listening to overall, or global, speech proficiency. Microscopic viewing, on the other hand, means looking for and listening in a more discrete, focal manner to specific attributes and problems that are part of the overall proficiency.

Three points must be made before moving from these introductory comments. First, whatever tool the clinician selects to assist in evaluating his patient's progress or proficiency—whether it is the Berlin criteria, the Wepman Scale, or another—its frequent application in the course of therapy can and should be used to modify and redirect the patient's course of therapy. In other words, charting or plotting progress simply for the sake of maintaining records is not enough.

Second, application of a preventive medicine approach to special problems works better than an approach designed to correct or to attempt to correct problems after they are firmly entrenched in the patient's communicative repertoire. For example, it is better to prevent the onset of loud stomal blast than to attempt to correct it once it is firmly entrenched. It is better to identify early in therapy the presence of a loud klunk and to attempt to reduce or eliminate it right away than to wait until it is habitual.

Third, in judging the laryngectomee's development of communication, it is useful to think in terms of (1) how he is progressing in esophageal voice, or phonatory development, and (2) how he is doing in developing speech skills. Initially our major concern should be the development of voice skills and only later should it be the integration of phonatory skills into the development of a high degree of speech proficiency.

A basic prerequisite for success in acquiring esophageal speech is the development early in therapy of strong basic foundations of voice. Basic foundations include *consistent vowel phonation, short latency,* and *adequate vowel duration.* In the early stage of esophageal voice instruction, the phonatory mechanism is often highly unstable. There is a natural tendency among newly laryngectomized patients to rush too quickly from vowels and syllables to sentences. The prudent esophageal speech instructor makes sure that the client develops good basic foundations of voice *before* moving into connected speech.

PROPERTIES OF SOUND

As stated at the start of this chapter, the ability to evaluate esophageal speech proficiency is based, in part, on a thorough understanding of the properties of sound. Consideration follows of each of the four properties of sound as they apply to the esophageal voice signal: duration, pitch, loudness, and voice quality.

Duration

The dimension of time or duration includes several components. Speech clinicians must consider selected components as they relate to the production of esophageal vowels, such as the time necessary to get air into the esophagus and the duration of the vowel itself on that air charge.

Consideration should be made of the point at which the patient attempts to initiate behavior that will result in an air charge. Early in therapy some patients may have a period of lip smacking, tongue moving, or searching behavior that they go through prior to recalling the starting point for initiating a successful air intake. At a second point the patient successfully starts the motor process that results in an esophageal air charge, with onset of phonation at a third point. The laryngectomee who spends 5 seconds from the time he wants to inflate the esophagus with air until perceived phonation will, in some instances, spend 4½ of those 5 seconds trying to figure out what to put where. The patient does not understand the mechanics for charging. It is therefore imprecise to say that this patient has a 5 second latency when, in fact, much of that time interval was spent in searching behavior.

An adequate duration of phonation is important. An esophageal speaker cannot say much on short, uncontrolled, staccato bursts of sound. Although some effective esophageal speakers can sustain a vowel on a single air charge for 5 or 6 seconds, a duration of 2 seconds or better is good and may be adequate for producing connected speech, especially if the speaker uses multiple methods of air charging. For example, consonant-linked injection may be the primary method of air charging, with standard injection a supplemental means of getting air.

Christensen and Weinberg (1976) investigated the duration characteristics of a number of representative vowels produced by ten esophageal and nine normal speakers. Overall, the vowel durations of the esophageal speakers were consistently longer than those of the normal speakers. The average vowel durations of /i/ and /a/ produced by esophageal and normal speakers were plotted as a function of consonant environment voicing differences; average vowel durations spoken in voiceless consonant environments were always longer for esophageal speakers than for normal speakers. In contrast, average vowel durations spoken in voiced consonant environments were generally comparable for the two groups.

Considering the average esophageal vowel durations for /i/ and /a/, the data show that esophageal vowel durations in voiced consonant contexts were always longer than those uttered in voiceless consonant environments. This last finding has clinical implications relative to therapy. Studies by Sacco, Mann, and Schultz (1967) and Marshall (1974) show that listener misidentification of consonant voicing contrasts in esophageal speech is a major contributor to reduced intelligibility. The laryngectomee intends to say "pie" and the listener perceives "by." The laryngectomee intends to say "tie" and the listener perceives "die." The laryngectomee will significantly improve the listener's perception of the voiced-voiceless distinction in cognate pairs if, for one thing, he shortens the vowel for a voiceless consonant and lengthens the vowel for the voiced counterpart. Christensen, Weinberg, and Alfonso (1978) measured the voice onset times (VOT) of a large number of stop consonant–initiated syllables produced by esophageal and normal speakers. They reported that esophageal speakers systematically varied VOT during the production of speech-sound categories having the same manner of articulation. Furthermore, average VOT associated with prevocalic voiceless stops of esophageal speakers were significantly shorter that VOT of normal speakers.

Pitch

Pitch is the psychological correlate of frequency. Most current data suggest that the average voice fundamental frequency of male esophageal speakers is about 65 hertz (Hz), or half that of normal male laryngeal speakers, and that the variation in average fundamental frequency among esophageal speakers is sizable. The average fundamental frequency level of esophageal speech is usually judged to be low, however, regardless of sex.

Some studies have looked at pitch in esophageal speech. Scragg, Martin, and Bliss (1976) have reported that neither basic esophageal pitch level nor degree of melodic intonation were significantly correlated to global ratings of proficiency in a group of 50 laryngectomized subjects. Curry and Snidecor (1961) pointed out that although the six superior esophageal speakers studied had greater frequency variability than normal speakers, they were judged perceptually as having a "restricted pitch range."

The ability of experienced listeners to evaluate inflectional directions of vowels produced by esophageal speakers was investigated by Podhoretz (1964). She reported that certain listeners were superior to other listeners in their ability to judge both consistently and in agreement with the inflectional direction attempted by the subject. Another finding was that listeners who were more consistent in their judgments tended more often to be in agreement with the subject's attempted directional inflection than did listeners who were less consistent.

Martin and Wiig (1968) investigated intonation contours of esophageal speech. Their findings agreed basically with those of Podhoretz. They also reported that the /2→/ intonation contour, a monotone, was the most characteristic intonation contour of esophageal speech across speaker proficiency levels. Furthermore, listener confusion and intonation contour disagreement among the judges were present, especially in judgments of superior esophageal speech. In many cases, what one sophisticated listener heard as an upward inflection in a syllable, word, or phrase, another heard as a downward or sustained tone.

Research by Stevens and Volkman (1940) showed that the pitch aspects of a stimulus below 100 Hz are greatly reduced when compared to frequencies at or above 100 Hz. Since the average fundamental frequency of esophageal speech is 65 Hz, the perception of small intonational changes might be difficult. There is no question that some laryngectomees can produce noticeable intonational changes in connected speech. However, awareness must be maintained of the difficulty inherent in reliable pitch perception in esophageal voice.

Smith, Weinberg, Feth, and Horii (1978) found that the magnitude of vocal jitter (expressed in either absolute or relative terms) present in sustained esophageal vowels was generally substantially larger than that observed in comparable speech utterances of normal speakers and those with vocal or laryngeal pathologic conditions.

Loudness

With respect to intensity or loudness, it should be recognized that the average level of loudness of the esophageal voice is reduced, as is the range of loudness. Blood (1981) reported that the level of esophageal speech in a consonant environment was approximately 9.4 decibels (dB) less than in normal speech. Furthermore, he will tend to have a range of about 20 dB, as opposed to a normal laryngeal speaker, who may make smooth intensity changes reaching up to 45 dB.

What tools do speech clinicians have available to evaluate basic loudness level and loudness variations in esophageal speech? Certainly none are specific to laryngectomees; however, objective indices of intensity can be obtained through the use of a sound level meter. The volume unit (VU) meter on a tape recorder can be used to help the patient monitor loudness, and a device called Talk Time with numbered and color-coded meters that can be adjusted to monitor loudness can also be of service. Certainly some esophageal speakers can increase their loudness.

Applying external pressure to the pharynoesophageal (PE) segment either digitally or with an elastic band quite frequently helps produce a louder noise. Damsté's (1958) suggestion of elongating the vocal tract by extending the neck may create a more elastic phonatory mechanism, thus increasing loudness. A laryngectomee who recently left the author's program after developing esophageal speech was dissatisfied with his level of loudness. Since he had a generally thick neck and extensive postradiation fibrosis, external pressure on the PE segment was not an answer to increasing loudness. He had undergone a radical neck dissection that, in his particular case, made any kind of elongation or stretching of the neck not feasible. His need for increased loudness of his esophageal voice was met by his use of a small microphone hooked onto his glasses and attached to an amplifier in his pocket.

Quality

Also important in evaluating esophageal speech is the matter of voice quality. How is voice quality judged? There are many adjectives to describe laryngeal variations in voice quality. How do you judge the quality of the esophageal voice? Does esophageal voice quality influence or contribute to ratings of overall proficiency? Acoustically, voice quality can be viewed in part through measurement of the periodicity of phonation. A skilled listener may be able to make perceptual judgments of periodicity by noting the consistency with which a vocal tone is produced. The more consistent the tone, generally the better the quality. The less consistent the tone, generally the poorer the quality. Shipp (1967) reported the tendency for better esophageal speakers to spend about 50 per cent of the total duration of a test sentence in periodic phonation, whereas the lower-rated speakers were only 38 per cent periodic. In short, the better-rated speakers put out a voice signal that was somewhat less noisy than that of the lower-rated speakers.

Damsté (1958) suggested a method to evaluate perceptually the periodicity of esophageal voices. He suggested slowing down a tape-recorded sample of a client's speech by a factor of 16 in order to hear the individual phonatory beeps and evaluate their regularity.

Damsté (1958) reported that an important characteristic of his group II speakers was the formation of a bulge in the ventral side of the pseudoglottis, in which secretions easily accumulate. All of these laryngectomees showed a common voice characteristic of a bubbling sound created by the tone passing through a layer of mucus secretions. Smith and co-workers (1978) reported that listeners were able to give reliable judgment of perceived vocal roughness of sustained vowel samples produced by esophageal speakers.

Does the quality of an esophageal voice contribute to or influence overall ratings of speech proficiency? This matter has received little if any attention in the literature. However, there is now preliminary evidence to support the contention that esophageal voice quality may be a more important variable than was thought.

Scragg and colleagues (1976) investigated the perceptual correlates of proficient esophageal speech. A panel of experienced judges rated speech samples from 50 male laryngectomees on a number of voice and speech attributes, as well as on global speech proficiency. The judges used a seven-point, equal-appearing intervals rating scale in which a rating of 1 represented poor voice quality, a rating of 7 represented excellent quality, and ratings between 1 and 7 reflected degrees in between.

Application of stepwise regression analysis to the data yielded the finding that the cluster of variables including phrasing, voice quality, overall rate, and articulatory proficiency accounted for 76 per cent of total variance in mean speech ratings. To a lesser extent, the absence or low levels of audible klunking was considered to have a positive effect on global speech ratings. Scragg and colleagues (1976) reported that their results have clinical implications for laryngectomees learning esophageal speech. In order to develop a high composite level of overall esophageal speech proficiency, it would seem reasonable to place clinical emphasis on those voice and speech attributes most highly associated with high overall speech ratings. Therefore, they recommend that clinical emphasis should be on the development of smooth phrasing, improved voice quality, acceleration of overall rate, and the elimination or reduction of klunking.

RATE OF SPEECH

Findings in the research literature concerning the relationship between the rate of esophageal speech and perceived speech proficiency have been generally consistent (Hoops and Noll, 1969; Scragg, et al., 1976; Shipp, 1967). They suggest that superior esophageal speakers tend to have a faster speaking rate than more poorly rated speakers.

Snidecor and Curry (1959) analyzed temporal aspects of the speech of six superior esophageal speakers. Their speaking rates ranged from 85 to 129 words per minute, with a mean of 113 words per minute.

Shipp (1967) related selected acoustical and perceptual measures to judgment of alaryngeal speech acceptability. The lower-rated speakers took 2⅓ seconds longer (7.92 versus 5.54 seconds) than the higher-rated speakers to read the 12 word test sentence. The six best speakers from Shipp's study had a mean duration of 4.39 seconds. The normal duration of this test sentence reported in a study of laryngeal speakers was 4.16 seconds. Shipp indicated that it was apparent that above-average speakers and the six best speakers in his study more closely approximated the normal rate, whereas below-average speakers took almost twice the time of normal laryngeal speakers to read the same sentence.

In spite of the general agreement in the literature, the speech pathologist who must retain laryngectomees is not given much information on how to approach rate clinically. Any esophageal speech instructor who has requested a laryngectomee to "speed up" or reduce overall speaking rate has seen a reduction in speech proficiency. It is apparent that a number of factors other than total speaking time are involved in rate. Factors of phrasing and pause time are elements influencing overall rate, and both are important to a listener's perception of esophageal speech effectiveness. Both Shipp (1967) and Hoops and Noll (1969) suggest a reduction in silence or pause time as a principal method of speeding up esophageal speech.

SELECTED SPECIAL PROBLEMS

Some laryngectomees develop audible or visible habits or mannerisms that detract from or interfere with effective communication. They include a loud klunk, multiple klunk, excessive stoma noise, and facial grimaces. These problems require early identification, evaluation, and remediation.

Loud Klunk

A loud klunk is associated with too rapid injection of air into the esophagus. The klunk appears when trapping air prior to phonation. The klunk is a distracting, prephonatory, audible accessory sound.

Multiple Klunk

Some esophageal speakers are not satisfied with a single loud klunk. They insist on being "multiple klunkers." A multiple klunk can occur when the esophageal speaker fears that a single injection, a single pump, will not give him enough air to say what he wants to say. So he injects two, three, or more times in rapid succession before attempting to speak.

Excessive Stoma Noise

Excessive stoma noise or stoma blast is another problem that society judges with considerable prejudice. Shipp (1967) reported that excessive stoma noise reduced rated speech acceptability significantly. Patients who inject air usually do not make stoma noise on inhalation of pulmonary air, but the stoma noise is heard on expulsion of esophageal air in synchrony with pulmonary exhalation. Laryngectomees who use the inhalation method of air intake have a tendency to produce excessive stoma noise on both inhalation and exhalation of pulmonary air.

Excessive stoma noise appears to have its origins in the laryngectomized patient's attempts to speak using air from the lungs, as was the case presurgically, instead of using esophageal air. It can also result from too much straining in an attempt to get the sound out, or attempting to achieve more vocal intensity than is actually required.

Patients have been seen for whom the basic underlying cause of loud stoma noise is a very small stoma. Even moderate air flow through a narrowed orifice can create disproportionately loud stoma noise in such patients. Patients with excessive stoma noise during quiet, relaxed pulmonary respiration, without speech attempts, should have their stoma examined for adequacy of size.

Facial Grimaces

The laryngectomee who makes unnecessary facial grimaces or head or body movements when he begins to talk or during air intake presents a visual component that distracts the listener and detracts from the overall effectivess of his speaking performance. The laryngectomee whose eye contact with the listener is poor has a correctable bad habit that influences communicative effectiveness.

It is clear that each of the special problems just discussed should be identified as early as possible in therapy and reduced or eliminated from the patient's communicative repertoire.

DEVELOPMENTAL RATING SCALES

Descriptive labels such as poor, average, good, and excellent for esophageal speech skills have limited usefulness. Unless the listeners or judges come from comparable experiential backgrounds, comparisons are difficult. For example, an average esophageal speaker in one study or clinic might well be a good esophageal speaker in another.

A number of authors have produced rating scales to classify esophageal speech development (Barton and Hejna, 1963; Berlin, 1963; Hyman, 1957; Robe, Moore, Andrews, and Holinger, 1956; Wepman, MacGahan, Rickard, and Shelton, 1953). The use of developmental rating scales corrects some of the inherent weakness in the use of descriptive labels. Some of the basic values of developmental rating scales, according to Wepman and co-workers (1953), are the following:

1. To provide a common frame of reference for discussing prognosis and progress.
2. To judge the stage of recovery at any given time.
3. To permit the patient to visualize progress; to foresee the stages through which he or she must go before achieving success.
4. To serve as a motivating device.

Accountability is a term that has increasingly crept into the profession's vernacular. Those speech clinicians who treat the communicatively handicapped are being asked to verify the efficacy of their therapeutic interventions. Being held accountable for treatment services has obvious implications from a professional viewpoint as well as from the viewpoint of third-party payment for our services. Accountability mandates careful record keeping and documentation. The laryngectomee who moves, in a reasonable period of time, from aphonia to proficient esophageal speech represents positive evidence in support of accountability, especially if that progress and product have been documented in some logical manner.

Wepman and colleagues (1953) published a seven-level descriptive scale ranging from no speech to automatic esophageal speech. They indicated that their scale is more than just a logical tool comprised of arbitrary levels. Rather, their scale reflects clinical observations made over many years of studying the development of speech after laryngectomy. Most patients were found to go through these stages in a natural progression in their growth to normal speech development. The Wepman scale incorporates the dual nature of the recovery process, namely, the progression of esophageal *sound* production and the acquisition of *speech* proficiency. The seven levels are as follows:

Level 7.   No esophageal sound production; no speech. A Level 7 rating means that the patient cannot produce esophageal voice either voluntarily or involuntarily.

Level 6.   Involuntary esophageal sound production; no speech. A Level 6 rating reflects belching ability, according to Wepman. Sound is uncontrolled and produced with effort. Many patients come to therapy at a Level 6. (New laryngectomees should always be asked during their intake exam, Have you ever belched after a meal since the operation?) Level 6 is important in that production of sound is possible.

Level 5.   Voluntary sound production part of the time; no speech. A Level 5 means that the patient has shown that he can occasionally produce esophageal sound voluntarily. Level 5 is largely characterized by inconsistency of esophageal sound production, with involuntary sounds being produced more frequently than voluntary sounds. Wepman believes that achievement of Level 5 is important prognostically because it indicates that (1) the musculature for sound production is present and capable of functioning and (2) voluntary control of esophageal voice is possible. Wepman believes that progress beyond this point is largely the product of practice and motivation.

Level 4.   Voluntary sound production most of the time; vowel sounds differentiated monosyllabic speech. The phrase "vowel sounds differentiated" simply means that the patient can now produce a variety of vowels. There is a tendency for the patient to hurry his production. Emphasis must still be on sound production, with speech attempts kept to a minimum.

Level 3.   Esophageal sound produced at will; single-word speech. The patient can produce esophageal sound whenever he wishes. Attempts have little or no continuity, but single words—especially short ones—are easily distinguished by the listener.

Level 2.   Esophageal sound produced at will with continuity; word grouping. At this stage, elongation of sound production permits words to be grouped in short phrases. There is still conscious effort involved in trapping air in the esophagus. There is still a tendency to hurry in order to produce more sound and more words on each attempt. The major aspect of this level is the continuity of production, even though it takes conscious effort.

Level 1.   Automatic esophageal speech. Patient speaks with continuity. One aspect more than any other characterizes his efforts: he is now able to speak without thinking of taking air down or bringing it up. Speech is effortless and, while hoarse in quality and somewhat lacking in volume, it is naturally and easily produced.

Robe and associates (1956) presented a seven-level scale as follows:

1. No sounds produced.
2. Partial control; single sounds under fair control.
3. Simple words produced.
4. Combines two or three words.
5. Some sentences used.
6. Sentences consistently used.
7. Fluent, nonhesitant speech.

Hyman (1957) reported on the development of a rating scale to evaluate and classify esophageal speakers. The evaluator rates each of five dimensions on a scale from very poor to excellent. The dimensions are as follows:

1. Fluency: preparation time; rhythm; phrasing; syllables per intake of air.
2. Intelligibility: articulation of consonants; syllable pronunciation; rate.
3. Loudness: adequate loudness for quiet surroundings; the ability to vary volume.
4. Quality: pleasantness; the flexibility to indicate changes in meaning.
5. Social Acceptability: freedom from accessory nonfunctional noises, facial mannerisms, blowing sounds, and labored trapping of air.

(1) Fluency	(2) Intelligibility	(3) Loudness	(4) Quality	(5) Social Accept- ability
Excellent				
Good				
Fair				
Poor				
Very Poor				

Date _________________________   Evaluator _________________________

The Barton-Hejna Rating Scale (Barton and Hejna, 1963) is similar to the Robe and co-workers (1956) scale presented earlier:

1. No sounds produced; cannot voluntarily produce belch.
2. Partial control of belch; production of occasional vowel sound, but inability to combine vowel and consonants to form words.
3. Some simple words of one or two syllables produced. No phrases.

4. Combines two or three words in phrases; but production is not smooth or well coordinated. Stops for obvious intake of air between phrases.
5. Some sentence usage; can carry through short sentences on one intake of air or produce phrases with only slight pauses between. Rhythm may be somewhat uneven with excessive air noises.
6. Quite good use of sentences, with only slight noise of production.
7. Very good speech. Even rhythm; almost imperceptible intake of air. Difficult to differentiate from a normal but hoarse voice.

Berlin (1963) and his colleagues published a series of clinically significant articles in which they quantified measurements of four skills involved in learning esophageal speech that were considered to bear a face validity relationship to adequate esophageal speech.

Curves of skill acquisition were charted for 38 laryngectomees enrolled in intensive therapy. The clinicians used a stop watch. On the last day of therapy, speech proficiency ratings were made and the 38 speakers were divided into two groups. One group consisted of 28 laryngectomees rated as good speakers; a second group of 10 were rated as poor speakers.

Berlin's Four Skills

1. *Ability to Phonate Reliably on Demand*

The patient was asked to inflate the esophagus and then say /a/. Twenty trials were administered and scores were translated into percentages. A successful phonation was defined as one lasting 0.4 second or longer. Patients who developed into good esophageal speakers were able to phonate virtually 100 percent of the time on demand after 10 to 14 days.

2. *Maintenance of a Short Latency Between Inflation of the Esophagus and Phonation*

To measure latency, the patient was asked to phonate the vowel /a/ as quickly as possible after an inflation. The examiner started the stop watch at a signal from the patient that he was beginning to inflate the esophagus. The watch was stopped as soon as the examiner perceived vocalization. The laryngectomee was given ten trials and mean times were recorded. The same 0.4 second criterion used in Skill 1 was employed for a successful phonation.

Patients who developed into good speakers were able to maintain a short latency of approximately 0.2 to 0.6 second between inflation and phonation by the eighteenth day.

It should be remembered that the laryngectomee's esophageal air reservoir can hold only an estimated 40 to 70 cubic centimeters (cc) of air. The air volume capacity of the esophagus is much smaller than that of the lungs. The laryngectomee must frequently reinflate the esophageal air reservoir while talking. The speed and ease with which the patient can reinflate the esophagus should be reflected in the smoothness and continuity of connected speech.

3. *Maintenance of an Adequate Duration of Phonation*

This skill refers to the maximum possible duration of the vowel /a/ on one inflation. To assess this skill, the patient was instructed to phonate a single /a/ on one air charge and sustained it for as long as possible. Patients who developed into good esophageal speakers were able to sustain /a/ for 2.2 to 3.6 seconds by the twenty-fourth day. Berlin (1963) noted that two patients who returned for follow-up demonstrated a substantial reduction in their duration measure; they were found to have recurrence of cancer in the esophageal area. He also noted that once a patient surpassed 1.8 seconds' duration on one air charge, the prognosis for developing esophageal speech was good.

4. *Ability to Sustain Phonation During Articulation*

The patient was asked to use only one inflation and to repeat the syllable /da/ as many times as possible without consciously reinflating. The patient was given five trials. Patients who developed good esophageal speech were able to phonate eight to ten plosive syllables per overt inflation after 25 days. Berlin felt that skill in this area would relate to (1) ability to coordinate phonation with articulation and (2) ability to use plosive injection.

Simpson and Martin (1975) presented results of a pilot study to objectify two of the Berlin skills: ability to phonate reliably on demand and adequate duration of phonation. Berlin's clinicians used a stop watch to increase those two skills. Simpson and Martin used an electronic apparatus that consisted of a voice-operated relay, a microphone, and an alternating current (AC) counter. This apparatus provided a digital readout of esophageal voice duration. It was used as an adjunct in therapy with four laryngectomees.

All four subjects completed Skill 1 (phonating reliably on demand) within the norm of 10 to 14 days described by Berlin (1963). Although none of the four subjects fell within the Berlin norm of a minimal mean duration of 2.2 seconds by 24 days for Skill 2 (adequate duration of phonation), three of the four subjects approximated the prognostic norm of 1.8 seconds. These three subjects subsequently became Wepman Level 1 esophageal speakers.

RESEARCH

Investigators in alaryngeal speech have employed various tools for quantifying the effectiveness of esophageal speakers. These tools include word and sentence intelligibility tests and global ratings of acceptability or proficiency. Specific tools that have been used to obtain overall, global ratings of acceptability include the psychophysical methods of equal-appearing intervals rating scales and direct magnitude estimation.

Selected Intelligibility Studies

Tikofsky (1965) studied the relative intelligibility of normal and esophageal speakers. He reported that the two groups differed in intelligibility to such an extent that there was only minimal overlap between the two populations, and the probability of such overlap occurring would be quite low. Therefore, for all practical purposes it would be best to treat the esophageal and normal speakers as two independent populations. The results of a few investigations concerned with measuring either word or sentence intelligibility of esophageal speech or global speech ratings of acceptability will be considered.

Mean word intelligibility scores for esophageal speech across these studies, with untrained listeners, ranged from a low of 54.9 per cent reported by Shames, Font, and Matthews (1963) to a high of 70.9 per cent reported by Masters (1970). Kalb and Carpenter (1981) stressed the influence of individual speaker characteristics on intelligibility, aside from the type of alaryngeal communication used. Mean sentence intelligibility scores in these studies ranged from 54 per cent with untrained judges in the Clayton (1976) investigation to 75.1 per cent with trained judges in the Hoops and Curtis (1971) investigation.

Word intelligibility scores were found to be significantly correlated with global ratings of acceptability in three studies, with an r of .86 in the Masters (1970) study. Sentence intelligibility scores and global ratings have been found to be significantly correlated, $r = .37$ by Hoops and Curtis (1971) and $R = .83$ by Clayton (1976). Word and sentence intelligibility scores were found to be significantly correlated, $r = .71$ (Clayton, 1976).

Global Ratings

Equal-Appearing Intervals

One of the most common techniques for evaluating data has been the method of equal-appearing intervals proposed by Thurstone and Chave (1929). This method involves the rating or sorting of stimuli by observers into one or another of various categories. The categories are arranged to represent increasing degrees of the attribute possessed by the stimuli to be scaled. The observer's task is to classify the stimuli into groups, and these groups are separated from each other by apparent "equal intervals."

Numerous investigators in the area of alaryngeal speech have employed this method to scale esophageal speech "proficiency" or "acceptability" on five-, seven-, and nine-point scales. For example, a seven-point scale might have a rating of 1 to reflect least proficient esophageal speech and a rating of 7 to reflect most proficient esophageal speech. Mean ratings are derived from listener judgments and are considered to reflect in quantitative terms global proficiency. For example, Shipp (1967) used a five-point equal-appearing intervals scale to measure alaryngeal speech acceptability. Ratings were correlated with various acoustical and perceptual measures.

Interjudge reliability has generally been high with this scaling method. It should be noted that although a group of unsophisticated listeners can usually reliably rate esophageal speakers with the method of equal-appearing intervals, the bases for their individual judgments are not clearly understood. Scragg and colleagues (1976) investigated the perceptual correlates of proficient esophageal speech. Fifty male esophageal speakers, rated as either Level 1 or 2 à la Wepman, served as subjects. The method of equal-appearing intervals was employed with sophisticated judges to obtain global ratings of proficiency as well as performance on ten factors. Results indicated that the cluster of variables, including phrasing, vocal quality, overall rate, articulatory proficiency, and klunking, accounted for 78 per cent of the variance in mean speech ratings.

Direct Magnitude Estimation

The psychophysical method of direct magnitude estimation was used to obtain numerical indices of overall esophageal speech development by Diedrich and Youngstrom (1966). With this method, listeners are presented with a baseline speech sample, and all subsequent judgments are proportionally less than, equal to, or greater than the baseline recording.

In conclusion, this chapter has to provided the reader with information on the properties of esophageal sound, selected special problems and examples of developmental rating scales to evaluate progress and esophageal speech proficiency.

QUESTIONS

1. What methods of air intake often have an associated prephonatory klunk?
2. What is the average voice fundamental frequency of male esophageal speakers?
3. What five attributes should receive attention in developing speaker proficiency?
4. When attempting to speed up the speech of a laryngectomee, what rate should serve as a target?
5. How does Wepman and co-workers' (1953) scale differ from that of Robe and associates?
6. State Berlin's (1963) data in terms of therapeutic goals for a client.
7. What average speaking rate in words per minute did Snidecor and Curry (1959) report for their 6 superior esophageal speakers?

REFERENCES

Barton, J., and Hejna, R. (1963). Factors associated with success or nonsuccess in acquisition of esophageal speech. *J. Speech Hear. Assoc.* (Virginia), *4*, 19–20.

Berlin, C. I. (1963). Clinical measurement of esophageal speech. I. Methodology and curves of skill acquisition. *J. Speech Hear. Dis., 28,* 42–51.

Blood, O. (1981). The interactions of amplitude and phonetic quality in esophageal speech. *J. Speech Hear. Res., 24,* 308–312.

Christensen, J. M., and Weinberg, B. (1976). Vowel duration characteristics of esophageal speech. *J. Speech Hearing Dis., 19,* 678–689.

Christensen, J. M., Weinberg, B., and Alfonso, P. J. (1978). Productive voice onset time characteristics of esophageal speech. *J. Speech Hear. Res., 21* 56–62.

Clayton, S. (1976). *Relationships among word and sentence intelligibility global ratings of esophageal speech skill.* Unpublished master's thesis, Michigan State University, East Lansing, MI.

Curry, E. T., and Snidecor, J. C. (1961). Physical measurement and pitch perception in esophageal speech. *Laryngoscope, 71,* 415–424.

Damsté, P. H. (1958). *Oesophageal speech after laryngectomy.* Groningen: Hoitsema.

Diedrich, W. M., and Youngstrom, K. (1966). *Alaryngeal speech.* Springfield, IL: Charles C Thomas.

Hoops, H. R., and Curtis, J. F. (1971). Intelligibility of the esophageal speaker. *Arch. Otolaryng., 93,* 300–303.

Hoops, H. R., and Noll, J. D. (1969). Relationship of selected acoustic variables to judgment esophageal speech. *J. Comm. Dis., 2,* 1–13.

Hyman, M. (1957). *Evaluation of Proficiency and Classification of Esophageal Speakers.* University of Miami, Florida School of Medicine Post-Graduate Class.

Kalb, M. B., and Carpenter, M. A. (1981). Individual speaker influence on relative intelligibility of esophageal speech and artificial larynx speech. *J. Speech Hear. Dis., 46,* 77–80.

Marshall, R. C. (1974). *Listener mis-identification of selected voiced and voiceless consonants of esophageal speakers.* Paper given at annual convention of American Speech and Hearing Association, Las Vegas, NV.

Martin, D. E., and Wiig, E. (1968). Intonation contours of esophageal speech. *The University of Michigan Speech and Hearing Science Research Reports.*

Masters, J. S. (1970). *Relationships among the acceptability, intelligibility, and acoustic measures of alaryngeal speech.* Unpublished doctoral dissertation, State University of New York at Buffalo.

Podhoretz, C. M. (1964). *Listener judgments of vowel inflections produced by selected esophageal speakers.* Unpublished master's thesis, Indiana University, Bloomington, IN.

Robe, E. Y., Moore, P., Andrews, A. H., and Holinger, P. H. (1956). A study of the role of certain factors in the development of speech after laryngectomy. I. Type of operation. *Laryngoscope, 66,* 173–186.

Sacco, P., Mann, M., and Schultz, M. (1967). Perceptual confusion among selected phonemes in esophageal speech. *J. Ind. Speech Hear. Assoc., 26* 19–33.

Scragg, M. P., Martin, D. E., and Bliss, L. A. (1976). *Perceptual correlates of proficient esophageal speech.* Paper presented at annual convention of American Speech and Hearing Association, Houston, TX.

Shames, G. H., Font, J., and Matthews, J. (1963). Factors related to speech proficiency of the laryngectomized. *J. Speech Hear. Dis., 28,* 273–287.

Shipp, T. (1967). Frequency, duration and perceptual measures in relation to judgments of alaryngeal speech acceptability. *J. Speech Hear. Res., 10,* 417–427.

Simpson, M. L., and Martin, D. E. (1975). The use of an electronic apparatus to develop early esophageal voice skills. *J. Michigan Speech and Hear. Assoc., 11,* 210–214.

Smith, B. E., Weinberg, B., Feth, L. L., and Horii, Y. (1978). Vocal roughness and jitter characteristics of vowels produced by esophageal speakers. *J. Speech Hear. Res., 2,* 240–249.

Snidecor, J. C., and Curry, E. T. (1959). Temporal and pitch aspects of superior esophageal speech. *Ann. Otol. Rhin. Laryng., 68,* 623–636.

Stevens, S. S., and Volkmann, J. (1940). The relation of pitch to frequency: A revised scale. *Amer. J. Psych., 53,* 329–353.

Thurstone, L. L., and Chave, E. J. (1929). *The measurement of attitude.* Chicago: The University of Chicago Press.

Tikofsky, R. S. (1965). A comparison of the intelligibility of esophageal and normal speakers. *Folia Phoniat., 17,* 19–32.

Wepman, J. M., MacGahan, J. A., Rickard, J. C., and Shelton, N.W. (1953). The objective measurement of progressive esophageal speech development. *J. Speech Hearing Dis., 18,* 247–251.

Chapter 11

Factors Influencing the Intelligibility of Alaryngeal Speech

Melvin Hyman

Intelligibility may be defined as the recognition of speech signals. For a speech signal to be intelligible both a speaker and a listener must be involved. If any distortion or interference of the speech signal is either caused by the speaker or perceived by the listener, there may be interference in intelligibility and, consequently, in the oral communication between them. Various aspects of speech such as articulation, loudness, pitch, rate, quality, auditory and visual cues, noise, and acceptability or effectiveness have been studied to determine their possible relationship to intelligibility. This chapter will present some aspects of speech and their relationship to the intelligibility of the alaryngeal speaker.

ARTICULATION

Articulatory scores have been found to be highly correlated with speech intelligibility scores among laryngeal-speaking subjects. Snidecor (1968) stated that "given reasonable loudness and quality, intelligibility or understanding is almost entirely a result of effective articulation" (p. 185). He emphasized the case for clear articulation for the esophageal speaker:

> First, the basic phonation of the cricopharyngeus can never be as clear as the voice from a normal larynx, so the vowels, semi-vowels, and diphthongs must be articulated with a reasonable amount of extra care. Second, the consonants, with special reference to the unvoiced (whispered) consonants, are formed in large part from bursal (mouth) and pharyngeal (throat) air, and the amount of air available is of course substantially less than that from a normal air stream. (p. 185)

Filter (1968) had judges rate recorded samples of connected esophageal speech on a five-point scale of effectiveness. Effectiveness was not operationally defined. Effectiveness ratings were compared with perceptual measures of intelligibility and articulation and with acoustical parameters of rate, fundamental frequency, and mean relative intensity. Results of the study showed that all measures were correlated with effectiveness ratings at the .5 level. Only articulation was significantly correlated with intelligibility. These results indicate that effectiveness ratings reflect a wide variety of perceptual and acoustical aspects of esophageal speech, whereas intelligibility as measured by a multiple-choice intelligibility test may be another way of saying "articulation."

Anderson (1950) investigated the relationship of several phenomena of esophageal speech to intelligibility. Judges determined the speakers' intelligibility by listening to them read multiple-choice intelligibility phrases. Intelligibility scores differed among the speakers. Elements of esophageal speech found to be related to high intelligibility were (1) intensity, (2) number of sounds produced correctly, and (3) duration of phonation.

Shames, Font, and Matthews (1963) measured intelligibility and articulation with the Harvard Sentence Intelligibility Test and the Harvard Phonetically Balanced Word Lists. Results indicated that articulation was significantly correlated with sentence intelligibility.

Anderson (1950), Di Carlo, Amster, and Herer (1955), and Hyman (1955) studied vowel and consonant production from most to least intelligible. According to Anderson and Hyman, the most to least intelligible sounds were vowels, affricates, laterals, glides, nasals, plosives, and fricatives. The study of DiCarlo and co-workers indicated the following order: glides, laterals, plosives, vowels, fricatives, and nasals. Except for the placement of vowels in DiCarlo and colleague's study, the three least intelligible types of sounds were the same in all three studies. Sound errors in the low intelligibility speakers were more numerous than in the high intelligibility speakers. Voiced-voiceless cognates were often confused.

The speech clinician should take into consideration the important relationship of accurate articulation to intelligibility of esophageal speech and the particular phonemes and features needing attention.

LOUDNESS

It is obvious that without adequate loudness, even for the laryngeal speaker, speech intelligibility is reduced or totally lacking. In studies by Hyman (1955) and McKinley (1960), good esophageal speakers were 6 to 7 decibels (dB) below the loudness level of laryngeal speakers in normal conversation. These speakers should have no difficulty in communicating in a one-to-one relationship with a distance of 6 to 9 feet separating the speaker and listener, or even a small group of listeners, in a quiet environment. When noise is introduced, however, it is another matter. The comparatively small volume of air available for speech and the very nature of the pseudoglottis make it difficult to speak above any sizable amount of noise. Several noise sources tend to mask the speech of the alaryngeal speaker and thus reduce the perception of his or her speech. Noise may occur from the klunking that accompanies the injection of air, from the stoma, from articulatory additions, and from the environment in which the speaker is talking.

Klunking.   Klunking is not an actual interference but more of a distraction to the listener during the injection phase and not during speech production. However, this distraction can be detrimental to oral communication.

Stoma Noise.   It is not a question of whether stoma air should be synchronized with speech attempts, since research indicates that most good esophageal speakers exhale through the tracheal stoma while speaking (Snidecor, 1968). It is a question of the amount of air escaping from the stoma. Some laryngectomees develop excessive stoma noise on exhalation that tends to mask the esophageal speech (Diedrich and Youngstrom, 1966; Shipp, 1967). Owing to the fact that this noise tends to be high frequency in nature, fricative sounds will suffer most. Because the fricatives and voiceless sounds are produced with air from the oral or pharyngeal cavities or both, they tend to be weak in intensity. A fairly loud stoma noise will mask out these weaker sounds.

Articulatory Additions.   Some laryngectomees substitute a clicking sound or another phoneme for the /h/ phoneme. These extraneous noises may distract or confuse the listener. It is better to omit the /h/ and let the listener's perception fill it in. Additional noises or vowels may be heard when the speaker produces consonant clusters. Instead of /blu/ (blue), the listener may hear /bəlu/; /kəlak/, instead of /klak/. The speech clinician should employ blending exercises to eliminate these extraneous noises. (See Chapter 9, The Intermediate Stage of Teaching Alaryngeal Speech.)

Environmental Noises.   Esophageal speakers, like laryngeal speakers, often find themselves in noisy environments. Noise and other interfering sounds emanating from an air conditioner, a phonograph recording, a television set, or an automobile or at a restaurant, a party, or a factory, and so on, will reduce the intelligibility of the laryngectomized speaker. Many of these noises are quite loud and of low frequency and will mask the low pitch levels of the speaker who, in addition, does not have the loudness capability to override the level of the noise.

Visual Cues for Laryngeal Speakers. The importance of visual cues in the intelligibility of normal speech in adverse listening conditions has been reported in the literature. Sumbly and Pollack (1954) reported on the visual contribution to the speech intelligibility of normal speakers. Oral speech intelligibility tests were conducted with and without supplementary visual observation of the speaker's facial movements. One speaker read, in varying order, test lists of 25 and 50 items constructed from 256 spondee words to listeners. The listeners were tested in groups of six. Half the listeners watched the speaker's facial movements as he spoke (auditory and visual presentation); the other half faced away from the speaker (auditory presentation only). Noise of uniform level per cycle for the frequency band of 20 to 10,000 hertz (Hz) mixed electronically with the speech signal was transmitted through tight-fitting headsets worn by each listener. The signal-to-noise ratio was varied by changing the speech level as the noise level was held constant. Results of the investigation indicated that the visual contribution to speech intelligibility of a laryngeal speaker was increased as the speech-to-noise ratio was decreased.

In an attempt to quantify further the visual contribution to speech intelligibility in a high-intensity environment of noise, Neely (1956) had laryngeal speakers read from a multiple-choice intelligibility test. The noise level from a random noise generator with an output of 100 dB introduced into the test room through loud speakers was ". . . sufficient enough to ensure that the only auditory speech cues heard by the listeners were those received through their earphones" (p. 1276). The speech signal received through the earphones was approximately 80 dB SPL. The results of the study were: (1) visual cues contributed approximately 20 per cent of the normal speaker's intelligibility, and (2) the effect on listener intelligibility scores within a 3 to 9 foot limit was not significant.

Visual Cues for Alaryngeal Speakers. In an initial study, Henry (1967) investigated the relationship of visual aspects of esophageal speech to esophageal speech intelligibility. Twelve male "good" esophageal speakers were recorded on videotape while reading a list of 27 words from a multiple-choice intelligibility test. Two conditions were used: audio and audiovisual. Thirty naive listeners marked a multiple-choice intelligibility check sheet as they watched and listened to the esophageal speakers on closed-circuit television. For the audio-only condition a similar group of 30 listeners determined the intelligibility of the speakers in a manner similar to that of the first group, as they heard but did not see the same 12 speakers reading the same test material. All the listeners were seated in a relatively quiet environment. The results indicated that the speakers were more intelligible by 16 per cent when listeners could see as well as hear them as opposed to just hearing them.

In a follow-up study, Neubert (1968) used the same prerecorded videotape employed by Henry. Two panels of 30 college students, considered to be naive listeners, judged the intelligibility of 12 prerecorded esophageal speakers under two conditions, audio and audiovisual. Both panels of listeners heard the speech stimuli in the presence of noise, concentrated in the speech frequencies extending from 500 to 2,000 Hz. The noise stimulus was presented at a zero signal-to-noise ratio. Results of the investigation revealed a 50 per cent increase in speaker intelligibility for the audiovisual condition.

In a pilot study, Neubert (1968), using the same experimental design except for changing the signal-to-noise ratio to -5 dB, found an 820 per cent increase in intelligibility when visual cues were introduced. The number of correct responses, however, was quite small even in the audiovisual condition.

Taking into account the importance of visual cues to the listener, Lauder (1969) recommends (1) standing close to the listener, (2) maintaining eye contact with the listener, (3) use of appropriate facial and body movements, and (4) use of pitch change and emphasis. Additions to this list for the laryngectomee should include the following: (1) avoid noisy environments when possible, (2) use amplification or an artificial larynx if necessary, and (3) open the mouth wider to take advantage of increased projection.

Loudness is an important aspect of intelligibility. Taking into account the upper age range of many of these patients, it is not unlikely that the spouse and friends may have hearing loss. Considering the limited loudness range (from 11 dB [Hyman, 1955] to 20 dB [Snidecor, 1968]), the alaryngeal speaker must take advantage of the aforementioned recommendations in order to communicate adequately with those in his environment.

PITCH

The average pitch level of esophageal speakers is between 60 and 90 Hz. The pitch range is between an octave and an octave and a half (compared to laryngeal speakers). Pitch level has not been found to be correlated with intelligibility for either alaryngeal or laryngeal speakers. Reduced vowel intelligibility among alaryngeal speakers has been attributed to the greater variability of their first and second vowel formants, resulting in the physical overlap of adjacent vowels (Snidecor, 1968).

Several studies have investigated the relationship of pitch to "acceptability" or "effectiveness." Martin, Noll, and Hoops (1969) used untrained listeners to rate samples of connected esophageal speech on a five-point scale of acceptability. The investigators compared most acceptable and least acceptable speakers on several acoustical parameters. Results indicated that the two groups of speakers did not differ significantly either on the basis of average fundamental frequency or on the number or extent of upward or downward inflections. The two groups did differ significantly on pitch standard deviations and on functional pitch ranges.

Shipp (1967) had untrained judges rate esophageal speech samples on a five-point scale of acceptability. The data indicated that the more closely alaryngeal speech approximates the characteristics of laryngeal speech (including pitch), the more highly it will be rated with regard to acceptability. Bennett and Weinberg (1973) reported that listeners rated vocal pitch as a frequent reason for perceiving esophageal speech as abnormal.

It thus appears that the higher the fundamental pitch and the more pitch variability the alaryngeal speaker can attain, the greater his acceptability to the listener.

QUALITY

The most frequent description of the quality of esophageal speech is "hoarse." In a study of broadband spectrograms, the striations of a normal speaker were regular in contrast to the irregular striations of an esophageal speaker (Snidecor, 1968). The formants of esophageal voice are resonant emphases of selected narrow bands of inharmonic broadband noise (Snidecor, 1968).

Bennett and Weinberg (1973) reported that the most frequent complaint of listeners in response to esophageal speech was that its quality did not sound normal. The aperiodic phonations or noise components of the voice are emphasized when the alaryngeal speaker increases loudness. Aside from the physical limitations attributed to the esophageal sphincter, a combination of optimal pitch and loudness along with optimal oral and pharyngeal muscle contraction may reduce the hoarseness and increase the acceptability of the voice.

RATE

The average esophageal speaker reads orally at an average rate of 120 words per minute as compared with the average rate of 160 words per minute of the laryngeal speaker (Snidecor, 1968). The relationship of rate to intelligibility and acceptibility has been studied by several investigators.

Hoops and Noll (1969) had untrained listeners rate samples of connected esophageal speech on a seven-point scale of effectiveness. The effectiveness ratings were correlated with several acoustical measures. Only rate was significantly correlated with effectiveness ratings (above .69).

Masters (1970) in a similar study found that acceptable speakers showed a higher rate of speech, more periodic phonation, and less aperiodic phonation. Intelligible speakers showed a higher rate of speech, more aperiodic phonation, and faster air intake.

Caution should be exercised concerning rate. Especially for the beginning esophageal speaker, rate often is stressed over articulation, phonation time, loudness, and control of respiratory air. More important for intelligible speech is satisfactory articulation, including voicing all sonant sounds, adequate loudness, and control of respiratory air.

SUMMARY

Intelligible alaryngeal speakers are those for whom the listener can correctly identify at least 90 per cent of their articulation, have adequate loudness for the situation, control respiratory air so that it does not mask their speech, and speak at a rate of approximately 120 words per minute. In addition, those who are judged most acceptable have pitch levels and inflection variations approximating those of the laryngeal speaker.

QUESTIONS

1. Contrast speech "effectiveness" with speech "intelligibility."
2. What is the most common type of consonant confusions produced by laryngectomized speakers?
3. What advice would you give to listeners who turn their head away from the speaker?
4. What effect might rate of speech have on intelligibility?

REFERENCES

Anderson, J. O. (1950). *A descriptive study of elements of esophageal speech.* Unpublished doctoral dissertation, Ohio State University, Columbus.

Bennett, S., and Weinberg, B. (1973). Acceptability ratings of normal, esophageal, and artificial larynx speech. *J. Speech Hearing Res., 16,* 608–615.

Di Carlo, L. M., Amster, W. W., and Herer, G. R. (1955). *Speech after laryngec-tomy.* Syracuse, NY: Syracuse University Press.

Diedrich, W. M., and Youngstrom, K. A. (1966). *Alaryngeal Speech.* Springfield, IL: Charles C Thomas.

Fieter, M. D. (1968). The relationship of acoustical parameters and perceptual ratings of esophageal speech. Paper presented at 44th Annual Convention of American Speech and Hearing Association, Denver, CO.

Henry, J. K. (1967). *An experimental study of the intelligibility of esophageal speakers with and without visual cues.* Unpublished master's thesis, Bowling Green State University, Bowling Green, OH.

Hoops, H. R., and Noll, J. D. (1969). Relationships of selected acoustical variables to judgments of esophageal speech. *J. Commun. Dis., 2,* 1–13.

Hyman, M. (1955). An experimental study of artificial larynx and esophageal speech. *J. Speech Hearing Dis., 20,* 291–299.

Lauder, E. (1969). A laryngectomee's viewpoint on the intelligibility of esopha-geal speech. *J. Speech Hearing Dis., 34,* 358–359.

Martin, D. E., Noll, J. D., and Hoops, H. R. (1969). A study of selected funda-mental frequency characteristics of esophageal speech. *J. Mich. Speech Hearing Assn., 5,* 59–74.

Masters, J. J. (1970). *Relationships among the acceptability, intelligibility, and acoustic measures of alaryngeal speech.* Unpublished doctoral dissertation, State University of New York at Buffalo.

McKinley, S. (1960). Correlates of stress patterns in esophageal speech. Unpub-lished master's thesis, Vanderbilt University.

Neely, K. K. (1956). Effects of visual factors on the intelligibility of speech. *J. Acoustical Soc. Amer., 28,* 1275–1277.

Neubert, L. A. (1968). *An experimental study of the intelligibility of esophageal speakers heard in the presence of speech noise with and without visual cues.* Unpublished master's thesis, Bowling Green State University, Bowling Green, OH.

Shames, G. H., Font, J., and Matthews, J. (1963). Factors related to speech proficiency of the laryngectomized. *J. Speech Hearing Dis., 28,* 273–287.

Shipp, T. (1967). Frequency, duration, and perceptual measures in relation to judgments of alaryngeal speech acceptability. *J. Speech Hearing Res., 10,* 417–427.

Snidecor, J. C. (1968). *Speech Rehabilitation of the Laryngectomized* (2nd ed.). Springfield, IL: Charles C Thomas.

Sumbly, W. H., and Pollack, I. (1954). Visual contribution to speech intelligibil-ity in noise. *J. Acoustical Soc. Amer., 26,* 212–215.

Chapter 12

Death and Dying

Paula A. Square

All professionals working with laryngectomized patients are eventually, if not frequently, confronted with the need to deal effectively with those who are terminally ill. Doctor Zwitman stated that, although the speech pathologist's role may be very limited, we should at least know how to approach the dying patient. In addition, we should be able to state clearly, as individuals and professionals, just what our roles are in such situations.

Much of the discussion of the group focused on the issue of the capabilities of the speech pathologist to provide counseling to the patient and his family during the dying period. The general consensus was that speech pathologists have neither the training nor the professional obligation to become involved in such activities. Social workers, psychologists, and clergymen are not only better trained but also are more professionally responsible in dealing with the circumstances that evolve for both the patient and family in the death process. Nevertheless, the speech pathologist may, either inadvertently or with great awareness and compliance, become more than superficially involved with the patient or his family during the final days of his life. Under such circumstances, just what is the speech pathologist's role? Does this role extend beyond the mere facilitation of communication? And how can we better prepare ourselves to deal effectively with the inevitability of the death of our patients?

Panel Participants: Helbert Damsté, Marshall Duguay, Melvin Hyman, Daniel Zwitman.

Doctor Damsté offered some concrete suggestions that seemed to help the audience better conceptualize their roles. He stated that it should be the primary goal of all members of the team working with the terminally ill to facilitate an anxiety-free attitude within the patient. In this vein, the speech pathologist as a communications specialist can play an invaluable role. In most instances, the information supplied by the physician is succinct and not fully understood by patients and their families. Doctor Damsté was of the opinion that speech pathologists can reduce the anxiety of their patients and families by expanding this information for the patient and answering questions. In addition, the speech pathologist may actively assist patients in the formulation of specific questions for their physicians. Although Doctor Damsté conceded that not all speech pathologists may possess the ability to provide these services, many do and should attempt to provide such services. By clarification of issues for the patient and reinforcement of independence, benefits resulting from aiding the patient in his communication with his physician, much of the anxiety of dying in an unfamiliar, sterile environment may be eliminated. Doctor Damsté cautioned, however, that at this stage the speech pathologist must shift from the role of "teacher," "protector," or "parent" and must communicate with the patient as adults communicate in daily life. This shift of role by the speech pathologist will, in addition, foster an attitude of independence within the patient. Lastly, Doctor Damsté emphasized that the speech pathologist must not abandon the dying patient with regard to treatment during this final days. Every attempt to provide technical means for communication should be made.

Doctor Duguay agreed with the position that, as speech pathologists, our role is defined to include only the territory of communication. He stated that we must be mainly concerned with our role to aid the patient with communication rather than counseling either the patient or the family. Speech pathologists are probably limited in both their abilities to understand and counsel the dying; it was implied by Doctor Duguay that although our intentions may be of the highest quality, we must not attempt to counsel the dying unless we have been specifically trained in this area.

Doctor Hyman opposed these positions. Because the speech pathologist has often become the one team member who has been involved with both the laryngectomee and his family over a period of time, he may be asked, either indirectly or directly, to counsel or at least listen throughout the dying process. Doctor Hyman conceded that the speech pathologist may not be the best person to counsel either the laryngectomee or his family; nevertheless, it is likely that some time throughout his career he will find himself in the position of being asked to assist. Doctor Hyman was of the opinion that the best contribution might be to counsel the family of the dying patient. By counseling the family the speech pathologist may help to influence in a positive manner the interactions between the patient and his family during the patient's final days.

Doctor Hyman cited the words of Kübler-Ross (1975) in describing five stages of dying: (1) denial and isolation, (2) agony, (3) bargaining with one's Creator, (4) depression, and (5) acceptance of death. It was suggested that the family should be familiarized with these stages so that they can fully realize, understand, and accept with the dying member the impending finality of life. By promoting an understanding of the death process among family members, the final stages of life for the patient may be less anxiety-ridden and more acceptable. In addition, Doctor Hyman suggested that families be encouraged to continue their normal activities of daily life. Furthermore, they must be encouraged to treat their dying family member as before; however, they must encourage discussions that will meet the emotional needs of the patient during the dying process.

Several audience members reacted to the apparent assumption that all dying patients and their families need counseling. Doctor Hyman stated that some patients and their families may not need help and that speech pathologists may rarely be called upon for assistance. Nevertheless, if we are called upon by a family during their hour of desperation, we should make ourselves available and be prepared to contribute positively to the situation. Doctor Zwitman suggested that we, as professionals, must definitely learn how to approach the dying patient; however, it must be a personal decision as to how much "counseling" we do. Paramount to the whole issue is the development of an appropriate approach to the dying patient and his family rather than the ability to counsel. Doctor Zwitman suggested that if we view ourselves more as visitors than as therapists, we may be more likely to approach the dying patient in a comforting and helpful way. By providing the patient with an opportunity to talk and to state his feelings, we may help facilitate a higher level of acceptance of death. Dying, however, is not a subject that everyone wants to hear about. If a dying patient is allowed the opportunity to express his feelings and emotions, a concurrent commitment to be available to the patient in his hours of need is made. Unless the speech pathologist is willing to accept the responsibilities of such a commitment, involvement beyond that of a communication specialist appears to be prohibited.

QUESTIONS

1. Who could be involved to help the dying patient meet his or her needs?
2. Damsté suggests what supportive role the speech pathologist might assume. Briefly, what is that role?
3. Hyman's suggestion of the role of the speech pathologist could be summarized how?

REFERENCES

Kübler-Ross, E. (1975). *Death, the final stage of growth.* Englewood Cliffs, NJ: Prentice-Hall.

Chapter 13

Advanced Stage of Teaching Alaryngeal Speech

Walter W. Amster

Surgical and surgical prosthetic voice restoration advances have significantly changed the usual treatment format for postlaryngectomy voice rehabilitation. The traditional three-stage hierarchy of instruction in alaryngeal speech—initial, intermediate, and advanced instruction—no longer may be operationally effective.

Increasing technological advances (Blom, Singer, and Hamaker, 1982; Panje, 1981; and Singer and Blom, 1980) allow for a readily available source of air directly from the trachea into the esophagus while minimizing the complications of aspiration. The major problem in the initial stage of voice rehabilitation after laryngectomy has been the development of voice through air-intake procedures (inhalation and injection). With the advent of endoscopic tracheoesophageal surgical techniques and the use of indwelling voice prostheses and tracheostoma valves, immediate air supply for voice production exists. Although these procedures are not being applied universally at the present time and there may be others forthcoming, their impact on voice restoration procedures is apparent. These advances portend an increasing luxury on the part of the clinician to focus on the refinement of voice quality and intelligibility in addition to more intensive concern with the pragmatic aspects of communication for the laryngectomized individual..

The term ''advanced stage'' has served to define that period of time used to increase length of utterance, eradicate inappropriate habit patterns, develop more precise articulation, increase loudness, and refine voice quality. Within the present context, this culminating stage should be expanded to incorporate increased attention to the social, psychological, and vocational issues relative to laryngectomy. Just as there is concern that premature interruption or cessation of treatment may account for a percentage of failure rate in the earlier stages of acquisition of alaryngeal speech, it may also be that treatment is ending prematurely in the later stages. In this regard, Cooper (1977) stated:

> The voice of the laryngectomized patient is sadly in need of the vocational rehabilitation efforts we afford the functional and organic voice disorders, such as nodes, polyps, contact ulcer, and myasthenia laryngis. Too often, the patient's demand for speech is abetted by those therapists who have little time, little patience, and little concern for a pleasing, well-modulated quality in the esophageal voice. The aphonia of the severe dysphonic whom we see is in no way thought to have terminated therapy because a moderate dysphonia now exists. Rather, we continue our vocal rehabilitation efforts until the voice is clear, easy, and well modulated. But, for the laryngectomized patient, we have no such goals at the outset of therapy. (p. 208)

Diedrich and Youngstrom (1966) and Amster and co-workers (1972) agreed that improvement in esophageal speech may continue for at least a 2 year period following surgery. The clinician's projections of what constitutes functional communication for the laryngectomized may be less than realistic. Perhaps speech pathologists need to ask the question posed by Greene (1980): "How good can speech become?" The answer to this question is a distinctly individual matter and not necessarily an arbitrary juncture determined by the clinician and based on traditional treatment patterns, available speech proficiency scales, and preconceived treatment expectations. What is presently labeled the advanced stage should in fact be considered the precursor to the final stage of therapy, which approaches the highest boundaries of communication proficiency achievable by the laryngectomized speaker.

Speech-language pathology must be judged, as are all sciences, by its commitment to research. It must further be judged by the application of research findings to the delivery of improved services. In this regard research data concerning the physiological processes involved in speech production after laryngectomy are available. This area has been the subject of considerable controversy for almost a century. The major issues have been (1) the site of the neo- or pseudoglottis, (2) the site of the air reservoir, and (3) the relationship between respiration and phonation relative to synchrony and asynchrony.

Information is also available concerning air intake; air volume; air flow; pharyngoesophageal muscle activity; pharyngeal and esophageal air pressures; movement patterns of the pharynx and pseudoglottis during phonation; and pitch, rate, and loudness factors.

With respect to the physiological processes involved in speech after laryngectomy, the application of our research knowledge to the speech-learning problems of the laryngectomized has been painfully slow. Although investigations have been relatively few in number, there does appear to be substantial agreement among individuals during research in this area. A sufficient body of knowledge is now accessible, the potential of which has not been fully realized.

Stetson (1937) stated:

> At first sight the efforts to make the ordinary expiratory movement for speech would seem to be just the wrong thing for esophageal speech. But intelligible speech cannot be made with an air supply exerting continuous pressure on the normal larynx or a substitute larynx, although that is a common assumption. The air pressure must fall to zero between the small groups of syllables and often between syllables, and a separate pressure pulse must be made for each syllable. The one available mechanism for syllable production is the normal respiratory mechanism. Records of excellent esophageal speech show that the subject breathes just as in normal speech. Syllable grouping, phrasing and accentuation are produced by just such expiratory movement as in normal speech. (p. 101)

Research indicates that the laryngectomized individual is capable of continuing his normal breathing and speech coordinations. It is most important that the treatment framework allow continuance of these coordinations, since it appears to be well established that the better or more intelligible laryngectomized speaker's breathing and speech coordinations approach closely those of the normal speaker.

Di Carlo, Amster, and Herer (1955), based on their research findings, stated:

> The laryngectomized speaker should learn to utilize the air supply to coincide with normal speech coordinations most efficiently, through proper intake and control of the air column for voice production. It would appear desirable to develop synchronous speech-breathing coordinations and voice control prior to the development of communicative speech. The process would emphasize "relaxation" techniques which would help develop more adequate control of the air column and voice production. During this process after adequate prolongation of voice has been established, the voice should be fused with articulatory movements into proper feet and accent patterns. (p. 166)

Cooper (1977) appears to be in agreement with this concept:

> This type of approach would help to establish rhythm and phrasing units prior to communicative speech. Under such conditions respiration and phonation would be closely associated and the entire process could be formulated within the framework of an adequate learning theory in which success with voice control would represent goal attainment and primary reinforcement. Primary and secondary reinforcement would facilitate

extension to the articulatory process. These results should culminate in a more satisfactory communication instruction situation whereby the mechanics of speech retraining would develop on a level of unawareness and would circumvent the acquisition of extraneous and unnecessary muscular behavior, which would provide distraction and enhance unintelligibility. (p. 166)

It would appear logical that if synchronous speech-breathing coordinations and voice control were established prior to the initiation of communicative speech, many of the problems now classified as requiring remediation in the advanced stages either would not be present or would be minimized. As Cooper (1977) stated:

> Often we neglect to afford a quality voice, or development of quality in voice for the laryngectomized. It is my view that quality is the essence and not a refinement that should be afforded the laryngectomized patient. Quality should be established at the beginning and not at the conclusion of therapy, since few patients are willing to develop a good voice once they have acquired some form of esophageal voice. We should not rush the patient into voice, but into an understanding of how to produce an efficient and well-modulated voice at the outset of therapy. It may slow down therapy at the beginning, and frustrate the patient not to speak earlier or faster, but the final result is much better and a goal to be sought, if excellence is sought. (p. 182)

The production of voice and the lengthening of voice with appropriate rhythm and phrasing prior to development of communicative speech should avoid a group of problems characteristic of inadequate speech after laryngectomy. Prevention of these problems would, of course, be desirable. If they do occur, they must be addressed as they occur in the early stages of voice development prior to their habituation. The extra efforts required at that time for the amelioration of these problems accomplish a twofold advantage: (1) the use of more socially acceptable speech and its psychosocial concomitants would further motivate the laryngectomee to employ this new communication tool to a greater and more rewarding extent, providing its own reinforcement, and (2) the time and effort required to change these habit patterns at a later stage once they are incorporated into the motor act becomes increasingly greater, and the accompanying frustration of the speaker may serve to deter communication and further improvement.

In general, the most prevalent problems presenting themselves during the development of speech and carried inappropriately into the advanced stage include grimacing, klunking, buccal speech, rapid rate, air escape from the tracheal stoma, inappropriate head and neck positions, neck and head jerking, inappropriate phrasing and rhythm resulting in word-by-word utterances, and inadequate articulation.

These habit patterns, which may interfere significantly with the intelligibility and social acceptability of speech, would appear to arise primarily from excessive tension and force brought about by premature attempts to communicate before the patient has developed voice that is controlled, fused synchronously with articulation, and molded into appropriate rhythm and phrasing patterns. The eradication or amelioration of these poor habit patterns if they are present in advanced stages would seem to be dependent on (1) relaxation and (2) reteaching and relearning of easy, effortless voice production.

Relaxation Considerations

Traditional treatment procedures employed in dealing with voice disorders include relaxation techniques to relieve excessive tension during voice production. Similar techniques may be used effectively with the laryngectomized who are employing a substitute vocal mechanism.

Moore (1971) provided an in-depth rationale for relaxation and presents procedures for its use in vocal rehabilitation. His discussion focused on relaxation of the voluntary muscles through techniques of "suggestion" and the progressive relaxation method developed by Jacobson (1934, 1938). Relaxation of the speech organs is assisted by relaxation of the large voluntary muscles in conjunction with Jacobson's procedures for "differential relaxation." The "chewing method" developed by Froeschels (1952) is also presented as a procedure for relieving excessive tension. The psychological status of the laryngectomee must be considered, since physiological relaxation alone would be unproductive.

Further discussion of relaxation techniques may be found in Van Riper and Irwin (1958) and Boone (1977). Application of relaxation methods for the laryngectomized has been described (Di Carlo, Amster, and Herer, 1955; Diedrich and Youngstrom, 1966; Greene, 1980; Snidecor, 1968). The potential for the application of biofeedback methodology as an aid to relaxation for the laryngectomee has not yet been fully realized.

Reteaching and Relearning Procedures

The second essential to the removal of inappropriate habits is the reteaching and relearning of easy, effortless voice production. The sequence should involve the stages of production, prolongation, and utilization of appropriate rhythm patterns without the urgency of communication.

Di Carlo (1971) delineated a hierarchy of teaching procedures that have their foundation in the work of Stetson's motor phonetics (1937, 1951) and the research of Di Carlo, Amster, and Herer (1955). These procedures are designed to assist the laryngectomee to perform voice production smoothly and economically with little effort of the articulatory organs while using the phrase movement coordinations of the non-laryngectomized speaker. The four stages of Di Carlo's hierarchy are designated (1) economy and ease of production, (2) prolongation of vocalization, (3) syllabication, and (4) rhythmic sequences.

In instructing the laryngectomee to produce voice easily and effortlessly, Di Carlo suggested use of "vowel coordinations" with the lips relaxed and an open conformation of the mouth with the tongue in rest position. The use of the vowel /ɑ/ facilitates production.

Upon achievement of adequate vowel production, prolongation of vocalization can then be pursued. Di Carlo (1971) stated:

> The purpose is to bring about rapid self-releasing and self-arresting coordinations of the vowel. The production of the vowel, the syllable nucleus, accompanies the syllable pulse and becomes audible via the voicing mechanism. Since a consonant does not precede or follow the vowel, the speech musculature must start or open (self-release) and stop or end (self-arrest) the syllable movement. A quick self-release and a quick self-arrest mean a longer time interval for the vocalization of the vowel. This work continues until the laryngectomee can prolong the vowel up to five or more seconds. (p. 47)

Once this goal has been achieved, the next stage is syllabication, which involves breaking up the prolonged vowel into separate syllables that are fused by accent patterns. The laryngectomee proceeds from two vowels with a spondaic accent pattern to three and four repetitions of the vowel with the same duration for each. All the other vowels and consonant-vowel-consonant combinations are presented as progress continues.

The final stage, rhythmic sequences, proceeds from short noun phrases and colloquial phrases to paragraphs, with specific attention to varied accent patterns and appropriate pause positions. The procedures of this reteaching-relearning hierarchy are, of course, equally applicable to the initial and intermediate stages of developing alaryngeal speech.

For those individuals who have received traditional laryngectomy, it may be necessary to evaluate the air-intake procedure used by the laryngectomee to determine whether it is the most appropriate method for the individual patient. If not, an eclectic approach to air-intake retraining techniques would then appear to be in order.

Berlin's (1963, 1965) list of early phonation skills as predictors of future communication adequacy is particularly useful in the early development of voice as well as in later stages. It includes the following: (1) phonation reliably on demand, (2) maintaining a short latency between inflation of the esophagus and vocalization, (3) maintaining an adequate duration of phonation, and (4) sustaining phonation during articulation.

If breathing and speech coordinations are appropriate and voice control is adequate, such voice would be fused synchronously with articulation, providing for acceptable rhythm and phrasing patterns. This should lessen the need for articulation retraining.

Cooper (1977) in discussing articulation stated:

> Articulation is a minor concern in the procurement of a new speaking voice. It is the voice itself which must be redefined and reaffirmed, not the articulation. Therefore, practice on mastery of the voice, of the basic sound until it is easily produced and controlled will enable the patient to use his normal articulatory process. (p. 213)

Some attention may be necessary with respect to the production of the nasal sounds /m/, /n/, and /ŋ/, as Greene (1980) and Diedrich and Youngstrom (1966) indicated. Diedrich and Youngstrom noted that a majority of laryngectomized subjects in their study "maintain velopharyngeal closure during the phonation of nasal sounds" (p. 35).

Di Carlo, Amster, and Herer (1955) found that nasals were the least intelligibly produced by laryngectomized speakers of the various sound categories.

The final stage of the treatment process should be that level at which we explore the question posed by Diedrich and Youngstrom (1966), Snidecor (1968), Cooper (1977), and Greene (1980) as to how effective the laryngectomized speaker can become. This question and possible methodologies for seeking answers have not yet been fully investigated.

The advanced stage should serve as a juncture for careful re-evaluation of the communicative status of the laryngectomized speaker. It is at this point that a realistic appraisal of future needs and the establishment of specific therapy goals are essential.

This extension of treatment into refinement aspects of communication is frequently not pursued. Speech pathologists, however, should be content until the farthest boundaries that the laryngectomized individual is capable of have been approached. Evaluation models by Wepman, MacGahan, Rickard, and Shelton (1953), Hyman (1953), Berlin (1963), and Creech (1966) should be used during this re-evaluation process and should be extended to include factors of pitch, rate, loudness, and quality as they function in more demanding communication situations.

Psychosocial Considerations

The adjustment process of the laryngectomized is of primary importance not only at the pre- and postoperative stages but also in the more advanced stages. Although a sense of accomplishment in having provided functional communication for the patient may be felt, it does not necessarily follow that the patient is equally satisfied. He realizes now that his voice, although serviceable, does not meet the esthetic standards met by his presurgical voice and that difficulties arise when he attempts to use it in acoustically poor environmental settings. Cooper (1977) discussed this issue:

> The vocal image is one of those keys that unlock the patient's desire, will, and ability to speak again effectively. The vocal image extensively prevails among laryngectomized patients. The laryngectomized patient is concerned with how he will sound. He compares the new sound or voice to the presurgical voice, judging the new sound for its ease, flexibility, durability, and aesthetic listenability. He is also concerned with how other people will accept the new sound. (p. 209)

Gardner (1966) spoke about the special problems of women in this regard. His subjects reported concern over the low pitch of the esophageal voice, which frequently caused them to be mistaken for men. Another problem the laryngectomee must confront is the generalization by people in the environment of the impairment to the total personality, a phenomenon not uncommon to other disfiguring or impairing diseases. This delusion prevails especially among men who now perceive their role as less than manly, which may eventually lead to impotence and unsatisfactory sex relationships. In discussion of psychological reactions to carcinoma of the larynx, Locke (1966) suggested that "surgical removal of the larynx is viewed by many patients as a form of castration."

Natvig (1983) found that premorbid adjustment patterns and personality traits were more important than social or situational factors in predicting success in esophageal speech acquisition.

For the preretirement age laryngectomee this period is one of decision with regard to vocational plans. The previous employment may no longer be possible in view of medical contraindications or communication demands.

Vocational counseling would seem to be imperative in conjunction with a speech rehabilitation program that would be specifically designed to meet the needs of the laryngectomee. Goldberg (1975), in evaluating vocational and social adjustment after laryngectomy, found that motivation, realism, rehabilitation outlook, and previous vocational plans were some of the factors that predicted postlaryngectomy vocational and social adjustment.

Richardson (1983) conducted in-depth interviews with 60 laryngectomized patients concerning employment, speech, and social functioning. Failure to work after surgery appeared to be initiated by the patient and was not related to high-level achievement in other areas.

The implications for developing positive attitudes through appropriate counseling are apparent. Through the provision of such services the vocational alternatives of the laryngectomee are broadened, and he may not be faced with forced retirement as his only option.

For the retired individual, restricted communication may mean restricted socialization and concomitant withdrawal and unproductivity. For this individual, as well, the exploration of communication throughout the rehabilitation process is urgent.

Aspects of Intelligibility and Social Acceptability

Intelligibility and social acceptability of speech may determine to a considerable extent whether the laryngectomee will make adequate postoperative psychosocial adjustment. As Di Carlo (1971) indicated, "The ultimate goal of speech therapy is to enable the laryngectomized individual to communicate orally with others" (pp. 50–51). The quality of that speech will determine the extent to which it is used as a successful and self-reinforcing communication tool. It is the mission of the advanced stage of the speech rehabilitation program to ensure that the quality of speech is optimal.

Diedrich and Youngstrom (1966), in attempting to answer the question of how effective the laryngectomized speaker can be, listed a number of criteria drawn from the available literature: (1) reliable phonation upon demand, (2) air intake at the speed of approximately ½ second, (3) short latency (about ⅕ second) between air intake and phonation, (4) four to nine syllables or vowel duration of 2 to 3 seconds per air intake, (5) rate in words per minute averaging 85 to 129, (6) phrase patterns that approximate the normal, (7) pitch level of 52 to 82 Hz with expectation of normal range, (8) intensity average of 6 to 7 dB below normal, (9) rhythm more normal and fewer nonrhythmic patterns, and (10) good intelligibility with 90 per cent of all consonant and vowel sounds produced correctly.

The characteristics of the superior esophageal speaker have been investigated extensively by Snidecor (1968) and his colleagues, who evaluated factors of pitch, rate, loudness, and quality. In-depth investigations of articulation factors are provided by Anderson (1950), Hyman (1953), and Di Carlo, Amster, and Herer (1955). In addition, the latter study explored the parameters of rhythm and phrasing patterns of high- and low-intelligibility laryngectomized speakers.

Shipp (1967), in reporting on judgments of alaryngeal speech acceptability, indicated that above-average acceptability ratings related to a higher mean fundamental frequency, a more rapid utterance of the test sentence, a greater proportion of periodic phonation, and a lesser proportion of both aperiodic phonation and silence. Accompanying these was the ability to inhibit respiration noise.

Shipp (1967) further indicated that

> these data appear to verify the notion that the more an alaryngeal speaker approximates the characteristics of the normal speaker, the more highly he is rated on acceptability. This judging characteristic applies even to the voice fundamental frequency as was noted before. The speaker who is able to complete an utterance in a short time does so by increasing the percentage of the utterance spent in periodic phonation with a reduction in the percentage of silence. Furthermore, the combination of these two factors appears to coexist with the speaker's ability to inhibit the respiratory noise from the tracheostoma. (p. 424)

Rate and phrasing and their relationship to speech proficiency were investigated by Hoops and Guzek (1974). Their results indicate that of 13 rate and phrasing factors considered, syllable per sentence per minute rate and interphrase pause time are predictive of judged esophageal speech proficiency.

Snidecor (1968) reported a maximal level of 85 dB for his superior esophageal speaker as compared with the 95 dB level for a normal speaker; the comparison was based on both speakers' sustaining the vowel /ɑ/. The normal speaker averaged smooth intensity changes from low to high and high to low from 35 to 45 dB. The esophageal speaker averaged only 20 dB for both the upward and downward intensity sweep. Snidecor noted that the potential intensity levels and variability are considerably less for the esophageal speaker than for the normal speaker. He continued, however, as follows:

> One must hasten to add that when continuous propositional speech is under consideration, sound pressure levels and variability are essentially the same for each speaker. In fifty-one words of propositional speech, on the basis of measuring peak values, the esophageal speaker has a mean value of 77 dB, the normal speaker of 79 dB. The method of peak measurement may slightly exaggerate values in continuous speech, but the relative values are stable and dependable. (p. 154)

Nichols (1968) suggested various procedures for esophageal voices that are deficient in loudness. These procedures involve use of the artificial larynx and a small amplifier system. He also discussed various physiological reasons for the differences in loudness levels between the laryngeal and alaryngeal speaker. In addition, he noted that the apparent loudness of voice is a function of the speaker's intelligibility. More highly intelligible voices does not require as much loudness for listener acceptability. Thus, improvement in intelligibility should also have an effect on apparent loudness.

Snidecor (1968) also discussed the factor of quality or wave-form information:

> Spectrographic analysis of esophageal voice revealed that although the voice contains a noise component up to a high-frequency region (6000 Hz), the harmonic components are still clear and easily distinguishable from each other. When the voice is high in pitch, the noise component is relatively great, and the pitch is unstable as noted in irregular, "vertical striations" of a wide-band sonogram. Such a high-pitched voice is usually produced with great strain. A narrow-band sonogram shows the general tendency that an increase in intensity is accompanied by a relative accentuation of high-frequency components. (p. 155)

Nichols (1968) and Shipp (1967) stressed the deleterious effect of respiratory noise on voice quality. Nichols also suggested that improvement in voice quality as well as intensity involves production of vowels that are "open, intelligible, clearly differentiated, and controlled" (p. 127). Such productions should contribute to the lessening of the harsh, hoarse voice characteristic of the esophageal speaker.

Swisher (1980), investigating oral pressure, vowel duration, and acceptability ratings of esophageal speakers using aerodynamic, acoustic, and perceptual measurements, indicated that esophageal speakers show significantly higher oral pressure and longer vowel duration when compared with laryngeal speakers. Esophageal speakers whose oral pressure and vowel duration are most like those of laryngeal speakers are judged to be the most acceptable speakers.

The acoustic characteristics of intended syllabic stress in excellent esophageal speakers were examined by McHenry, Reich, and Minifie (1982), who found that excellent esophageal speakers are capable of producing some correlates of primary syllabic stress in a fashion remarkably similar to but somewhat less consistent than normal speakers.

Weinberg and his associates in a series of related investigations (Angermeier and Weinberg, 1981; Christensen and Weinberg, 1981; Gandour and Weinberg, 1983; Gandour, Weinberg, and Garzione, 1983; Scarpino and Weinberg, 1981; Weinberg, Horii, Blom, and Singer, 1982; Weinberg, Horii, and Smith, 1980) have contributed significantly to the identification of specific aspects of linguistic, perceptual, and production factors involved in esophageal and tracheoesophageal speech. The application of psychoacoustical measures used in these studies has provided definitive direction for future research in alaryngeal speech.

Implications of Surgical-Prosthetic Approaches

Since the advent of tracheoesophageal puncture (TEP) surgery (Singer and Blom, 1980), investigations have revealed that the availability of a pulmonary air supply enhances rapid development of postlaryngectomy speech. Robbins, Fisher, Blom, and Singer (1984) compared and quantified the acoustic characteristics of 15 subjects who had undergone the TEP method of postlaryngectomy vocal rehabilitation with 15 esophageal speakers and 15 laryngeal speakers. Measures of frequency and duration for the three speaker groups revealed the superiority of tracheoesophageal speech with respect to factors of intensity, frequency, and rate. They noted that tracheoesophageal speech is more similar to normal speech than is esophageal speech in their investigation.

Wood, Rusnov, Tucker, and Levine (1981) indicated that 92 per cent of the 30 patients who received TEP were able to produce significantly better voice when compared with their preoperative postlaryngectomy voice.

Donegan, Gluckman, and Singh (1981) agreed that TEP with use of the Blom-Singer prosthesis is a major development in neoglottic surgical reconstruction. However, they reported some difficulties experienced by their subjects, including inability to manage the prosthesis in the home, anatomical problems, and inability to produce fluent speech. They further stated that although TEP is currently the most effective technique for voice restoration, it may not be applicable for all laryngectomized patients. They underscored the need for careful patient selection.

Although for the most part the preponderance of research supports TEP as the method of choice in postlaryngectomy voice rehabilitation, there are significant considerations that may affect the advanced stage of treatment. Perhaps the greatest inherent danger to the patient lies in too early dismissal from treatment, providing opportunities for problems to emerge that may eventually delimit effective use of the prosthetic device. A careful, long-range program of monitoring patients with respect to possible complications in the use and care of the prosthesis and tracheostoma breathing valve is essential. The readily available pulmonary air supply and the subsequent esophageal voice production does not ensure fluent speech or communication adequacy. Factors of quality of voice, pitch, rate, loudness, and articulation should constitute the refinement process provided in the advanced stage for tracheoesophageal speakers, esophageal speakers, and those using artificial larynxes.

Conclusions

The research information available regarding voice factors and speech after laryngectomy indicates that the excellent or superior esophageal speaker approaches the norm for the laryngeal speaker. Where there is disparity, various modifications and voluntary manipulations of intake, voice control, and voice-articulation fusion processes permit closer approximation to these norms.

In this vein, the research evidence presents a mandate to clinicians to involve the laryngectomized speaker in a well-formulated refinement process incorporating careful evaluation of the factors of pitch, rate, loudness, quality, phrasing, rhythm, and articulation. Treatment models for this process are available, since these are the factors commonly explored and remediated in working with individuals with intact larynges but presenting a variety of voice disorders. Van Riper and Irwin (1958), Fairbanks (1960), Moore (1971), Greene (1980), Cooper (1977), Fox and Blechman (1975), Boone (1977), Shanks and Duguay (1984), and Stemple (1984) provide excellent sources for therapy rationale and procedures.

The advanced stage of treatment for the laryngectomized speaker should be a period of carefully controlled experimentation, goal establishment, and determination of the outer limits of communication efficiency. It should be stressed that the development of these goals should be based on the best available clinical and research evidence. The supportive benefits of group membership at this stage as well as during the earlier stages are well recognized. The tailoring of the clinical model should include situations that approximate the social and vocational activities in which the individual may be involved once the rehabilitation period is completed. The conclusion of the treatment process should be based on decisions made by the patient and the clinician when both feel that optimal communication has been achieved.

QUESTIONS

1. Amster recommends placing early emphasis on respiratory patterns and on voice quality, reserving focus of attention on issues of refined vocal skills later in therapy. What do you believe regarding these alternatives and what is the rationale for your belief?
2. DiCarlo (1955, 1971) is cited as advocating extending duration of phonation before a laryngectomee is moved into syllable, word, or phrase production. What disadvantages do you see in following this advice?
3. Does your clinical experience agree or disagree with Diedrich and Youngstrom (1966), who indicate that nasal sounds are often produced inadequately by laryngectomized speakers?
4. What might account for the development of keeping the velopharyngeal port closed during /m/, /n/, and /ŋ/? (The answer is not in the chapter.)
5. What vocal factors should receive consideration in an advanced stage of training?

6. If you were to counsel your clients on vocational aspects of life, what would you be attempting to do and how would you accomplish this?
7. What factors contribute to "quality speech" for the laryngectomized?
8. Describe the data you think must have led Hoops and Guzek (1974) to pose a relationship between interphrase pause time and speaker proficiency?
9. How well should a client speak before terminating speech instruction?

REFERENCES

Amster, W. W., Love, R. J., Menzel, O. J., Sandler, J., Sculthorpe, W. B., and Gross, F. (1972). Psychosocial factors and speech after laryngectomy. *J. Commun. Dis., 5,* 1–18.

Anderson, J. O. (1950). *A descriptive study of elements of esophageal speech.* Unpublished doctoral dissertation, Ohio State University, Columbus, OH.

Angermeier, C. B., and Weinberg, B. (1981). Some aspects of fundamental frequency control by esophageal speakers. *J. Speech Hear. Res., 24,* 85–91.

Berlin, C. I. (1963). Clinical measurement of esophageal speech: I. Methodology and curves of skill acquisition. *J. Speech Hear. Dis., 28,* 42–51.

Berlin, C. I. (1965). Clinical measurement of esophageal speech: III. Performance of non-biased groups. *J. Speech Hear. Dis., 30,* 174–183.

Blom, E. D., Singer, M. I., and Hamaker, R. C. (1982). Tracheostoma valve for post-laryngectomy voice rehabilitation. *Ann. Otol. Rhinol. Laryngol., 91,* 576–578.

Boone, D. R. (1977). *The voice and voice therapy* (2nd ed.). Englewood Cliffs, NJ: Prentice-Hall.

Christensen, J. M., and Weinberg, B. (1981). Fricative duration in esophageal speech. *J. Commun. Dis., 14,* 127–131.

Cooper, M. (1977). *Modern techniques of vocal rehabilitation.* Springfield, IL: Charles C Thomas.

Creech, H. B. (1966). Evaluating esophageal speech. *J. Speech Hear. Assoc., 7,* 13–19.

Di Carlo, L. M. (1971). Advanced stage of teaching. In S. Rigrodsky and J. Lerman (Eds.), *Therapy for the laryngectomized patient.* New York: Teachers College Press.

Di Carlo, L. M., Amster, W. W., and Herer, G. R. (1955). *Speech after laryngectomy.* Syracuse: Syracuse University Press.

Diedrich, W. M., and Youngstrom, K. A. (1966). *Alaryngeal speech.* Springfield, IL: Charles C Thomas.

Donegan, J. O., Gluckman, J. L., and Singh, J. (1981). Limitations of the Blom-Singer technique for voice restoration. *Ann. Otol. Rhinol. Laryngol., 90,* 495–497.

Fairbanks, G. (1960). *Voice and Articulation Drillbook* (2nd ed.). New York: Harper and Brothers.

Fox, D. R., and Blechman, M. (1975). *Clinical management of voice disorders.* Lincoln, NE: Cliff Notes.

Froeschels, E. (1952). Chewing method as therapy. *Arch. Otolaryngol., 56,* 427–434.

Gandour, J., Weinberg, B., and Garzione, B. (1983). Perception of lexical stress in alaryngeal speech. *J. Speech Hear. Res., 26,* 418–424.

Gandour, J., and Weinberg, B. (1983). Perception of intonational contrasts in alaryngeal speech. *J. Speech Hear. Res., 26,* 142–148.

Gardner, W. H. (1966). Adjustment problems of laryngectomized women. *Arch. Otolaryngol., 83,* 31–42.

Goldberg, R. L. (1975). Vocational and social adjustment after laryntectomy. *Scand. J. Rehab. Med., 7,* 1–8.

Greene, M. C. L. (1980). *The voice and its disorders* (4th ed.). Philadelphia: Lippincott.

Hoops, H. R., and Guzek, T. J. (1974). The relationship of rate and phrasing to esophageal speech proficiency. *Arch. Otolaryngol., 100,* 190–193.

Hyman, M. (1953). *An experimental study of the relative pressure, duration, intelligibility, and aesthetic aspects of the speech of artificial larynx, esophageal and normal speakers.* Unpublished doctoral dissertation. Ohio State University, Columbus, OH.

Hyman, M. (1971). Intermediate stage of teaching alaryngeal speech. In S. Rigrodsky and J. Lerman (Eds.), *Therapy for the laryngectomized patient.* New York: Teachers College Press.

Jacobson, E. (1934). *You must relax.* New York: McGraw-Hill.

Jacobson, E. (1938). *Progressive relaxation.* Chicago: University of Chicago Press.

Locke, B. (1966). Psychology of the laryngectomee. *Milit. Med., 131,* 539–599.

McHenry, M., Reich, A., and Minifie, F. (1982). Acoustical characteristics of intended syllabic stress in excellent esophageal speakers. *J. Speech Hear. Res., 25,* 564–573.

Moore, P. G. (1971). *Organic voice disorders.* Englewood Cliffs, NJ: Prentice-Hall.

Natvig, K. (1983). Laryngectomees in Norway. Study No. 3: Pre- and postoperative factors of significance to esophageal speech acquisition. *J. Otolaryngol., 12,* 332–333.

Nichols, A. C. (1968). Loudness and quality in esophageal speech and the artificial larynx. In J. C. Snidecor (Ed.), *Speech rehabilitation of the laryngectomized.* Springfield, IL: Charles C Thomas.

Panje, W. (1981). The production of voice following total laryngectomy. The Voice Button. *Ann. Otol., Rhinol. Laryngol., 90,* 116–120.

Richardson, J. L. (1983). Vocational adjustments after total laryngectomy. *Arch. Phys. Med. Rehab., 64,* 172–175.

Robbins, J., Fisher, H. B., Blom, E. D., and Singer, M. I. (1984). A comparative acoustic study of normal, esophageal, and tracheoesophageal speech production. *J. Speech Hear. Dis., 49,* 202–210.

Scarpino, J., and Weinberg, B. (1981). Junctural contrasts in esophageal and normal speech. *J. Speech Hear. Res., 24,* 120–126.

Shanks, J. C., and Duguay, M. (1984). Voice remediation and the teaching of alaryngeal speech. In S. Dickson (Ed.), *Communication disorders: Remedial principles and practices* (2nd ed.). Glenview, IL: Scott Foresman.

Shipp, T. (1967). Frequency, duration, and perceptual measures in relation to judgments of alaryngeal speech and acceptability. *J. Speech Hear. Res., 10,* 412–427.

Singer, M. I., and Blom, E. D. (1980). An endoscopic technique for restoration of voice after laryngectomy. *Ann. Otol. Rhinol. Laryngol., 89,* 529–533.

Snidecor, J. C. (1968). *Speech rehabilitation of the laryngectomized* (2nd ed.). Springfield, IL: Charles C Thomas.

Stemple, J. C. (1984). *Clinical voice pathology: Theory and management.* Columbus, OH: Charles E. Merrill.

Stetson, R. H. (1951). *Motor phonetics: A study of speech movement in action.* Amsterdam: North-Holland Publishing.

Stetson, R. H. (1937). Oesophageal speech: Method of instruction after laryngectomy. *Arch. Neerl. de Phon. Exp., 13,* 95–110.

Swisher, W. E. (1980). Oral pressures, vowel durations, and acceptability ratings of esophageal speakers. *J. Commun. Dis., 13,* 171–181.

Van Riper, C., and Irwin, J. V. (1958). *Voice and Articulation.* Englewood Cliffs, NJ: Prentice-Hall.

Weinberg, B., Horii, Y., Blom, E. D., and Singer, M. I. (1982). Airway resistance during esophageal phonation. *J. Speech Hear. Dis., 47,* 194–199.

Weinberg, B., Horii, Y., and Smith, B. E. (1980). Long-time spectral and intensity characteristics of esophageal speech. *J. Acoust. Soc. Amer., 67,* 1781–1784.

Wepman, J. M., MacGahan, J. A., Rickard, J. C., and Shelton, N. W. (1953). The objective measurement of progressive esophageal speech development. *J. Speech Hear. Dis., 18,* 247–251.

Wood, B. G., Rusnov, M. G., Tucker, H. M., and Levine, H. L. (1981). Tracheoesophageal puncture for alaryngeal voice restoration. *Ann. Otol. Rhinol. Laryngol., 90,* 492–494.

Chapter **14**

Tracheoesophageal Fistulization for Voice Restoration: Presurgical Considerations and Trouble-Shooting Procedures

Zilpha T. Bosone

The person who has a laryngectomy loses one component of the act of talking: the ability to generate sound. One way to generate sound is with an artificial larynx; another is with the pharyngoesophageal (PE) segment or junction. Until recently, the only way to activate the PE segment was to insufflate the esophagus via the mouth, the nose, or both (''air charging''). The esophagus holds approximately 80 cubic centimeters (cc) of air, on which the average esophageal speaker can produce four to six syllables before having to insufflate again.

Voice restoration for laryngectomees was revolutionized in 1979 when Dr. Mark Singer, an otolaryngologist, and Dr. Eric Blom, a speech pathologist, reported a new surgical procedure described as a ''tracheoesophageal puncture'' (Singer and Blom, 1979). The purpose is to provide lung air for esophageal speech. A small fistula is created in the wall between the trachea and the esophagus. The opening is maintained by a silicone prosthesis that acts as a one-way valve. When the stoma is occluded, the prosthesis allows lung air to pass into the esophagus while preventing food and liquid from entering the trachea. The puncture can be reversed by removing the prosthesis.

There are many advantages in having over 2,000 cc of lung air available for esophageal speech: (1) a spontaneous expansion of the loudness range, (2) an increase in pitch variation, and (3) an extension of the duration of sound (Robbins, Fisher, Blom and Singer, 1984; Singer, 1983). Clinical experience also suggests that improvement in sound quality is attained earlier than with regular esophageal speech. In addition, tracheoesophageal fistulization (TEF) speech is compatible with other forms of alaryngeal speech; that is, it does not prevent the alternate use of regular esophageal speech or an artificial larynx.

A variety of surgical procedures, adaptations, and prosthetic devices have evolved around TEF since the Singer-Blom surgery and Blom-Singer prosthesis of 1979. Some of these are described by Singer and Blom (1981), Singer, Blom, and Hamaker (1981, 1983), Panje (1981), Spofford, Jafek, and Barcz (1984), Henley-Cohn (1981), Shapiro and Ramanathan (1982), and Annyas, Nijdam, Escajadillo, Mahieu, and Leever (1984). Changes can be expected to continue. Therefore, this section will present the topic from a generic approach that extends across all surgical procedures and prostheses. After a brief review of the salient presurgical considerations, the emphasis will be on trouble-shooting procedures. It is incumbent on the reader to keep abreast of the literature and to be scholarly and open to new developments.

PATIENT SELECTION

Selection of a candidate who will benefit from TEF surgery requires consideration of certain mental and physical prerequisites.

Mental Requirements

The candidates must want the surgery. They should not be motivated solely by pressure from professionals, family, peers, or other outside influences. Patients frequently desire TEF surgery because they are dissatisfied with their present methods or method of communication or because they wish to add to their communication repertoire. The good esophageal speaker falls into the last category. Unfortunately, there are references in the literature that suggest that suitable candidates are those who have failed to learn good esophageal speech (Donegan, Gluckman, and Singh, 1981; Knapp and Panje, 1982; Lyons, 1983; and Mitchell, Kirkland, and Morrison, 1981), implying that good esophageal speakers might not be considered. However, the advantages are so impressive that even the most proficient esophageal speaker has something to gain from a TEF procedure.

Candidates should have good mentation. They should be able to follow instructions for the care and use of the prosthesis. They should be reliable in making and keeping appointments, and they should be able to accept responsibility for maintaining good hygiene.

Physical Requirements

One of the most important requirements for a successful TEF procedure is a functioning sound generator. The PE segment can be evaluated by an esophageal air insufflation test described by Singer and Blom (1980) and Taub (1981). This test was originally performed by van den Berg, and reported by Damsté, van den Berg, and Moolenaar-Bijl (1956) and Damsté (1958). The purpose of this test is to estimate whether sound can be produced without remedial procedures. A small catheter, 12 or 14 Fr, is inserted transnasally into the upper esophagus. The clinician blows air into the catheter in an attempt to elicit esophageal sound. Ease of blowing and the quality and duration of sound are subjectively evaluated. It is not necessary to administer this test to a good esophageal speaker, as it can be assumed that the PE segment is able to produce satisfactory sound. Another method used to evaluate the PE segment is radiography (Vincent, Robbins, Walsh, and Vaughn, 1984). The patient swallows contrast material, and the structures and functioning of oral, pharyngeal, and esophageal areas are observed for abnormalities during resting, swallowing, and if possible, attempts at phonation.

There should be no evidence of cancer recurrence, and the trachea must be in good condition, with no tracheitis or ulceration. The required stoma size may vary with the procedure but should not be smaller in diameter than a #8 laryngectomy tube. If necessary, a stoma revision can be done at the time of the fistulization (Panje, VanDemark, and McCabe, 1981).

Alcohol abuse can be a major deterrent to efficient use and responsible care of a TEF (Donegan, Gluckman, and Singh, 1981; Johns and Cantrell, 1981; Schuller, Jarrow, Kelly, and Miglets, 1983). In a 1983 study of 20 patients who had Singer-Blom procedures, alcohol abuse and stoma size (too small or too large) had the highest correlations with lack of success in developing speech (Schuller et al., 1983).

Manual dexterity and good vision are necessary because the prosthesis is small and the entrance to the fistula is inside the stoma. If the patient does not possess these attributes, the procedure may still be done if there is a family member willing to accept the responsibility for cleaning and inserting the prosthesis.

Pulmonary function must be adequate to support sound generation. Panje (1981) has stated that "patients with excessive lung disease who cannot generate moderate stomal pressure against the surgeon's thumb, asthmatics, or patients who cough excessively with stomal capping do not appear to be candidates" (p. 119) for TEF procedures.

Factors not considered contraindications to TEF procedures include diabetes, neck dissection, and radiation therapy.

TIMING

Initially, TEFs were done only as secondary procedures after complete recovery from the most recent surgery (laryngectomy, stoma revision, neck dissection, and so on) or radiation treatment. Panje and colleagues (1981) suggested waiting as long as 3 to 6 months after radiation treatments. Now, however, TEFs are also being performed as part of the primary laryngectomy, (Annyas et al. 1984; Maves and Lingeman, 1982; Panje, 1981; Singer, Blom, and Hamaker, 1983).

THE ROLE OF THE SPEECH PATHOLOGIST

The literature emphasizes the need for the speech pathologist and surgeon to work together with TEF patients. The speech pathologist should be involved in the presurgery testing to determine candidacy. The speech pathologist should also be able to fit the prosthesis and to train the patient to insert, clean, and care for the prosthesis and fistula. The patient will require varying amounts of instruction in order to achieve maximal benefits from the surgery. Treatment should cover stomal occlusion, production of sound, improvement of sound quality, and speech intelligibility. Workshops, seminars, and courses are available for the speech pathologist interested in acquiring clinical skills for treating TEF patients and learning of new developments.

Tracheoesophageal fistulization procedures are not yet common. Therefore, if there is trouble with the fistula or the prosthesis after the patient has been discharged, the patient is likely to find that many physicians, speech pathologists, and hospital personnel are unfamiliar with the diagnosis and treatment of postfistulization problems. For this reason, an important function of the speech pathologist is to instruct each patient in trouble-shooting procedures. Such information allows the patient either to resolve the problem or to know when the help of the physician or speech pathologist is needed.

TROUBLE-SHOOTING

Trouble-shooting involves two processes: (1) identifying the cause of the problem and (2) taking steps toward remedying it. The remainder of this section will describe symptoms, indicate causes, and offer suggestions for resolving typical complaints that may arise after surgery. Because the information is of practical value, it is presented in an informal manner in order to facilitate its application.

Poor or No Sound

These symptoms could be caused by problems with the fistula, the prosthesis, or the sound generator.

Fistula

The fistula may be closed. The fistula closes in a direction from the esophagus to the trachea, that is, from back to front. The fistula is closed when:

1. No sound can be produced either with the prosthesis in place or removed (open fistula).
2. No saliva or other liquids pass through the open fistula (prosthesis removed) on swallowing. To check for leaking on swallowing, the observer shines a light on the open fistula site. The patient is asked to swallow saliva. If there is no leakage, the patient is asked to take a small sip of water and hold it in the mouth until asked to swallow. The observer waits a few seconds after the swallow for the water to clear the esophageal end of the fistula. If there is still no leakage, the amount of liquid swallowed is gradually increased. If fluids do not leak through the fistula, it is a reasonable assumption that at least the esophageal end of the track has closed. Occasionally a patient will be encountered whose fistula structure allows swallowing without leaking, even though the fistula is open. This is rare.
3. The prosthesis protrudes from the fistula and cannot be pushed back into place, nor can a catheter be inserted through the fistula into the esophagus.

Causes

1. Wearing a prosthesis that is too short and does not extend into the esophagus.
2. Unnoticed partial or total extrusion of the prosthesis, especially during the night or with coughing.
3. Failure to insert the prosthesis into the fistula. Occasionally when the prosthesis is inserted, it slips across the fistula entrance and down the back wall of the trachea. The patient may proceed with the taping or whatever procedures are necessary for insertion and not notice what has happened. When the stoma is occluded, the person will be able to make sound, shunting air through the open fistula; that is, until the fistula closes. There will probably be leaking into the trachea on swallowing, but not everyone experiences this. The lesson here is that the patient must check for correct placement of the prosthesis after insertion.

4. Misalignment of the fistula. This occurrence is rare. It probably happens during the fistulization surgery. The tissues forming the wall between the esophagus and the trachea are capable of sliding against each other. When the fistula is created, the tissues may slip out of alignment against pressure from the needle, scalpel, or other instrument used to make the opening. At some point after surgery, these tissues may resume their normal alignment. Since the entrance of the fistula will no longer be in a line with the exit, the effect is closure. Neither the prosthesis nor a catheter will be able to be inserted into the esophagus. In fact, there is a danger of entering the fascia between the tissues of the wall when using a catheter or similar device to probe open the closure.

Suggestions

If the fistula is closing, the object is to try to get something into the fistula to keep it open, or, if it has already closed, to open it by penetrating the newly closed tissue. Catheters can be used for this purpose. Plastic catheters are stiffer and consequently more penetrating than red rubber catheters and are therefore preferable for opening the fistula. The responsible patient should be taught how to use the catheters to open a closed fistula and should have a complete set of catheters at home and in the car.

Start with a catheter that is the same size as that used to stent the opening for the prosthesis being worn; for example, a 14 or 16 Fr for a 16 Fr prosthesis. Insert it into the fistula as far as it will go. One can assume that the catheter is in the esophagus if it passes easily and without discomfort to the patient to within 10 to 13 centimeters (cm) of the distal end. If it does not enter the esophagus, apply continuous and mildly forceful pressure for several minutes. If the catheter does not penetrate through to the esophagus, try the next smaller size catheter, using the same procedure. It may be necessary to go down to a 10 Fr or smaller in order to penetrate the closure.

Opening a closed fistula can take some time, so do not be in a hurry. The newly closed tissue should give way first and keep the catheter from creating a new tunnel. However, the danger of entering the fascia when attempting to reopen the fistula, especially if the tunnel is misaligned, must always be kept in mind. It is rare to have a fistula as long as 4 cm, so if any catheter has been inserted a distance of 4 cm and has not entered the esophagus, it is probably slipping between the muscles of the wall. The patient will complain of discomfort that can become severe if the probing continues. Once the fascia has been entered, the catheter will almost inevitably continue to follow the same path every time it is inserted. Probing must stop immediately in order to avoid infection and other complications. There should be no significant pain or discomfort on probing with the catheter, and little or no bleeding. Mainly, the patient will be aware only of the pressure being exerted against the tissues.

If the catheter does enter the esophagus, a knot should be tied about 10 cm from the distal end to prevent leakage and the catheter taped to the side of the neck. If it is the patient who has opened the fistula, the patient should contact the physician or speech pathologist as soon as possible for further advice. The fistula can be up-stented with a size larger catheter each day until the size that is compatible with the size of the prosthesis is reached. Sometimes the up-stenting can proceed faster by skipping a size.

If the catheter can be inserted only part of the way, the fistula may still be salvageable if the patient keeps the catheter inserted as far as it will go and proceeds immediately to the physician, speech pathologist, or emergency room, taking all the supplies needed for use with the tracheoesophageal fistula, including prostheses, catheters, tape and other adhesives, inserters, and so on. There are other procedures that the physician may wish to try.

If the fistula is open, it has to be determined whether poor or no sound is due to the prosthesis or the sound generator.

Prosthesis

The prosthesis is at fault if there is poor sound or no sound with the prosthesis in place but satisfactory sound when the prosthesis is removed (open fistula).

Causes

The air-flow port by which tracheal air enters the prosthesis may be blocked. It may be blocked by a plug of mucus or blocked because the prosthesis was inserted upside down. The prosthesis may be right side up, but it may be seated so deeply into the fistula that the air-entry port is partially or totally occluded. Excessive digital pressure on the stoma may not only push the prosthesis into the fistula and cover the air-flow port but can also narrow the esophagus , producing a subsequent restriction in air flow.

The esophageal end of the prosthesis may not be opening well, thereby inhibiting or preventing air flow into the esophagus. The end is frequently stuck together on new prostheses. Mucus can also cause the opening to stick. If a prosthesis is too long or too much digital pressure is used for stoma occlusion, the esophageal end of the prosthesis may be pushed into the esophageal wall, restricting opening. If the prosthesis is too short and completely contained within the fistula, air exit may be limited.

Suggestions

The proper size prosthesis must be selected. If it is new, it should be checked and, if necessary, the esophageal end should be pried open to assure it can open properly. The prosthesis is inserted right side up and kept clean. Excessive pressure should be eliminated when occluding the stoma. The rule should be "complete but gentle" closure. With many patients, a forward movement of the stoma occurs as air expands the esophagus. The finger covering the stoma should also rock forward, following the movement of the neck while maintaining a good seal over the stoma. The problems associated with a deep-seated prosthesis can sometimes be remedied by taping the prosthesis with the bottom tilted upward or by placing the air-entry port at any angle that would improve air flow.

Sound Generator

The sound generator is the same as that used for esophageal speech, that is, the PE segment or junction. The sound generator is involved if the sound is poor or absent with the prosthesis in or out of the fistula and the fistula has not closed.

Causes

It has been hypothesized and studies using nerve block and esophageal insufflation testing have suggested that the sound generator will not function well if the resistance to air flowing through it is too low or too high (Bosone-Crouch, 1974; Chodosh, Giancarlo, and Goldstein, 1984; McGarvey and Weinberg, 1984; Singer and Blom, 1981).

1. If the resistance is too low, the sound will be quiet and breathy or absent.

   Suggestion.   The solution for low resistance is to apply digital pressure on the outside of the neck. The two variables to consider are the location of the pressure point and the amount of pressure to be used.
2. If resistance is too high, sound production will be effortful and the result may be no sound, intermittent sound, or short sound. Interestingly, the PE segment can be too resistant for good sound generation, but the patient will not complain of swallowing problems. On the other hand, when a patient complains of food or liquid "hanging up" in the throat, be alert for a problem with the sound generator.

   Suggestion.   Generally a sound generator that is highly resistant to air flow will be recognized prior to fistulization, and remedial procedures will be undertaken at that time. If the tissues forming or surrounding the sound generator are highly resistant to air flow, dilation (bouginage) may be tried. Remarkable success has been seen by the author with one or a series of dilation treatments. In order to evaluate the effect of the treatment, each dilation should be followed immediately by renewed attempts to make sound, either via the TEF or with an esophageal insufflation test. If satisfactory sound is obtained, the sound provides a model for the patient to emulate in practice. Initially successful results may be followed in a few days by a return to high resistance; therefore, repeated dilations may be necessary. Ideally the effects of the dilation will be long term, but some patients will need periodic treatments in order to maintain a satisfactory opening.

A patient may exhibit mild muscular spasm in the sound generator. Resistance to air flow increases with the spasm (Singer and Blom, 1981). The patient is generally aphonic during the spasm. Patients can often learn to ease into and through these moments while maintaining sound. The situation is not unlike coping with a moment of stuttering. That is, through experience they seem to sense the imminent onset of the spasm. They are taught that at this moment they should reduce the effort used to speak, reduce loudness and sometimes rate, and ease through the spasm. Initially they may not be able to sustain sound but only effect the behavioral changes. Sound resumes as the spasm leaves. As time goes on, however, speech can become functionally fluent.

When the PE segment is highly resistant to air flow, the treatment alternative is pharyngeal myotomy. This surgery has been done as part of the primary laryngectomy (Singer, Blom, and Hamaker, 1983; Spofford, 1984) and as a secondary procedure (Singer and Blom, 1981; Chodosh et al., 1984). The surgery is especially useful in relieving severe muscular spasm. Pharyngeal myotomy, as done by Dr. Mark Singer, involves incising the inferior pharyngeal constrictor (the inferior border of which is the cricopharyngeus muscle) and the middle pharyngeal constrictor (Singer and Blom, 1981).

Leaking

When the patient swallows liquids, some of the fluid may enter the trachea and cause coughing. There are two sites for leaking: (1) *around* the prosthesis and (2) *through* the prosthesis. It is essential to determine which site is involved because the solutions are different.

How to Test

One way to determine the location of the leak is to add a drop or two of dark food coloring to a glass of water. Most of the cotton from the tip of a 6 inch cotton-tipped applicator is removed and this end is placed inside the prosthesis worn by the patient. The cotton tip is inserted just beyond the port of entry for tracheal air; or if the prosthesis does not have a separate tracheal air flow port, the applicator is inserted beyond any opening in the prosthesis through which the liquid could leak out before touching the cotton. The patient is asked to take a small sip of the colored water and to hold it in the mouth until told to swallow. The examiner turns a light on the stoma and sits in a position to see the prosthesis clearly, including the underside. The patient is asked to swallow and the examiner watches for any trace of the colored liquid. If some is seen, it will be coming from *around* the prosthesis, because the inside of the prosthesis is blocked with the cotton. If no colored liquid is seen, the applicator is removed from the center of the prosthesis. If the tip is tinged with the food coloring, the leak was *through* the prosthesis.

Causes

1. The prosthesis may leak because it is old and worn out, faulty, or too long. If the prosthesis is too long, the esophageal end may become damaged, and it will leak prematurely. It is a good idea for the clinician to keep track of how long each prosthesis lasts and to check the fit occasionally. It is not unusual to have to change to a prosthesis of a shorter length as time goes on. A patient may or may not complain of throat discomfort when the prosthesis is too long.

   Suggestion. The solution for a prosthesis that leaks is to replace it. Care should always be taken to make sure the prosthesis is the proper size.

2. If the leaking is around the prosthesis, it means the walls of the fistula no longer fit snugly around the prosthesis. This sometimes occurs when no specific reason can be identified. It may happen with some patients simply from wearing a prosthesis over time. A prosthesis that is too long can also contribute to the enlargement of the fistula, especially at the esophageal end.

   Suggestion. One procedure for controlling leakage around the prosthesis is to have the patient remove the prosthesis before going to bed and replace it with a catheter that is the next size smaller than the one used to stent the present fistula; for example, a 12 Fr catheter is used as a stent for a patient who was originally stented with a 14 Fr catheter. The catheter is maintained in place overnight or until there is no leaking around the catheter on swallowing liquids.

If the patient has not been wearing a prosthesis with a retention collar, a change to this design may be sufficient to prevent esophageal leakage.

A quick and easy remedy for reducing the lumen of the fistula is electrocauterization (Singer and Blom, 1980; Singer, Blom, and Hamaker, 1981). Electrocauterization promotes scarring and thereby narrows the diameter of the fistula. The procedure is done by the physician. One treatment is usually sufficient to achieve the desired result.

Coughing Out a Prosthesis

Causes

1. A prosthesis without a retention collar is easier to dislodge than one with a retention collar.

    Suggestion. With the advent of the retention collar, seldom does a patient cough out a prosthesis. Nonetheless, an attempt should be made to hold in the prosthesis during coughing and to check to see it is in place afterward.

2. Improper taping can be responsible for extruding the prosthesis on coughing.

    Suggestion. If taping is essential for prosthesis retention, it is important to use only the tape specifically recommended for that purpose. The tape should be applied according to the directions that come with the prosthesis. It is helpful if the tape is placed close to the edge of the stoma in order to reduce the "play" in the movement of the prosthesis.

Stoma Noise

Stoma noise during speech after TEF is the result of an air leak when the stoma is occluded. It is a common occurrence in the initial stages of training. If the patient is able to use a tracheostoma valve (Blom, Singer, and Hamaker, 1982), there should be no problem with stoma noise.

Causes

1. The patient may have the idea that it is necessary to push a large amount of air through the prosthesis in order to generate sound. There is also a tendency to feel that the sound is not loud enough.

As a result, the patient inhales deeply and exhales forcefully, causing excessive pressure and concomitant air leakage around the finger occluding the stoma.

Suggestion.   A reduction in depth and force of respiration will resolve stoma noise related to loudness and excessive effort.

2.   Stoma noise can also be caused by inadequate occlusion of the stoma. If the peristomal area is not dry (e.g., tracheal discharge has not been completely wiped off), it is difficult to obtain a good seal and stoma noise will result. Sometimes the finger used for occlusion is not large enough or not angled correctly for an adequate seal. Occasionally the stoma is too large for a good seal without stoma noise.

Suggestion.   When the problem is inadequate occlusion of the stoma, the patient should experiment with other fingers and various positions on the stoma. Normally, the fingers of the nondominant hand are used for stoma occlusion, but the patient may have to resort to using the dominant hand if that is the only way to obtain a good seal.

When the stoma is large, the patient should try occluding over a plastic foam cover. There are also voice prostheses built into silicone tracheostoma tubes or vents (Perry, Cheesman, and Eden, 1982; Shapiro and Ramanathan, 1982; Spofford, 1984). These tracheostoma tubes have an outer peristomal flange that can provide a good seal in two ways. A tracheostoma tube size can be selected with an opening small enough for the finger to seal against it. Also, pressure from the finger should effectively seal the flange against the peristomal skin, resulting in a functionally smaller stoma.

Maintaining an Airtight Seal on the Tracheostoma Valve

When a valve replaces manual occlusion of the stoma, the most common problem is maintaining the seal between the housing for the valve and the peristomal skin (Blom et al., 1982).

Causes

1.   Improper procedures used in preparing the skin.

Suggestion.   It is important to follow the directions that come with the valve; for example, cleaning the peristomal area with alcohol. It may also be helpful to apply up to three coats of liquid adhesive, allowing each coat to dry about 3 minutes between applications and before attaching the housing. Occasionally a patient is unable to use the tracheostoma valve because of an allergic reaction to the adhesives. The manufacturer of the valve may have suggestions about other adhesives to try.

2. Improper procedures used in applying the housing to the skin.

Suggestion. The housing must be positioned correctly; that is, the opening in the housing must be centered over the stoma, preferably not occluding any of it. The housing must conform to the contour of the peristoma area. Sometimes this can be difficult when the stoma is deep-set between prominent sternocleidomastoid muscles. Discharge from the trachea should not be allowed to accumulate around the inside of the housing, especially after coughing. The discharge loosens the adhesive.

Attention should be paid to the location of air leaks under the valve housing, and particular care taken with that spot the next time the housing is put on. Recurring air leaks in the same location should draw attention to something unique about that location. Perhaps a concave area should be pulled outward as the housing is attached in order to assure good contact between the adhesive backing and the skin. If the air leak recurs around the neck strap (or straps) of the prosthesis, it may be helpful to shorten the strap so that it does not extend beyond the edge of the housing. The clinician can also experiment with different ways of taping or not taping the strap to the skin before applying the housing (e.g., using double-faced tape, using only a small strip of paper tape over the strap, or using a liquid adhesive applied to the strap. The addition of paper tape over the housing may provide some extra protection from air leaks, especially during initial use.

3. High air pressure behind the valve. Excessive back pressure can be related to air-flow resistance in the PE segment or the prosthesis, deep breathing, emotional speech, or coughing. Back pressure closes the valve and places a strain on the seal of the housing, and by doing so, is the major cause of failure in effective use of tracheostoma valves (Blom, Singer, and Hamaker, 1982).

Suggestion. The valve should be removed from the housing prior to coughing not only to reduce the strain on the housing but to prevent eversion of the diaphragm and to eliminate the need for cleaning the valve. Patients can often learn to resist the impulse to cough until either the sensation goes away or it is convenient to remove the valve and cough.

Air-flow resistance in the PE segment may be approached with behavior modification, dilation, or pharyngeal myotomy, as discussed earlier. Air-flow resistance in the prosthesis may be reduced

50 per cent or more by changing to a low-resistance type of prosthesis. This change alone could significantly increase the patient's chance of success in wearing a tracheostoma valve (Weinberg and Moon, 1984). Deep breathing can be modified with training. The patient needs to be aware of the effect of emotional speech on the PE segment, possibly making it more resistant to air flow and consequently increasing back pressure to the valve.

Reversing Tracheoesophageal Fistulization

There are several ways to promote closure of the fistula, should this become necessary or desirable. The fistula will close from the esophageal end forward. Only the esophageal end has to close to prevent leaking on swallowing. The length of time it takes for this closure varies from a few hours to several days.

The esophageal end of the fistula can be left free to close if the patient is fitted with a prosthesis that is at least two sizes smaller than the one being worn. The prosthesis must not have a retention collar. The patient will not be able to use the short prosthesis for speech but should be able to eat and drink without leaking while the esophageal end of the fistula closes. A short "dummy" prosthesis may be substituted for this purpose. Once the esophageal end of the fistula has closed, the prosthesis can be removed and the rest of the fistula should close spontaneously.

Another method to facilitate closure is to instruct the patient to remove the existing prosthesis just before going to bed, leaving the fistula open. Leaks into the trachea from swallowing during the night are not likely to be a problem during sleeping, and by the next morning the fistula should have at least begun to close.

Closure of the fistula may also proceed in graduated steps by stenting with one size smaller catheter (down-stenting) each night until reaching a 10 or 8 Fr catheter. At that point, the catheter is removed and the fistula is left open until closure occurs.

To check on the progress of the closure, the prosthesis is removed and the patient is asked to produce sound by shunting air through the open fistula. If no sound is produced, the patient should proceed to swallow a small sip of water and be observed for leakage. If there is no leaking with a small sip, larger amounts should be swallowed while the patient is monitored for leaking. No sound and the absence of leaking on swallowing liquids means the esophageal end of the fistula has closed. If there is only a small leak on swallowing water, the clinician may still consider leaving the fistula to close spontaneously. Solid foods can generally be swallowed without a problem, and liquids can be mixed with solid foods until no leak occurs.

If the fistula fails to close within a few days, electrocauterization can usually complete the process. It generally takes only one treatment, but occasionally more are required.

The information provided in this chapter is based on personal experience with patients and, therefore, should serve as a core of knowledge that can be used to resolve many common problems. However, the relatively new field of tracheoesophageal fistulization is developing rapidly through increasing world-wide interest and research. Practical information derived from experience with currently available prostheses and procedures will be affected most significantly. Therefore, concerned professionals are cautioned to be attuned to new developments and to be flexible in their approach to problems.

QUESTIONS

1. List four items that should be in a curriculum designed to teach a person to use a prosthesis adequately.
2. Refute the statement, "Nothing can be done for one whose tracheoesophageal fistula (TEF) has become too small after inadvertent loss of the prosthesis."
3. A patient who has just had a prosthesis placed in his TEF fails to produce sound even when the clinician successfully occludes the stoma. What are some possible causes of this failure?
4. How might a functional spasm of the PE segment be treated?
5. How do you test for possible leaks of liquid around and through a prosthesis?
6. List two basic causes of stomal noise when using a prosthesis.
7. Why use a stoma button with TEF patients? (List two possible reasons.)

REFERENCES

Annyas, A. A., Nijdam, H. F., Escajadillo, J. R., Mahieu, H. F., and Leever, H. (1984). Groningen prosthesis for voice rehabilitation after laryngectomy. *Clin. Otolaryngol., 9,* 51–54.

Blom, E. D., Singer, M. I., and Hamaker, R. C. (1982). Tracheostoma valve for postlaryngectomy voice rehabilitation. *Ann. Otol. Rhinol. Laryngol., 91,* 576–578.

Bosone-Crouch, Z. (1974). *The relationship of intraluminal swallowing, resting, and phonation pressures, to esophageal phonation "goodness" and maximum duration of phonation.* Unpublished doctoral dissertation, University of Kansas, Lawrence, KS.

Chodosh, P. L., Giancarlo, H. R., and Goldstein, J. (1984). Pharyngeal myotomy for vocal rehabilitation postlaryngectomy. *Laryngoscope, 94,* 52–57.

Damsté, P. H., van den Berg, J., and Moolenaar-Bijl, A. J. (1956). Why are some patients unable to learn esophageal speech? *Ann. Otol. Rhinol. Laryngol., 65,* 998–1005.

Damsté, P. H. (1958). Oesophageal speech after laryngectomy. Groningen, Netherlands: Gebr. Hoitsema.

Donegan, J. O., Gluckman, J. L., and Singh, J. (1981). Limitations of the Blom-Singer technique for voice restoration. *Ann. Otol. Rhinol. Laryngol., 90,* 495–497.

Henley-Cohn, J. (1981). New technique for insertion of laryngeal prosthesis. *Laryngoscope, 91,* 1957–1959.

Johns, M. E., and Cantrell, R. W. (1981). Voice restoration of the total laryngectomy patient: The Singer-Blom technique. *Otolaryngol. Head Neck Surg., 89,* 82–86.

Knapp, B. A., and Panje, W. R. (1982). A voice button for laryngectomees. *AORN Journal, 36,* 183–193.

Lyons, R. J. (1983). Surgical implants: voice prostheses. *AORN Journal, 37,* 1369–1380.

Maves, M. D., and Lingeman, R. E. (1982). Primary vocal rehabilitation using the Blom-Singer and Panje voice prostheses. *Ann. Otol. Rhinol. Laryngol., 91,* 458–460.

McGarvey, S. D., and Weinberg, B. (1984). Esophageal insufflation testing in nonlaryngectomized adults. *J. Speech Hearing Dis., 49,* 272–277.

Mitchell, F. B., Kirkland, R. H., and Morrison, W. V. (1981). The Blom-Singer endoscopic technique under local anesthesia for restoration of voice after laryngectomy. *J. Tennessee Med. Assoc., 74,* 867–869.

Panje, W. R. (1981). Prosthetic vocal rehabilitation following laryngectomy. *Ann. Otol. Rhinol. Laryngol., 90,* 116–120.

Panje, W. R., VanDemark, D., and McCabe, B. F. (1981). Voice button prosthesis rehabilitation of the laryngectomee: additional notes. *Ann. Otol. Rhinol. Laryngol., 90,* 503–505.

Perry, A., Cheesman, A. D., and Eden, R. (1982). A modification of the Blom-Singer valve for restoration of voice after laryngectomy. *J. Laryngol. Otol., 96,* 1005–1011.

Robbins, J., Fisher, H. B., Blom, E. D., and Singer, M. I. (1984). A comparative acoustic study of normal, esophageal, and tracheoesophageal speech production. *J. Speech Hearing Dis., 49,* 202–210.

Schuller, D. E., Jarrow, J. E., Kelly, D. R., and Miglets, A. W. (1983). Prognostic factors affecting the success of duckbill vocal restoration. *Otolaryngol. Head and Neck Surg., 91,* 396–398.

Shapiro, M. J., and Ramanathan, V. R. (1982). Trachea stoma vent voice prosthesis. *Laryngoscope, 92,* 1126–1129.

Singer, M. I. (1983). Tracheoesophageal speech: voice rehabilitation after total laryngectomy. *Laryngoscope, 93,* 1454–1465.

Singer, M. I., and Blom, E. D. (1979). *Tracheoesophageal puncture: A surgical-prosthetic method for postlaryngectomy speech restoration.* Third International Symposium on Plastic and Reconstructive Surgery of the Head and Neck, New Orleans, LA.

Singer, M. I., and Blom, E. D. (1980). An endoscopic technique for restoration of voice after laryngectomy. *Ann. Otol. Rhinol. Laryngol., 89,* 529–533.

Singer, M. I., and Blom, E. D. (1981). Selective myotomy for voice restoration after total laryngectomy. *Archives of Otolaryngology, 107,* 670–673.

Singer, M. I., Blom, E. D., and Hamaker, R. C. (1981). Further experience with voice restoration after total laryngectomy. *Ann. Otol. Rhinol. Laryngol., 90,* 498–502.

Singer, M. I., Blom, E. D., and Hamaker, R. C. (1983). Voice rehabilitation after total laryngectomy. *J. Otolaryngol., 12,* 329–334.

Spofford, B. (1984). *Tracheoesophageal fistula speech: A guide for the head and neck surgeon.* Denver: University of Colorado Medical Center, Department of Otolaryngology—Head and Neck Surgery.

Spofford, B., Jafek, B., and Barcz, D. (1984). An improved method for creating tracheoesophageal fistulas for Blom-Singer or Panje prostheses. *Laryngoscope, 94,* 257–258.

Taub, S. (1981). Air-bypass voice prosthesis for vocal rehabilitation of laryngectomees. *Ear Nose Throat J., 60,* 42–54.

Vincent, M. E., Robbins, A. H., Walsh, M., and Vaughn, C. (1984). Evaluation of Blom-Singer voice prosthesis. *AJR, 143,* 745–750.

Weinberg, B., and Moon, J. (1984). Aerodynamic properties of four tracheoesophageal puncture prostheses. *Arch. Otolaryngol., 110,* 673–675.

Chapter 15

Pre- and Postoperative Anatomical and Physiological Observations in Laryngectomy

Daniel E. Martin

This chapter is a discussion of anatomical and physiological factors as they relate to the speech rehabilitation of the laryngectomized. Emphasis will be on physical factors that may influence the successful acquisition of esophageal speech. The literature concerned with speech rehabilitation following laryngectomy indicates a growing concern about the number of patients who fail to respond successfully to existing speech therapy procedures. This problem is exacerbated by steady increases in the number of laryngectomy operations performed annually in the United States.

Statistical data from the Surveillance Epidemiology and End Results (SEER) Program of the National Cancer Institute Report on Cancer Incidence and Mortality in the United States for 1973 to 1976 (1978) indicates an average age-adjusted incidence rate for laryngeal cancer of 4.6 per 100,000 population. Furthermore, the American Cancer Society (1984) estimated 11,150 new cases of laryngeal cancer in the United States for 1984. Among the permanent surgical sequelae of laryngectomy, loss of the ability to produce voice is the single most debilitating handicap (King, Marshall, and Gunderson, 1971; Locke, 1966; Reed, 1961; Wallen, 1966). This problem has far-reaching implications that affect both the communicative and the emotional functions of verbal communication. The literature suggests that the approximate number of laryngectomees who fail to attain satisfactory proficiency with esophageal speech ranges from 10 per cent (Hunt, 1964) to 60 per cent or more

(Martin, 1963). The generalizability of many of the findings reported is substantially reduced because of methodological differences between studies in research design and variability among criterion measures for rating success or failure. Nevertheless, average estimates place the number of esophageal speech failures at approximately one third (Snidecor, 1968). There is a need for increased understanding of the factors that operate to interfere with speech acquisition in certain laryngectomy patients. It is frequently not possible to pinpoint the exact cause or causes of speech failure or failure to develop a high level of proficiency. Most likely there are multiple coexisting factors that determine esophageal speech success or failure. These factors may include physical factors, psychosocial factors, economic factors, and other unknown factors. Although early identification of proven negative prognostic factors must be strived for, the situation becomes more complex when the abilities of some individuals to overcome what appear to be significant obstacles and attain successful speech rehabilitation are considered.

Major features of the laryngectomy operation include total removal of the larynx and creation of a permanent tracheostoma. Since the laryngectomee is a neck breather, mouth-to-mouth resuscitation would be of no value in an instance of respiratory or cardiac arrest. It is quite evident that with the removal of the larynx the individual has lost his voice-producing mechanism. There are certain additional, associated changes that occur after surgery. For example, the nonlaryngectomee inhales air through the nose and mouth in such activities as smelling, sniffing, tasting, sipping, and snoring, all of which are altered by laryngectomy because it precludes the movement of air into the lungs through the throat and mouth or nose. Similarly, pulmonary exhalation normally involves moving air from the respiratory tree through the pharynx and into the nose and mouth en route to the atmospheric air outside the body. Exhaling air through the nose and mouth is involved in activities such as speaking, whistling, sneezing, nose blowing, gargling, snoring, spitting, puffing out the cheeks, emitting a Bronx cheer, snorting, and sighing. Any of these activities may be altered by the laryngectomy, since it precludes the movement of air from the lungs out through the throat and mouth or nose.

The risk of aspirating food or liquid is eliminated by the surgical tie-off between the pharynx and the trachea, but there is an increased risk of aspirating water at the stoma during activities such as showering and swimming, against which the laryngectomee must take precautions. For example, patients might consider boating with people who own yachts rather than rowboats, which are less stable. Similarly, they will have to guard against the entry of insects, dust, and fumes into the lungs. The use of a stoma cover helps prevent entry of unwanted foreign materials into the stoma.

BASIC PROCESSES IN SPEECH PRODUCTION

Most early course work in the field of speech pathology includes a description of the four basic processes involved in speech production, namely, respiration, phonation, resonation, and articulation.

A review of speech production from the point of view of an integrated systems approach follows. Laryngectomy involves not only removal of the voice-producing mechanism but also elimination of the continued use of the trachea and the lungs to supply air for speech (if users of pneumatic artificial larynxes and specialized surgical reconstruction procedures to restore voice are excluded).

The structures involved in each of these four basic processes for the laryngeal speaker stand in contrast to those of the alaryngeal speaker. (Alaryngeal speaker here specifically means the esophageal speaker.) The speech-producing mechanism of the laryngeal speaker has four major components: power supply in the form of a respiratory mechanism (lungs), a phonatory or voice-producing mechanism (vocal cords), a resonatory mechanism (vocal tract), and an articulatory mechanism (articulators). What structures are involved in esophageal speech production and how they differ from structures used in laryngeal speech will be considered, as will how the laryngectomy itself and possible associated surgery may influence the production of esophageal speech.

Pulmonary respiration can be designated as breathing used to sustain life, and phonic respiration, as that used for voice production. The esophagus functions as the new reservoir for phonic respiration in esophageal speech. The esophagus is located posterior to the trachea. The esophagus is an elastic structure, capable of being charged with air by various methods of air intake. The esophagus is usually in a collapsed position during the resting state in both laryngeal and alaryngeal speakers. The pulmonary vital capacity of a normal nonlaryngectomized adult male is in the neighborhood of 3500 to 4000 cubic centimeters (cc) of air. Contrast that figure with the estimated 40 to 80 cc air volume capacity of the esophagus. Clearly esophageal speakers have comparatively little air available for voice production. Their development of the ability to parcel out and regulate esophageal air flow and to replenish esophageal air frequently is considered critical to the development of effective esophageal speech. It has been reported that only the upper one third to one half of the esophagus is inflated during air intake by good or superior esophageal speakers. In any event, it is the esophagus and not the stomach that serves as the primary air reservoir in esophageal voice.

A question that has emerged with periodic regularity in the literature pertains to the relationship between pulmonary and phonic respiration in esophageal speakers. Is an esophageal speaker's intake and expulsion of air for speech purposes in synchrony or asynchrony with pulmonary function? Snidecor and Isshiki (1965) have given evidence that synchrony and asynchrony occur not only in different speakers but in the same speaker. As a generalization, there is frequently synchrony for both major methods of air intake. However, patients using the standard injection method of air intake are asynchronous more frequently than those who use the inhalation method.

The lower or distal esophageal sphincter (cardiac sphincter) has been investigated in relation to esophageal speech. Wolfe, Olson, and Goldenberg (1971) employed pressure and radiographic instrumentation to ascertain whether a relationship exists between distal esophageal sphincter failure and the ability to master esophageal speech. Seven of 13 laryngectomees in their study had hiatal hernia and spontaneous reflux or regurgitation during fluoroscopy. Six of the 7 had either no esophageal speech or developed poor esophageal speech. The other 6 without hiatal hernia symptoms were considered good esophageal speakers. The authors indicated that there is a relationship between distal esophageal sphincter competence and the ability to acquire good esophageal speech. If hiatal hernia is found, they recommended the use of an artificial larynx or surgical reconstruction to prevent difficulties that might be encountered in the patient's attempt to develop esophageal speech.

The upper or proximal esophageal sphincter (cricopharyngeus sphincter) is an important element in the new voice-producing mechanism of the esophageal speaker. The late Dr. Nathaniel Levin of the University of Miami Medical School is given credit for radiologically identifying the cricopharyngeus muscle as an essential vibratory element in esophageal voice. Consideration has been given to the importance of anatomical and physiological features of the postlaryngectomy esophagus that might determine its ability to function as an efficient air reservoir (Dey and Kirchner, 1961; Wolfe et al., 1971; Winans, Reichbach, and Waldrop, 1974).

Winans and co-workers (1974) applied intraluminal manometry techniques to study the esophagus and its sphincters in 20 laryngectomees and 20 controls. The resting cricopharyngeus sphincter pressure was found to be significantly lower (13 mm Hg) in laryngectomees with fluent esophageal speech than in those unable to develop esophageal speech (30 mm Hg). Furthermore, good talkers had significantly higher gastric pressure (18 mm Hg) than those unable to acquire speech (11 mm Hg). The investigators suggested that patients having difficulty mastering air intake might benefit by mechanical dilation of the cricopharyngeal area if manometric studies revealed unusually high pressures. This author wants to be very careful to point out that several investigators, including Salmon (1965), have studied relationships among pharyngeal pressures, the esophageal sphincters, and good or poor esophageal voices and have not obtained significant correlations.

What is the new vibrator or neoglottis for esophageal speech? The older view was that the cricopharyngeus alone served as the new sound generator. Subsequent radiological research by Diedrich and Youngstrom (1966) expanded that view. The current view is to consider the pharyngoesophageal segment (PE sphincter) as the neoglottis. The PE sphincter is considered to contain the cricopharyngeus muscle as well as additional muscle tissue. Diedrich and Youngstrom noted that the PE segment is most often at the level of the fifth and sixth cervical vertebrae. Furthermore, they indicated that if the cervical levels from four to seven are grouped, the PE segment will fall there over 90 per cent of the time. Damsté (1958) has pointed out that in good esophageal speakers the shape of the neoglottis is fairly regular or at least less indefinite than in poor speakers.

Up to this point the structures examined have been involved in phonic respiration and phonation in the laryngectomee; a consideration of changes in the resonatory mechanism of the laryngectomee follows. Research findings reported by a number of independent investigators (Kytta, 1964; Rollin, 1962; Sisty and Weinberg, 1972) consistently indicated that removal of the larynx results in altered vowel cavity transmission characteristics. More specifically, the data indicated that vowel formant frequencies for esophageal speakers are generally higher than those for normal laryngeal speakers. Differences in tongue position and mouth opening per se would not fully explain that effect. Sisty and Weinberg (1972) present an acoustically derived hypothesis that total laryngectomy results in a shortening of the effective vocal tract length. If the laryngectomee undergoes more extensive surgery involving pharyngectomy or partial glossectomy, even more substantial changes in the resonance process might be reasonably anticipated.

Articulation in esophageal speech is of concern. Various investigations have indicated that the intelligibility of esophageal speech is poorer than that of normal laryngeal speech. For example, Creech (1966) reported a mean overall intelligibility for esophageal speech of 60 per cent and a mean intelligibility of 82 per cent for excellent esophageal speech. Diedrich and Youngstrom (1966) in pre- and postoperative studies reported that tongue mobility is not restricted after a laryngectomy. Noll and Torgerson (1967) conducted a cineradiographic investigation of tongue postures in esophageal speakers. They reported a lower and more posterior tongue posture in the more proficient esophageal speakers.

Some question exists as to whether surgical factors influence the development of esophageal speech. A number of studies have concluded that the surgery per se is not a major factor influencing esophageal speech acquisition. Putney (1958) reported that type of neck incision, extensive surgical removal, method of pharyngeal closure, and amount of adjacent cervical tissue excised were not significantly related to speech success. Similarly, Robe, Moore, Andrews, and Holinger (1956) concluded that type of surgery had no demonstrable effect on the relative excellence of the speech result or the amount of speech training necessary to achieve satisfactory results. Simpson, Smith, and Gordon (1972), on the other hand, described in detail four types of surgical reconstruction techniques they employed in a series of laryngectomees. They reported that the type of surgical reconstruction of the hypopharynx was correlated with the resulting radiological appearance and with the efficiency of the esophageal voice achieved. They reported that of the four techniques, one was shown to give significantly superior results. (It is the author's personal opinion that the premise that surgical factors are not all that significant in the development of esophageal speech has been accepted too readily. He thinks more research needs to be conducted similar to the Simpson, Smith, and Gordon investigation before any final determination can be made.)

Diedrich and Youngstrom (1966) presented a list of physical conditions that may prevent or retard the acquisition of esophageal speech. Some of the conditions they list are cicatrix, recurring fistulas, innervation disorder, postradiation fibrosis, esophageal stenosis, recurrence of carcinoma, hernia, senility, colostomy, aerophagia, abdominal surgery, hearing loss, palatal dysfunction, pulmonary disease, and cricopharyngeal spasm.

This discussion of the specific physical factors that may slow down or prevent the development of proficient esophageal speech is approached from the context of certain elements within the postsurgical evaluation. The basic goal of the initial speech evaluation is to assess comprehensively the patient's assets and liabilities and to assemble and integrate sufficient data from multiple sources to establish a realistic plan of treatment. What are some of the kinds of useful information one can glean from the typically voluminous medical and surgical reports, including the discharge summary, the operative report or reports, pathology reports, radiotherapy reports, general medical history, and others?

INFORMATION FROM MEDICAL AND SURGICAL REPORTS

First, the discharge summary generally gives a nice overview of the problem in terms of what has been done, what follow-up procedures have been established, and what subsequent treatment procedures are planned. Information from medical reports on clinical staging of the patient's tumor is useful. Speech pathologists should have a working knowledge of the clinical staging to indicate the size and extent of spread of the patient's tumor. The operative report or reports should be examined with a fine-toothed comb, prior to the initial speech evaluation if at all possible, for knowledge of what structures were removed and what structures remain. Did the patient undergo a simple laryngectomy, or did he undergo associated surgeries including unilateral or bilateral radical neck dissection? If there was radical neck dissection, was the spinal accessory nerve sacrificed or saved? If it was sacrificed, the evaluator can be on the lookout for the need for referral for physical or occupational therapy to handle the accompanying shoulder dysfunction problem. Some patients undergo even more extensive surgery involving the tongue and various maxillofacial structures. If, for example, the patient underwent total laryngectomy and partial glossectomy, the involvement with articulation as well as the involvement of the tongue in the standard injection process for air intake must be considered. If the patient's cancer resulted in resection of the upper portion of the esophagus and possible gastric pull-through operation or colonic interposition, then the nature of the PE segment has been changed and the patient may develop a colonic voice* or require use of an artificial larynx to communicate.

Speech pathologists should have a working knowledge of information in the pathology report regarding the grading of the tumor and whether any neck nodes were positive. The pre- and postoperative radiotherapy reports will provide important information on the patient's program of radiation therapy. Patients who have undergone preoperative radiotherapy frequently experience complications postsurgically, including wound breakdown, retarded tissue healing, and the formation of fistulas. Masters, Berry, and Pepa (1974), in a pilot investigation, described an apparent trend showing that radiation therapy may cause physiological changes in the esophagus that may limit the patient's ability to acquire esophageal speech. Furthermore, laryngectomees who have undergone radiotherapy may have postradiation fibrosis. This may

---

*Colon transplant was used to replace the excised esophagus. Voice using the colon is noted as colonic voice. Wertz, R. T., Keith, R. L., and DeSanto, L. (1973). Speech after laryngo-esophagectomy with colon transplant. *Journal of Speech and Hearing Disorders, 38,* 495–501.

mean hardened neck tissues that do not accept penetration of the tone from certain or all neck-type artificial larynxes. Such patients may require a cheek placement of a neck-type device or use of an electronic or pneumatic mouth-type artificial larynx. Furthermore, there are patients whose esophageal voice skills begin to deteriorate at some point after the onset of postoperative radiotherapy. Their esophageal speech instruction might need to be temporarily delayed until the swelling goes down and the tissues soften.

Physical Conditions Influencing Esophageal Speech Development

Any physical conditions that limit the ability of the mouth of the esophagus to open up and permit the esophagus to receive an air charge or that limit the ability of the PE segment to vibrate in a fairly periodic manner can interfere with esophageal speech development. For example, cicatrix, defined as the fibrous tissue left after wound healing, if located in the region of the neoglottis, can be detrimental. Furthermore, van den Berg and Moolenaar-Bijl (1959) reported patients with cricopharyngeal spasm who had up to 10 cc or more of water pressure recorded in their esophagus. The underlying basis for cricopharyngeal spasm is complex, since emotional tension has been reported to be a contributor to this condition. Mechanical dilation of the esophagus by the physician or relaxation therapy by the speech pathologist or both can be of assistance in selected cases. The condition of stenosis, or narrowing, of the upper esophagus can also be a detriment.

Damsté (1958) indicates that accumulation of mucus above the esophagus is an important cause of aperiodicity in the alaryngeal speech signal. Air is forced in a highly irregular way through a varying thick layer of secretions that accumulates in a diverticulum or pocket, creating gurgle voice quality. Berlin (1963) reported that a significant reduction in the duration of esophageal phonation can be an indication, in some cases, of recurrent cancer in the esophageal area.

Berlin (1964) reported that patients having palatal weakness, perhaps as a postoperative complication or as part of advancing age, may not be able to generate adequate intraoral pressure to inject air into the esophagus. Patients with such palatal difficulty should probably be switched to the inhalation method of air intake. Furthermore, patients are occasionally encountered who were born with a congenital cleft palate; although repaired, they had inadequate palatopharyngeal function. Such patients are a challenge to the speech pathologist, the surgeon, and the maxillofacial prosthodontist. Inadequate palatopharyngeal functioning, from whatever cause, can interfere with both esophageal speech and use of an artificial larynx. There is a considerable reduction in the speech intelligibility of patients with palatopharyngeal problems using a neck-type or mouth-type electronic artificial larynx.

With respect to the impact of a colostomy on esophageal speech, a few laryngectomized patients were seen by the author who developed excellent esophageal speech and subsequently underwent a colostomy. These patients were generally able to maintain their prior level of esophageal speech skill. The author has not had any experience with patients who had undergone a colostomy prior to entrance into the speech program.

Atypical location and irregular configuration of the tracheostoma may make it difficult to use a pneumatic artificial larynx or at least may require the use of adaptive coupling. Ill-fitting dentures can interfere with the injection process of air intake as well as with articulation.

There is clinical and research evidence that diminished auditory sensitivity and discrimination can significantly alter the prognosis for successful acquisition of esophageal speech (Martin, Hoops, and Shanks, 1974). Altered hearing can affect not only self-monitoring of excessive stomal noise but also monitoring of precise speech articulation during esophageal speech production. Miraglia del Giudice, Amorelli, and Perella (1961) reported conductive hearing loss occurring as a sequela to laryngectomy.

Kahane and Irwin (1975) studied hearing sensitivity and stoma noise in 90 male esophageal speakers ranging in age from 30 to 90 years. The 90 subjects were subdivided into six groups by decade and evaluated with respect to high-frequency hearing, hearing in the speech frequencies, stoma noise production, and duration of therapy. Speech frequency hearing sensitivity (mean threshold at 500, 1000, and 2000 Hz) and high-frequency hearing sensitivity (mean threshold at 2000, 4000, and 8000 Hz) were assessed at the onset of speech therapy. Hearing sensitivity curves, representing the better ear at each frequency, were generated. Stoma noise ratings were based on a six-level scale. Esophageal speech ratings were based on the Wepman scale (Wepman, MacGahan, Rickard, and Shelton, 1953) and were obtained from each patient on dismissal from therapy.

Their results showed slight to moderate high-frequency hearing losses, as represented by mean hearing sensitivity in the better ear, in speakers in the sixth decade and above; these mean thresholds did not exceed 60 dB even in the oldest age group (80 to 89 years). Mean speech frequency hearing losses did not exceed 30 dB, even in the oldest age group.

Audible stoma noise accompanied the speech of all speakers with the exception of the youngest age group (30 to 39 years). Stoma noise was reported to be progressively more distracting with increasing age. Yet mean stoma noise ratings were never so prominent as to mask part (rating 5) or all of the sentence produced (rating 6).

A trend for older laryngectomees to be enrolled in therapy significantly longer than younger laryngectomees was evident throughout the entire age range and especially noted in patients over 50 years old.

Kahane and Irwin (1975) stated that although cause and effect could not be attributed to the relationships investigated, these measures were found to be highly correlated ($r = .90$) and also showed no reversal in trend. This intercorrelation appears to be clinically significant. It represents a constellation of characteristics warranting close scrutiny. High-frequency hearing losses were found among the majority of esophageal speakers 60 years of age or older. The older speakers also displayed higher stoma noise ratings than younger speakers. Since stoma noise is a predominantly high-frequency acoustic signal, modification of its output would be expected to be less successful in persons with poor hearing in the high frequencies than in those with better thresholds. Futhermore, the greater the production of stoma noise, the poorer the obtained speech proficiency ratings, and consequently the longer the duration of therapy required in an attempt to develop proficient esophageal speech. The investigators concluded that hearing sensitivity appears to be a critical element in esophageal speech rehabilitation and that audiometric assessment of each laryngectomee is imperative.

The factor of age at surgery appears to be related to some extent to esophageal speech acquisition, although disagreement as to the nature and extent of the relationship exists. A laryngectomee with a history of senility associated with advancing arteriosclerosis offers significant complications to the rehabilitation process.

Pulmonary disorders such as emphysema or asthma may contraindicate the use of a pneumatic artificial larynx. They may also contraindicate use of the inhalation method of air intake for esophageal speech.

In summary, anatomical and physiological changes after laryngectomy have been applied to the traditional model of speech production involving respiration, phonation, resonation, and articulation. An understanding of data from multiple medical and surgical reports should set the stage for a probing initial evaluation in which the clinician anticipates and looks for certain factors based on overall knowledge of the patient's disease and treatment modalities employed. An understanding of what components of the speech mechanism have been altered and what limitations exist can be of immeasurable assistance to the overall planning of rehabilitation. An understanding of physical conditions that may have a detrimental effect on restoration of communication sets the stage for possible needed medical maneuvers as well as for diagnostic therapy and the establishment of realistic expectations.

QUESTIONS

1. Contrast the amount of air available to laryngeal and alaryngeal speakers (using standard esophageal voice processes) and indicate what implications this has for phonation.
2. What is the physical basis for gurgle voice quality in esophageal speech?
3. Why might laryngectomees using the inhalation method of air charge be inclined to demonstrate synchrony between phonic and physiological respiratory patterns?
4. Identify two major findings of Winans and colleagues' (1974) study and indicate why each seems important in terms of physiology of phonation.
5. Identify two major findings of Kahane and Irwin (1975) and discuss their implications for esophageal speech development.
6. Identify five potential factors that might lower patients' prognosis for developing esophageal speech.

REFERENCES

American Cancer Society (1984). *Cancer Facts and Figures.* New York: Author.

van den Berg, J., and Moolenaar-Bijl, A. J. (1959). Cricopharyngeal sphincter, pitch, intensity, and fluency in oesophageal speech. *Practica Oto-Rhino-Laryngologica, 21,* 291–315.

Berlin, C. I. (1963). Clinical measurement of esophageal speech. I: Methodology and curves of skill acquisition. *J. Speech Hearing Dis., 28,* 42–51.

Berlin, C. I. (1964). Hearing loss, palatal function and other factors in postlaryngectomy rehabilitation. *J. Chron. Dis., 17,* 677–684.

Creech, H. B. (1966). Evaluating esophageal speech. *J. Speech Hearing Association* (Virginia), *7,* 13–19.

Damsté, P. H. (1958). *Oesophageal speech after laryngectomy.* Groningen: Hoitsema.

Dey, F. L., and Kirchner, J. A. (1961). The upper esophageal sphincter after laryngectomy. *Laryngoscope, 71,* 99–115.

Diedrich, W. M., and Youngstrom, K. A. (1966). *Alaryngeal speech.* Springfield, IL: Charles C Thomas.

Hunt, R. B. (1964). Rehabilitation of the laryngectomee. *Laryngoscope, 74,* 382–395.

Kahane, J. C., and Irwin, J. A. (1975). *Comparison of hearing sensitivity and stoma noise in 90 esophageal speakers.* Paper presented at the annual convention of American Speech and Hearing Association, Washington, D.C.

King, P. S., Marshall, R. C., and Gunderson, H. E. (1971). Management of the older laryngectomee. *Geriatrics, 26,* 112–118.

Kytta, J. (1964). Finnish oesophageal speech after laryngectomy. Sound spectrographic and cineradiographic studies. *Acta Otolaryngol.* (Stockholm), Suppl. 195, pp. 1–93.

Locke, B. (1966). Psychology of the laryngectomee. *Military Medical Journal, 131,* 593–599.

Martin, D. E., Hoops, H. R., and Shanks, J. C. (1974). The relationship between esophageal speech proficiency and selected measures of auditory function. *J. Speech Hearing Res., 74,* 80–85.

Martin, H. (1963). Rehabilitation of the laryngectomee. *Cancer, 16,* 823–841.

Masters, J. J., Berry, R. A., and Pepa, L. D. (1974). *The effect of radiation therapy on the acquisition of esophageal speech.* Paper presented at the annual convention of American Speech and Hearing Association, Las Vegas.

Miraglia del Giudice, E., Amorelli, A., and Perella, F. (1961). Audiometric findings in laryngectomees. *Arch. Ital. Laryng., 69,* 277–292.

National Cancer Institute (1978). SEER Program: *Cancer incidence and mortality in the United States 1973–1976.* Washington, DC, NIH Publication No. 81-2330. Biometry Branch, Division of Cancer Cause and Prevention.

Noll, J. D., and Torgerson, J. K. (1967). A cinefluorographic observation of the tongue in esophageal speakers. *Folia Phoniat., 19,* 343–350.

Putney, F. J. (1958). Rehabilitation of the post-laryngectomized patient; specific discussion of failures; advanced and difficult technical problems. *Ann. Otol. Rhinol. Laryngol., 67,* 544–549.

Reed, G. F. (1961). The long-term follow-up care of laryngectomized patients. *J. Amer. Med. Assoc., 175,* 980–985.

Robe, E. Y., Moore, P., Andrews, A. H., Jr., and Holinger, P. H. (1956). A study of the role of certain factors in the development of speech after laryngectomy. I. Type of operation. *Laryngoscope, 66,* 173–186.

Rollin, W. J. (1962). *A comparative study of vowel formants of esophageal and normal-speaking adults.* Unpublished doctoral dissertation, Wayne State University, Detroit.

Salmon, S. J. (1965). *Pressure variations in the esophagus, pharyngo-esophageal constriction and pharynx associated with esophageal sound production.* Unpublished doctoral dissertation, State University of Iowa, Iowa City.

Simpson, I. C., Smith, J. C. S., and Gordon, T. (1972). Laryngectomy: The influence of muscle reconstruction on the mechanism of oesophageal voice production. *J. Laryng. Otol., 86,* 961–990.

Sisty, N. L., and Weinberg, B. (1972). Formant frequency characteristics of esophageal speech. *J. Speech Hearing Res., 15,* 439–448.

Snidecor, J. C. (1968). *Speech rehabilitation of the laryngectomized.* Springfield, IL: Charles C Thomas.

Snidecor, J. C., and Isshiki, N. (1965). Air volume and air flow relationships of six male esophageal speakers. *J. Speech Hearing Dis., 30,* 205–216.

Wallen, V. (1966). Rehabilitation of the laryngectomy patient. *Military Medicine, 131,* 137–144.

Wepman, J. M., MacGahan, J. A., Rickard, J. C., and Shelton, N. W. (1953). The objective measurement of progressive esophageal speech development. *J. Speech Hearing Res., 18,* 247–251.

Winans, C. S., Reichbach, E. J., and Waldrop, W. F. (1974). Esophageal determinants of alaryngeal speech. *Arch. Otolaryng., 99,* 10–14.

Wolfe, R. B., Olson, J. E., and Goldenberg, D. D. (1971). Rehabilitation of the laryngectomee: The role of the distal esophageal sphincter. *Laryngoscope, 81,* 1971–1978.

Chapter 16

The Effect of the Laryngectomy on Pseudoglottis Function: Is There Need for Surgical Improvement?

Daniel H. Zwitman

The patient's ability to use esophageal speech depends on a small band of muscles that was never intended for vocalization. These muscles are described anatomically as the upper esophageal sphincter (UES) and to their function during speech as the pseudoglottis. Previously these fibers had been responsible for the horrendous sound mischievously produced when the teacher's back was turned or for the inappropriate eructation at the holiday dinner table, much to the family's chagrin. Now these same muscles are called upon to become the vibratory source of speech, a formidable task for such an unillustrious structure.

In laryngectomy the muscles that compose the pseudoglottis are excised and sutured together. Although at first glance it might be assumed that it would be simple to relate surgical technique to pseudoglottis function, variables such as postsurgical radiation and psychological anomalies confound these attempts; besides, certain past studies that purported to study this relationship concluded that it was of little significance anyway. It is apparent that the primary focus of today's research has been on the secondary surgical procedure such as myotomy of the cricopharyngeus and pharyngeal constrictor muscles (Chodosh, Giancarlo, and Goldstein, 1984) or tracheosophageal shunt (Singer and Blom, 1980; Panje, 1981), with limited attention directed to the laryngectomy. Nevertheless, the point that clearly needs to be made is that further research is *still* required to determine whether there are surgical procedures that will create a more reliable and efficient pseudoglottis. The purpose of this chapter is to identify specific areas that require exploration.

ANATOMY AND PHYSIOLOGY OF THE PSEUDOGLOTTIS

The pseudoglottis, or upper esophageal sphincter (UES), is located at the junction of the inferior pharyngeal constrictor and the esophagus. Cadaver dissection clearly isolates these muscles, but the circular fibers of the esophagus are continuous with the inferior constrictor; in other words, there is no definite demarcation between esophagus and pharynx. A circular band of tissue, known as the cricopharyngeus muscle, comprises the lowest part of the inferior constrictor. Although in some anatomy textbooks the cricopharyngeus muscle is not even mentioned, it is clearly distinct from the inferior constrictor. Fibers of the inferior constrictor travel posteriorly from the sides of the larynx to insert medially into the pharyngeal raphe, whereas the fibers of the cricopharyngeus muscle are circular in formation. They leave the cricoid cartilage on one side and form a circular band running around to the other side without posterior insertion into the raphe. Immediately in back of the larynx and attached to it is the front wall of the esophagus. The front esophageal wall is bordered laterally by the cricopharyngeus and the inferior constrictor muscle at the points of their attachment to the larynx. It is made up of thin but strong tissue essentially free of muscle fibers.

The cricopharyngeus muscle remains tonically contracted in the resting condition, but during the act of swallowing it allows the food brought down by the pharyngeal muscles to empty into the esophagus. In the case of the laryngectomee, it is hoped that the cricopharyngeus muscle will relax for the far less substantive injection of air and then return to a contracted state to be used for a vibratory source when air is ejected. Whether the laryngectomee is taking in air by way of the inhalation method or pressing air into the esophagus by using a glossal press or glossopharyngeal press, it is the perfectly timed opening and closing of the cricopharyngeus muscle and its adjacent fibers that will affect the quality and usefulness of the esophageal sound.

EFFECT OF THE LARYNGECTOMY ON PSEUDOGLOTTIS FUNCTION AND SPEECH ACQUISITION

Diedrich and Youngstrom (1966) listed approximately 30 reasons why a laryngectomized person might not acquire esophageal speech, but there is continuing controversy as to the relative importance of each of these reasons. Perhaps no other variable has received as much attention as surgery and its possible effect on esophageal speech, owing to the fact that surgery directly alters the eventual pseudoglottis because the inferior constrictor and cricopharyngeus muscle are transected when the larynx is removed. A large T-shaped defect remains in the hypopharynx and esophageal mucosa, and this defect is sutured closed by approximating the cut ends of the muscles at the midline.

Prior to the mid-1950s there was considerable support for reconstructing the cricopharyngeal sphincter to make it as intact as possible (Guttman, 1935; Levin, 1952; Mason, 1950). Crowe and Broyles (1938) made an attempt not to violate *any* of the hypopharynx or esophagus, but a very narrow field procedure suitable only for small lesions resulted. These tumors can now be effectively radiated or resected with a partial laryngectomy.

Those who favored preserving the musculature of the upper esophageal sphincter suffered a formidable setback when Robe, Moore, Andrews, and Holinger (1956) found that neither a narrow- nor a wide-field laryngectomy correlated with speech excellence in the patients they examined. This conclusion was supported by Putney (1958) after reviewing the surgical procedures employed in a large number of patients. He determined that the type of neck incision, method of pharyngeal closure, and amount of adjacent cervical tissue excised had no appreciable effect on speech proficiency. Moreover, Diedrich and Youngstrom (1966) observed no relationship between the quality of speech and the type of surgical field. Nevertheless, in *none* of these studies was the cricopharyngeus muscle isolated and the percentage of muscle preserved correlated with speech proficiency. More substantive information was forthcoming when Simpson, Smith, and Gordon (1972) examined surgical reconstruction of the cricopharyngeus and its effect on speech acquisition and in a controlled study verified that matching the cut ends of the pharyngoesophageal mucosa was a critical operative step with respect to future speech development. Furthermore, they attempted to preserve as much of the pharyngoesophageal tissue as possible during surgery, as authors prior to 1950 had recommended.

MANOMETRICAL, RADIOGRAPHIC, AND ELECTROMYOGRAPHIC STUDIES OF THE PSEUDOGLOTTIS

To achieve a better understanding of the effect surgery has on the function of the pseudoglottis, techniques such as intraluminal manometry, radiography, and electromyography (EMG) have been employed. Dey and Kirchner (1961) examined the reconstructed UES at rest and during swallowing by manometry and concluded that normal sphincteric closure was absent. Using infusion intraluminal manometry, Winans, Reichbach, and Waldrop (1974) found that resting cricopharyngeal sphincter pressure was significantly lower in laryngectomees than in normal speakers but was measurable at 13 millimeters of mercury (mm Hg) for good speakers and 30 mm Hg for poor speakers (normals measured 39 mm Hg). Welch, Luckmann, Ricks, Drake, and Gates (1979), using a circumferential probe, determined that reduced but higher sphincteric pressure (50 mm Hg) than that Winans had found was measurable after surgery; however, they did not make a comparison between poor and excellent esophageal speakers. Additional information is required about manometrical differences between poor and good esophageal speakers. At the present time, it appears that reduced UES pressure is a characteristic of the pseudoglottis for all laryngectomees but laryngectomees with the least pressure are the most proficient speakers.

Radiographic data clearly demonstrate a functioning pseudoglottis that in good esophageal speakers remains in a tonic state at rest but during phonation opens, closes, and vibrates as air passes in and out of the esophagus (Diedrich and Youngstrom, 1966).

EMG studies by Shipp (1970) and Shipp, Deatsch, and Robertson (1970) also supported the concept of active inferior constrictor and cricopharyngeus musculature during esophageal speech maneuvers. During a glossopharyngeal press to force air into the esophagus, injection noise and a short burst of activity from one or both muscles occurred simultaneously, followed by phonation. In other words, air is injected in a controlled manner in contrast to the act of swallowing, where an *inhibition* of cricopharyngeus activity allows food to pass through the upper sphincter. Shipp further compared inadequate and adequate speakers and found that the ability to contract cricopharyngeus muscle differentially when injecting and ejecting air was characteristic of proficient speakers. He concluded that "although surgery is thought to affect neither the innervation nor the blood supply of this muscle, it was apparent that substantial differences existed among subjects in their ability to control cricopharyngeus muscle activity during alaryngeal phonation" (p. 192).

RESEARCH AREAS PERTINENT TO SPEECH ACQUISITION

The optimal surgical procedure that results in the most efficient esophageal speech remains unknown, but this is likely because of a lack of knowledge, not because the nature of the surgical regimen has no bearing on speech acquisition. Even with the limited data presently available, definite directions for future study can be identified. Two areas are particularly important: (1) surgical techniques to facilitate speech acquisition and (2) protection of the neural control of the UES during surgery.

SURGICAL TECHNIQUES TO FACILITATE SPEECH ACQUISITION

As previously discussed, manometrical data indicate that reduced UES pressure is common among most laryngectomees when compared with normals and that laryngectomees who have lower sphincteric pressure are better speakers. This information is in concert with the opinions on postsurgical results presented prior to 1950 and to the research conducted by Simpson and associates (1972) that supported leaving the UES intact with as much tissue and fiber as possible for maximal speech benefit. Gates and Hearne (1982) further supported this concept when they found that among the 53 laryngectomy patients they studied, those who required dilations of the UES were unable to acquire esophageal voice. Only one of their esophageal speakers had dysphagia, whereas 50 per cent of the nonspeakers had swallowing difficulties. Moreover, the success rate for esophageal speech acquisition was almost five times greater among patients whose tumor location was identified as glottic or supraglottic than among patients whose tumor was located in the pyriform sinus. They concluded that a possible reason for this difference is that in surgery for pyriform sinus cancer, the amount of pharyngeal mucosa available for esophageal closure is much less.

It is possible to expand one step further the concept of leaving the UES as intact as possible. In the traditional laryngectomy, resection of the larynx is accomplished by transection of the pharynx, which starts inferiorly at the cricopharyngeus muscle and continues upward along the posterior border of the thyroid cartilage. After the larynx is removed, the remaining ends of the esophagus and pharynx are sutured together in a multilayer closure to form an enclosed port (Lore, 1973) (Fig. 16–1). A modification of this procedure, proposed by Tom Calcaterra, M.D., UCLA School of Medicine, further preserves the UES in its preoperative state when safety margins permit. First, the most anterior fibers of the cricopharyngeus are transected at the point at which they are attached to the cricoid cartilage. The anterior wall of the esophagus still remains attached to the posterior aspect of the larynx but is then bluntly separated from the cricoid cartilage. The result is a completely enclosed esophagus at the level of the cricopharyngeus muscle. The ends of the cricopharyngeus muscle are then sutured together over the front wall of the esophagus, because to leave these ends free would likely result in too

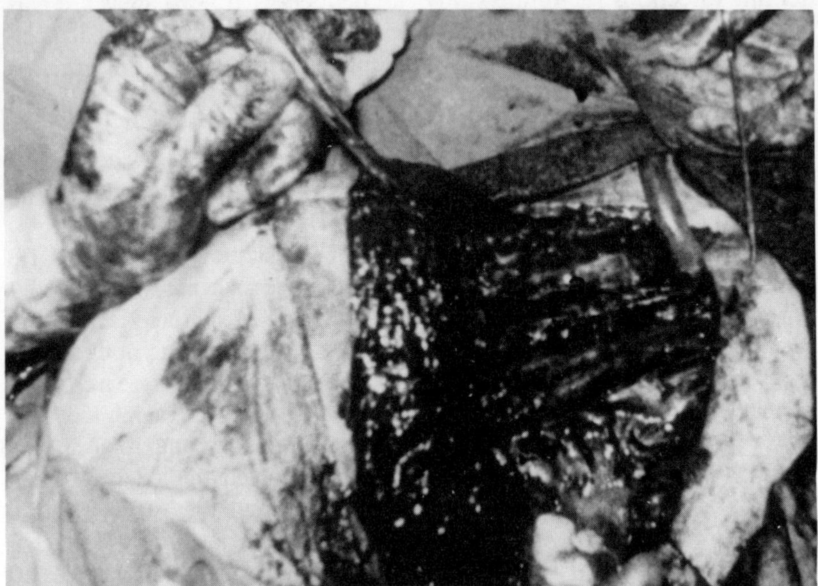

Figure 16–1. Pharyngoesophageal closure (A) after laryngectomy.

little sphincteric pressure for speech. Since the inner integrity of the esophagus is preserved by the anterior esophageal wall, there is less concern for fistulas, and the ends of the cricopharyngeus muscle can be approximated with less esophageal tissue than would have been required in the multilayer closing usually employed when the esophagus is incised. The author's experience with this procedure is that a "tight" esophageal sphincter is always avoided and the chances of speech acquisition are improved significantly. It is difficult to isolate the multiple variables that influence esophageal speech acquisition, but it appears that an intact UES after surgery provides the laryngectomee with the best chance for esophageal speech.

Protection of the Neural Control of the Upper Esophageal Sphincter (UES) During Surgery

Another area of particular importance is the neural control of the UES. Because the UES is composed of different combinations of pharyngeal and esophageal musculature, neural innervation of these muscles likely requires multinerve participation, which is accomplished primarily via three nerves. The *recurrent* nerve runs superiorly along the esophageal-tracheal sulcus and ends in the larynx but not before sending multiple neural branches to the UES prior to reaching the cricoid cartilage and larynx. The external branch of the *superior laryngeal* nerve descends on its way to the cricothyroid muscle, with multiple nerve fibers branching into the inferior constrictor and cricopharyngeus muscles before it reaches the larynx. The *pharyngeal plexus,* lying mainly over the middle constrictor, innervates most of the pharynx, including the inferior constrictor.

The specific role of these nerves on UES function has been the subject of considerable controversy, yet this information is important since neural innervation to the UES may be cut during the laryngectomy. With regard to the recurrent nerve, Hoover (1955), Conley (1960), Lund and Ardran (1964), and Ellis (1971) have rejected a commonly held belief that the parasympathetic supply that relaxes the UES during swallowing travels by way of the recurrent nerve (Asherson, 1962; English, 1976; Hollinshead, 1954). They based their conclusion, however, on the fact that patients with unilateral and bilateral vocal fold paralysis, usually following a thyroidectomy, do not have abnormalities of the cricopharyngeal sphincter. This may well be true, but in a thyroidectomy every attempt is made to *protect* the recurrent nerve, and surgeons may be more successful in saving the innervation to the cricopharyngeal sphincter than the nerve supply to the vocal folds.

There is greater concurrence that the sympathetic nerve supply that contracts the UES sphincter during inactivation is carried by way of the superior cervical ganglion (English, 1976; Palmer, 1976). However, there are those who disagree (Parrish, 1968).

The superior laryngeal nerve's effect on the UES has also received considerable attention. Conley (1960) reported that excision of both superior laryngeal nerves in a composite resection that includes the base of the tongue but not the larynx definitely compromises the act of swallowing. Schobinger (1958), Ogura, Saltzstein, and Spjut (1961), Mladick, Horton, and Adamson (1971), and Balfe and co-workers (1982) also reported that their patients frequently had swallowing difficulty associated with spasm of the cricopharyngeus muscle or pharyngeal dysmotility after extensive operations on the oropharyngeal region, including total and supraglottic laryngectomy, resection of the oral pharynx and hypopharynx, and partial or total glossectomy.

The author's cadaver dissections reveal that the recurrent and superior laryngeal nerves are positioned in such a way that they may or may not be transected before the branch to the UES leaves the nerve. The recurrent nerve starts sending branches to the UES at a lower level, approximately at the second or third tracheal ring, before it inserts into the larynx. Rohen and Yokochi (1983) isolate this branching well in their anatomy text (Fig. 16–2). The larynx is resected away from the pharynx

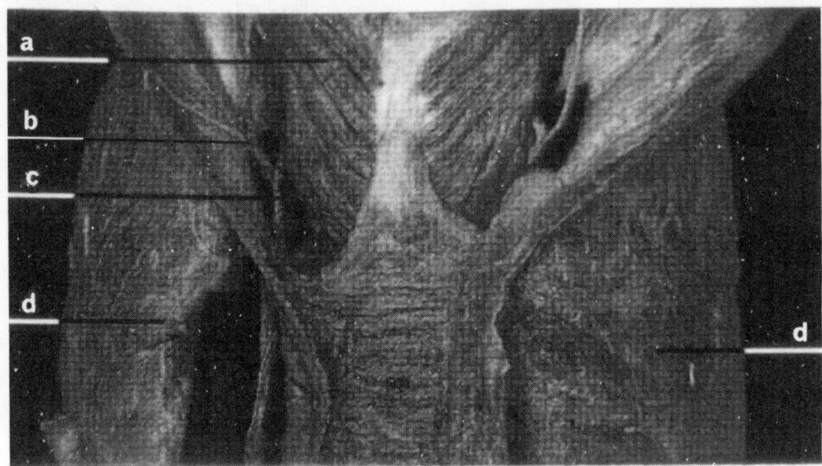

Figure 16–2. Branch of the recurrent nerve to the upper esophageal sphincter: A, posterior cricoarytenoid muscle. B, Recurrent nerve branch. C, Recurrent nerve. D, Thyroid gland. (From Rohen, J. W., and Yokochi, C. [1983]. *Color atlas of anatomy* [p. 146]. New York: Igaku-Shoin.

at the same level as, or below, the cricopharyngeus muscle; therefore, recurrent fibers may or may not continue to innervate this muscle after the laryngectomy. Likewise, the external branch of the superior laryngeal nerve is in a lateral position to the pharyngeal wall, running downward and forward from the back of the neck. There is no one particular site where it is transected during surgery. Although its innervation of the cricothyroid muscle is severed during surgery, its insertion into the cricopharyngeus muscle can be spared. In contrast, since the pharyngeal plexus is mainly located away from the surgical site, innervation of the pharyngeal complex is likely to continue intact after the operation.

The need is apparent for a study that compares speech acquisition of laryngectomees in whom all nerve innervation of the UES has been left intact with laryngectomees who have had one or both recurrent and superior laryngeal nerves transected before the branch to the sphincter occurred.

CONCLUSION

Current surgical protocol appears to dictate that secondary surgical procedures will likely be necessary after a laryngectomy. So strong is this conviction that some surgeons are recommending the inclusion of otherwise secondary procedures as part of the primary operation. It appears that the general opinion supported in the 1950s that care and preservation of the UES is unnecessary still has a definite impact on current procedure.

In reality, the relationship between the laryngectomy and esophageal speech acquisition remains an open issue. Two directions that require investigation have been discussed. It has been determined that UES pressure is reduced after the laryngectomy and that laryngectomees with some, but less, pressure are the best speakers. By leaving the UES as intact as possible, can its function during speech be improved? A surgical procedure that preserves the cricopharyngeus muscle in its preoperative state is proposed.

There appears to be a definite relationship between the amount of neural control of the UES after surgery and esophageal speech acquisition, and this control is different in speech than in swallowing since it is operative through the injection-ejection cycle. Is neural control preserved better by leaving the recurrent and superior laryngeal branches to the cricopharyngeus muscle intact? An argument in favor of isolation and preservation of the neural innervation to the UES during the laryngectomy has been presented in this chapter.

QUESTIONS

1. What is one consideration not investigated by authors reporting no correlation between surgical procedures and eventual speech proficiency?
2. Relate resting pressures within the PE segment to degree of speech proficiency patients may acquire.
3. Reiterate Shipp's (1970) findings related to electromyographic activity of the cricopharyngeus during injection versus swallowing.
4. What would you speculate might be the effect on voice production of cutting off the innervation to the PE segment during laryngectomy?

234   Daniel H. Zwitman

REFERENCES

Asherson, N. (1962). The vagaries of dysphagia. *Proc. Roy. Soc. Med., 55*, 117.

Balfe, D. M., Koehler, R. E., Setzen, M., Wayman, P. J., Baron, R. L., and Ogura, J. H. (1982). Barium examination of oesophagus after total laryngectomy. *Radiology, 143,* 501–508.

Chodosh, P. L., Giancarlo, H. R., and Goldstein, J. (1984). Pharyngeal myotomy for vocal rehabilitation post laryngectomy. *Laryngoscope, 94,* 52–57.

Conley, J. J. (1960). Swallowing dysfunctions associated with radical surgery of the head and neck. *Arch. Surg., 80,* 601–612.

Crowe, S. J., and Broyles, E. N. (1938). Carcinoma of the larynx and total laryngectomy. *Ann. Otol. Rhinol. Laryngol., 47,* 865–889.

Dey, F. L., and Kirchner, J. A. (1961). The upper esophageal sphincter after laryngectomy. *Laryngoscope, 71,* 99–115.

Diedrich, W. M., and Youngstrom, K. A. (1966). *Alaryngeal speech.* Springfield, IL: Charles C Thomas.

Ellis, F. H., Jr. (1971). Upper esophageal sphincter in health and disease. *Surg. Clin. N. Am., 51,* 553–565.

English, G. M. (1976). *Otolaryngology.* New York: Harper and Row.

Gates, G., and Hearne, E., (1982). Predicting esophageal speech. *Ann. Otol. Rhinol. Laryngol., 91,* 454–457.

Guttman, M. R. (1935). Tracheopharyngeal fistulization: A new procedure for speech production in the laryngectomized patient. *Trans. Am. Laryngol. Rhinol. Otolaryngol. Soc., 41,* 219–226.

Hollinshead, W. H. (1954). *Anatomy for surgeons.* New York: Harper Bros.

Hoover, W. B. (1955). Observations on the hypopharynx and cricopharyngeus area. *Ann. Otol., 64,* 874–897.

Levin, N. M. (1952). Speech rehabilitation after total removal of the larynx. *J. Amer. Med. Assn., 149,* 1281–1286.

Lore, J. M. (1973). *An atlas of head and neck surgery, Vol. 2.* Philadelphia: W. B. Saunders.

Lund, W. S., and Ardran, G. M. (1964). The motor nerve supply of the cricopharyngeal muscle. *Ann. Otol., 73,* 599–612.

Mason, M. (1950). The rehabilitation of patients following surgical removal of the larynx. *J. Laryngol. Otol., 64,* 759–770.

Mladick, R. A., Horton, C. E., and Adamson, J. E. (1971). Cricopharyngeal myotomy: Application and technique in major oral-pharyngeal resections. *Arch. Surg., 102,* 1–5.

Ogura, J. H., Saltzstein, S. L., and Spjut, H. J. (1961). Experiences with conservation surgery in laryngeal and pharyngeal carcinoma. *Laryngoscope, 71,* 258–276.

Palmer, E. D. (1976). Disorders of the cricopharyngeus muscle: A review. *Gastroenterology, 71,* 510–519.

Panje, W. R. (1981). Prosthetic voice rehabilitation following laryngectomy. *Ann. Otol. Rhinol. Laryngol., 90,* 116–140.

Parrish, R. M. (1968). Cricopharyngeus dysfunction and acute dysphagia. *Can. Med. Assoc. J., 99,* 1167–1171.

Putney, E. J. (1958). Rehabilitation of the post-laryngectomized patient. *Ann. Otol. Rhinol. Laryngol., 67,* 544–549.

Robe, E. Y., Moore, P., Andrews, A. H., Jr., and Holinger, P. H. (1956). A study of the role of certain factors in the development of speech after laryngectomy: 1. Type of operation. *Laryngoscope, 66,* 173–186.

Rohen, J. W., and Yokochi, C. (1983). *Color atlas of anatomy.* New York: Igaku-Shoin.

Schobinger, R. (1958). Spasm of the cricopharyngeal muscle as cause of dysphagia after total laryngectomy. *Arch. Otolaryng., 67,* 271–275.

Shipp, T. (1970). EMG of pharyngoesophageal musculature during alaryngeal voice production. *J. Speech Hearing Res., 13,* 184–192.

Shipp, T., Deatsch, H. H., and Robertson, K. (1970). Pharyngoesophageal muscle activity during swallowing in man. *Laryngoscope, 80,* 1–16.

Simpson, I. C., Smith, J. C. S., and Gordon, M. T. (1972). Laryngectomy: The influence of muscle reconstruction on the mechanism of oesophageal voice production. *J. Laryngol. Otol., 86,* 961–990.

Singer, M., and Blom, E. (1980). An endoscopic technique for restoration of voice after laryngectomy. *Ann. Otol. Rhinol. Laryngol. 89,* 529–532.

Welch, R. W., Luckmann, K., Ricks, P. M., Drake, S. T., and Gates, G. A. (1979). Manometry of the normal upper esophageal sphincter and its alterations in laryngectomy. *J. Clin. Invest., 63,* 1036–1041.

Winans, C. S., Reichbach, E. J., and Waldrop, W. F. (1974). Esophageal determinants of alaryngeal speech. *Arch. Otolaryngol., 99,* 10–14.

Chapter 17

Appropriate Covering for the Tracheal Stoma Area

Dan Kelly

Recently while shopping at a local department store, I overheard the comment, "Hey man, look at that hole in that sucker's neck. That's gross!" I glanced up to see a middle-aged man dressed in slacks and open-neck shirt with an uncovered stoma, greeting people in the store. I thought to myself at the time, "Well, he asked for it." On the other hand, almost weekly I get comments from my own patients like, "My God, Doctor, how can I ever go into public with this?" (pointing to the stoma); "I never knew I would be like this. . . . I never really understood before the surgery"; "I get embarrassed when I have to cough . . . and there is some phlegm hanging from my stoma." These and hundreds of similar statements have been made by patients. The statements reflect the concern, embarrassment, anxiety, and frustration experienced by the individual who must now breathe from an opening in his neck. These feelings are honest and reflect the predicament in which neck-breathing persons find themselves after surgery.

Whether you are yourself a neck breather, or the spouse, sibling, relative, friend, or professional who must deal directly with a neck-breathing patient, it is important that you keep in mind the wide range of feelings, concerns, and attitudes you have in relationship to physical differences. You will recall your mother or father telling you when you were a child that it was not polite to stare at someone in a wheelchair or at someone who limped. As you became older, those words were vividly recalled but you still found it necessary at times to take a long stare at a handicapped person, often trying to avoid his glance. It is important to understand that not everyone is adept at being comfortable with physical

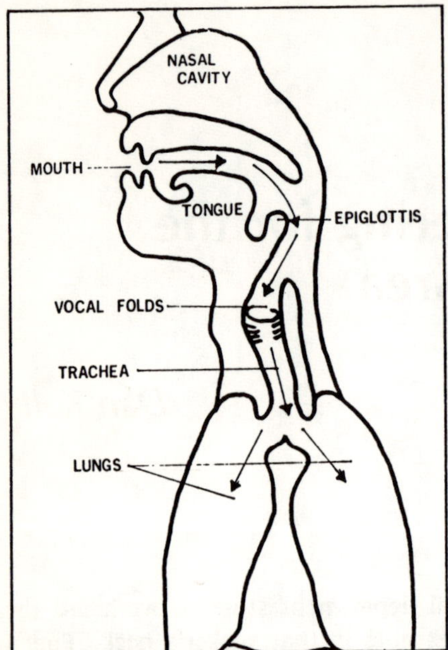

Figure 17–1. Normal breathing pattern before surgery.

differences. Although good manners are certainly appropriate, they entail consideration for other people. Some persons who become neck breathers experience self-imposed guilt because of their newly created physical difference. This is the guilt imposed on self when an adult rule or moral code is broken. Whereas young children are quite accepting of physical differences, as adults our attitudes are tainted by the unknown and the different. Some patients feel powerless to overcome their physical difference. Although the fact that neck breathers have a hole in their neck cannot be changed, they can attractively cover up the stoma and neck area in an appropriate way so as to permit them to function more successfully as persons.

Before surgery air is taken in through the nose, the mouth, or both (Fig. 17-1). Contained in the nose are small hairs and a moist mucous lining. The hair and mucous lining act as a filter and keep airborne particles from passing to the lungs. The air is also warmed and moistened as it swirls through the nose and throat regions on its route to the lungs. From the nose and mouth the air passes to the back of the throat just behind the tongue. The air then travels past the epiglottis, which sits on the upper part of the larynx. The larynx contains the false vocal folds

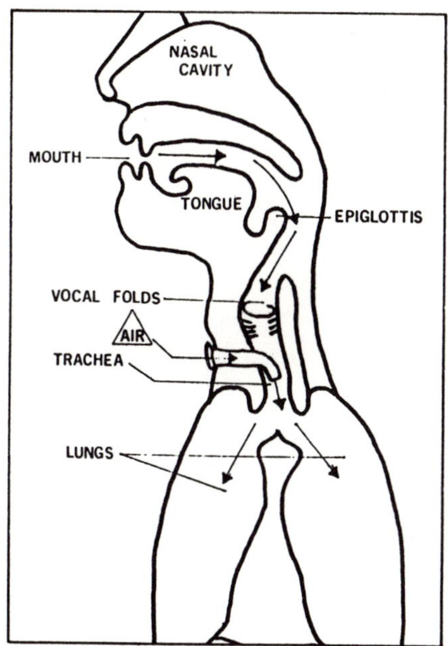

Figure 17–2. Breathing pattern after tracheostomy.

and the true vocal folds. The air passes between both the false vocal folds and the true vocal folds and enters the trachea. From the trachea the air goes to the lungs in the chest. When air is breathed out, the pathway is just reversed. The air in the lungs goes to the trachea and from the trachea past the true and false vocal folds and epiglottis to the back of the throat. From the back of the throat the air is expelled either through the nose or the mouth. During the course of 1 hour the average individual at rest repeats this process approximately 960 times.

After tracheostomy or laryngectomy the pathway for breathing is greatly changed (Figs. 17–2 and 17–3). The outside air now enters through an opening in the neck called a stoma. The air passes through the stoma into the trachea and enters the lungs. The air for breathing no longer must pass through the nose, mouth, and back of the throat to reach the lungs. In a sense, because the larynx and associated tissue has been removed or bypassed, the pathway for breathing has been shortened. Most patients have little if any difficulty adapting to this change in their breathing pathway. Because the air does not pass through the nose, however, it is no longer filtered by the hair follicles nor warmed and moistened by the lining of the nose and throat regions.

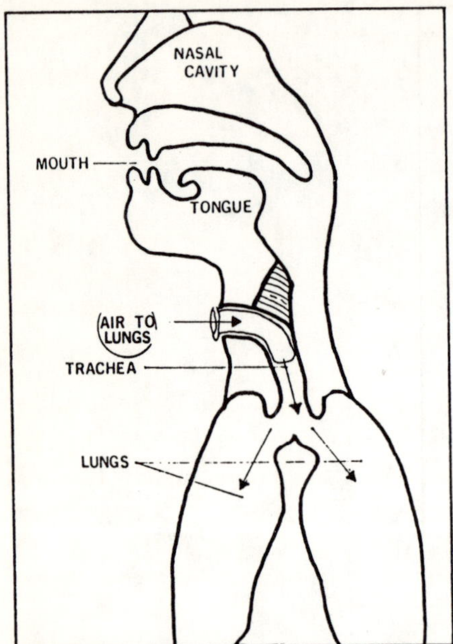

Figure 17–3.   Breathing pattern after laryngectomy.

As a result of becoming a neck breather the individual inherits a number of problems associated with having to breathe through an opening in the neck. Among these are reflex coughing, encrustations, secretions, mucus, aspiration of foreign matter, and discharge. As mentioned earlier, the air is no longer filtered, warmed, and moistened by the nose. The lack of these functions contributes greatly to the amount of crusting around and within the tracheal stoma area. The encrustation restricts the breathing pathway and makes it difficult for the individual to breathe easily. Because the natural protective mechanisms of the breathing pathway have been lost, it becomes necessary that neck breathers take special precautions to protect their trachea and lungs.

Before leaving the hospital, patients usually receive instruction in proper self-care from the nursing staff. This includes removal, cleansing, and reinsertion of tracheal tube cannulas, suctioning to maintain a clear tracheal airway, and methods for removing crust from the stoma and tracheal areas. Individuals vary, however, in the manner and degree in which they manage coughing. Before surgery, the individual simply covered his mouth and turned his head when coughing. This behavior was practiced over and over, year after year, and closely supervised by parents and peers. After surgery the patient must now learn to cover the stoma area to prevent mucus or phlegm from being expelled unknowingly. Early after surgery this is one of the most difficult changes to become accustomed to. For the individual who experiences long and frequent episodes of reflexive coughing, it can become frustrating and quite embarrassing awkwardly to cover the mouth only to find that discharged mucus or phlegm was deposited on the shirt collar, the front of a blouse, or—God forbid!—on an unsuspecting listener or bystander.

Surgery produces a significant change in the outward appearance of the neck-breathing individual. First and foremost is the presence of a permanent opening in the neck (stoma) that was not present before surgery. Although functional for life support (breathing), it is quite awkward in appearance and location. Located in the front of the body near the head region, the stoma is easily seen. The uncovered stoma is a quick "attention getter." It signifies that the person is physically different. As a result, most persons coming into contact with a patient openly displaying a stoma do not know how to respond. They are often dismayed and offended by the person's appearance. Their reaction is often one of avoidance and rejection. Some patients have required more extensive surgical procedures to close the neck area successfully. When it becomes necessary to remove tissue from one area of the body and reattach it to the neck region (pedicle), individuals must endure prolonged periods of unsightly tissue masses that easily call attention to the person. Likewise, the reactions of others to an uncovered pedicle and stoma may be even more devastating.

For individuals who experienced a breakdown in tissue and have developed a fistula, even more problems of appearance, hygiene, and care of the neck region are involved. Compression bandages are often required to assist in the closing of a fistula. Fistulas also produce varying degrees of leakage, which is unsightly on the neck. It often takes from several weeks to many months for a fistula to close. During this time the patient must continue to carry out his daily functioning. Coping with a fistula in addition to a stoma can be quite perplexing. Appropriate neck coverings can reduce the embarrassment and obviousness of awkward-appearing neck bandages and fistula leakage.

The feelings and anxieties individual neck-breathing persons have with regard to their appearance or the associated problems of having to breathe through a stoma are not to be minimized. Some individuals view their stoma as a significant and overwhelming physical disfigurement. Some persons have strong feelings of inferiority, inadequacy, and guilt, whereas still others spend endless hours worrying about having a stoma. The catastrophe of having a stoma frequently turns out to be, however, less horrible in reality than it was in their imagination. All of the worrying in the world cannot change the fact that some persons must become neck breathers if they are to survive. Many of the feelings expressed result from the neck breathers knowing and sometimes fearing that they must go back into a less than understanding society, that they must interact with people much as they did before surgery. However, with an obvious hole in one's neck, this is a most difficult task. Looks and stares can hurt!

Much of how people feel about themselves as well as how others perceive them is gained through the manner in which they present themselves. Their manner, the words they say, how they say them, how they look, and the clothes they wear determine to a great extent how others will perceive them. Neck breathers should give special attention to their appearance, particularly to how the stoma is covered (see Appendix 17–A). By covering the neck and stoma area the neck-breathing individual can present himself in an attractive and comfortable manner. In addition, neck covers help keep dust and other foreign materials from entering the lungs, assist in filtering and warming inhaled air, increase the humidity of the air around the stoma, aid in preventing crusting, protect against involuntary discharge, and provide a socially acceptable appearance.

Some neck breathers become anxious at the thought of covering their stoma for fear of suffocation. This is a totally unfounded fear. If the stoma opening is of adequate size and is kept clean and uncongested, there is virtually no difficulty breathing when the stoma cover is in place. Likewise, neck covering will not interfere with learning esophageal speech or with the use of the neck-type artificial larynx. Neck coverings should be worn at the onset of treatment so that training in the use of neck-type artificial larynxes can take into account the various neck coverings worn by the patient. Neck coverings can be modified to accommodate placement problems in using the neck-type artificial larynxes as well as for those individuals with more extensive neck involvements such as pedicles and flaps.

Dust, small insects, lint, and water can be easily sucked into the lungs through an open stoma. For individuals who are exposed to subfreezing temperatures it becomes extremely important that the stoma be covered in attempt to warm the air before it passes to the lungs.

After many years of dealing with head and neck cancer patients in rehabilitation programs in which little if any attention was given to the outward physical appearance of patients, it has become abundantly clear that assisting the neck breather to cover the stoma is of significant importance in the total rehabilitation effort. Programs of rehabilitation for the laryngectomized patient have focused on recovery of some form of oral communication. When the time came to address the covering of the airway (stoma), more times than not, patients were told to obtain the customary crocheted "bib" from the local cancer society or to purchase one of the commercially available coverings. When the patient returned nicely attired in meticulously pressed slacks, open neck sport shirt, blazer, and an unbleached cotton bib, something just did not seem right!

Since assisting patients develop appropriate neckwear was an important part of the rehabilitation program of the Speech and Hearing Institute at the University of Texas, staff members were determined to develop neck coverings appropriate to the stated needs of patients and to present the neckwear in a consistent and understandable manner. Furthermore, examples were made available for patients to examine and suitable neck coverings were made available to the patient at the earliest possible moment after surgery.

Two kinds of neckwear were developed: (1) *fashion covers,* which may be co-ordinated to go with the patient's current wardrobe, and (2) *undercovers,* which are designed to be worn under the fashion pieces. Patterns are available for fashioning formal, informal, sport, leisure, evening, and sleep neckwear. Not only was a set of full-sized patterns to be used in making the various neck covers developed, but step-by-step pattern instructions were developed for each pattern. The instructions contain information on (1) materials needed, (2) suggested fabrics, and (3) step-by-step check-off directions for construction.

If you are an individual who must now breathe through an opening in the neck, give special attention to your appearance. If you choose to use cosmetic aids such as described here, it should not be based on dislike of what you are covering up but for reasons of personal fulfillment.

QUESTIONS

1. List reasons you can think of for *not* covering the stoma and then list reasons posed by Kelly as well as your own reasons for using some form of stoma cover.
2. Defend either statement: "Laryngectomized instructors *should* use stoma covers." "Laryngectomized instructors *should not* use stoma covers."
3. Differentiate between "fashion covers" and "undercovers."

APPENDIX 17–A.   DICKEY STYLE NECK COVER WITH BIAS ROLLED NECKBAND

This cover can be made two ways. All of the fabric can be cut on the bias or only the neckband can be cut on the bias. (The *neckband* must be cut on the bias.)
If only the neckband is cut on the bias:
  Materials Needed:
    ⅔ yard of 45 inch wide fabric
    2 inch strip of Velcro to match fabric
    Thread to match fabric
    Optional: 5 inch piece of soutache braid
  Suggested Fabrics:
    Cotton   Chino
    Cotton polyester blends   Lightweight knits
    Challis
  Directions: Check (✔) steps as completed
    _________ Cut 2 pieces from pattern 6A.
    _________ Using tailor's tacks, mark "opening" markings (A and B), points at which soutache braid is attached, and Velcro placement.
    _________ Cut 1 piece from pattern 6B, *on the bias.*
    _________ Using tailor's tacks, mark fold line.
    _________ Fold neckband along fold line, with *right* sides together.
    _________ Stitch ⅜ inch seams on each short end of band.
    _________ Trim corners.
    _________ Turn right side out.
    _________ Using a dull instrument (such as the cap to a ballpoint pen), push material out at corners to obtain a "square corner."
    _________ Press.
    _________ Baste raw edges together.
    _________ With right sides together, pin neckband to notched edge of one 6A piece; match notches.
    _________ Machine stitch neckband to 6A piece.
    _________ Press seam toward body.
    _________ Pin the two 6A pieces right sides together.
    _________ Stitch from A to B in direction of arrows, leaving opening. (Be careful not to catch neckband in stitching.)
    _________ Trim corners; clip curves.
    _________ Turn right side out.
    _________ Using a dull instrument (such as the cap to a ballpoint pen), push material out at corners to obtain a "square corner."
    _________ Press seam allowance of raw edge to inside.
    _________ Pin and machine stitch loose edges together.
    _________ Adjust to fit neck; attach Velcro.
    _________ Attach soutache braid as marked, if desired.

---

*From Kelly, D. H., and Welborn, P. (1980). *The cover-up: Neckwear for the laryngectomee and other neck-breathers.* San Diego: College-Hill Press.

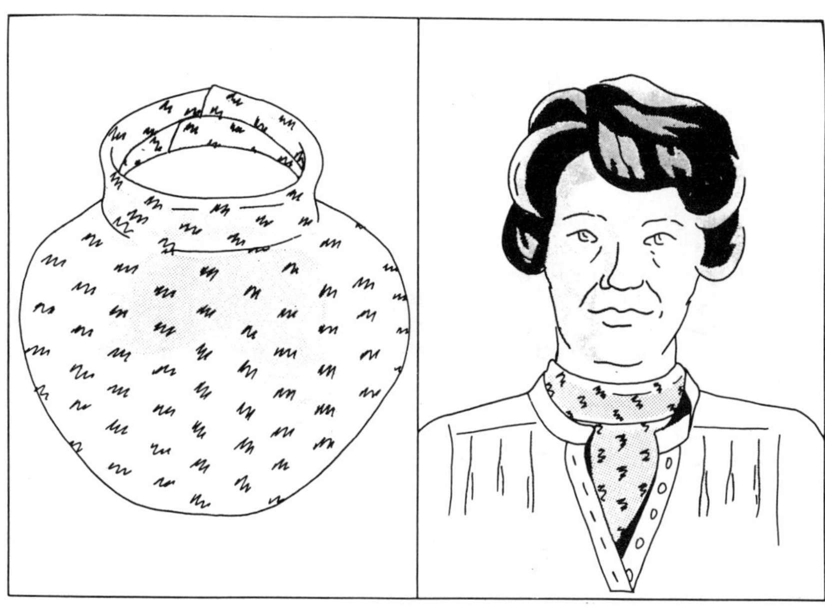

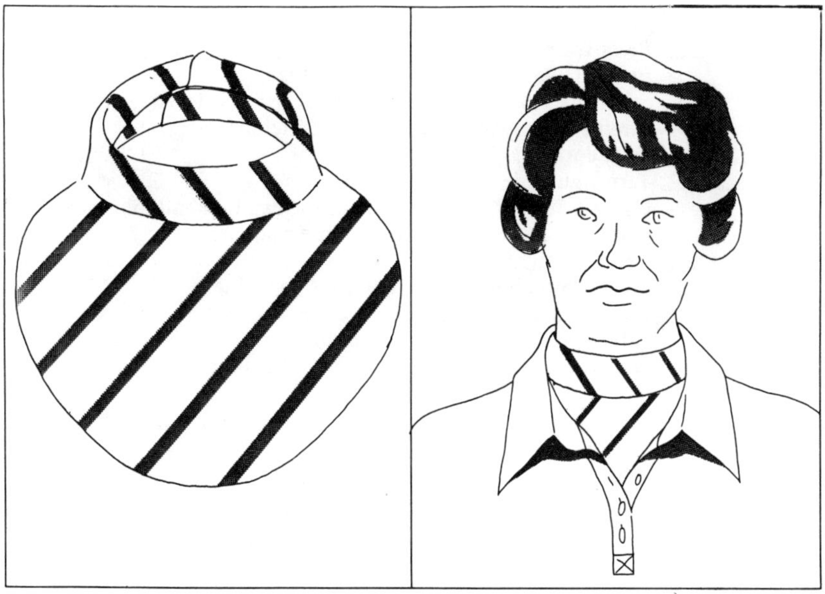

Completed Dickey Style Neck Covers.

If all of the fabric is cut on the bias:
  Materials Needed:
    1 yard of 45 inch wide fabric
    2 inch strip of Velcro to match fabric
    Thread to match fabric
    Optional: 5 inch piece of soutache braid
  Suggested Fabrics:
    Cotton   Chino
    Cotton polyester blends   Lightweight knits
    Challis
  Directions: Check (✔) steps as completed
    _________ Cut 2 pieces from pattern 6A, *on the bias*.
    _________ Using tailor's tacks, mark "opening" markings (A and B), points at which soutache braid is attached, and Velcro placement.
    _________ Cut 1 piece from pattern 6B, *on the bias*.
    _________ Using tailor's tacks, mark fold line.
    _________ Fold neckband along fold line, with *right* sides together.
    _________ Stitch ⅜ inch seams on each short end of band.
    _________ Trim corners.
    _________ Turn right side out.
    _________ Using a dull instrument (such as the cap to a ballpoint pen), push material out at corners to obtain a "square corner."
    _________ Press.
    _________ Baste raw edges together.
    _________ With right sides together, pin neckband to notched edge of one 6A piece; match notches.
    _________ Machine stitch neckband to 6A piece.
    _________ Press seam toward body.
    _________ Pin the two 6A pieces right sides together.
    _________ Stitch from A to B in direction of arrows, leaving opening. (Be careful not to catch neckband in stitching.)
    _________ Trim corners; clip curves.
    _________ Turn right side out.
    _________ Using a dull instrument (such as the cap to a ballpoint pen), push material out at corners to obtain a "square corner."
    _________ Press.
    _________ Press seam allowance of raw edge to inside.
    _________ Pin and machine stitch loose edges together.
    _________ Adjust to fit neck; attach Velcro.
    _________ Attach soutache braid as marked, if desired.

Chapter 18

Current Concepts of Laryngeal Transplantation and Reinnervation

Bruce W. Pearson

THE FIRST HUMAN LARYNGEAL TRANSPLANTATION

In 1969 newspapers around the world reported the first transplantation of a human larynx. Dr. Paul Kluysens in Belgium had placed a cadaver larynx into a patient at the time of a laryngectomy for cancer. On closer analysis it appears that just the internal parts of the larynx were transplanted. Clinical observations subsequently suggested that they were accepted, but they did not acquire movement; the patient still required his tracheotomy for an airway. Less newsprint was devoted to the fact that the patient developed a recurrence of his cancer and died of it within a year of the transplant.

Assuming an adequate resection of the original cancer, it may be speculated that the recurrence of this patient's cancer was hastened by the immunosuppression required to maintain the transplant. Immunosuppressive drugs interfere with host lymphocytes so that they will not reject a graft from someone else. But we now believe they also interfere with tumor recognition and rejection. Patients on immunosuppression after kidney transplantation, for example, have an incidence of malignancy that is up to 30 times normal.

The Donor Problem

What are the problems faced in trying to replace a larynx that has been taken out because of cancer? Particularly what are the problems faced in trying to use somebody else's larynx? Live donors are not available, of course, so the donor would be recently deceased. This is in contrast to many of the successful kidney transplants, which involve a living kidney; donors have two kidneys and can part with one.

The Blood Supply Problem

Even if the process of consent and immediate postmortem organ procurement were streamlined so that a "revivable" laryngeal transplant was accessible, to continue life in the patient recipient, the transplant would have to acquire a blood supply. The muscles, nerves, mucosa, and other living components depend on oxygen and nutrients being brought to them and metabolic waste products being carried away. Tissues such as muscle and mucosa have a high metabolic rate, and they need to be richly perfused with blood to live. Other tissues, such as cartilage, can survive on a meager blood supply that just nourishes them by diffusion. Because of the necessity of perfusing muscles in the transplanted larynx, surgical vascular anastomosis would be required. Small (2 to 3 mm) blood vessels the size of the superior thyroid artery and vein have been successfully anastomosed using painstaking microsurgical techniques. Microvascular operations are lengthy, but if the only major barrier to laryngeal transplantation were in providing a blood supply, the technical solution to laryngeal replacement would lie within our grasp.

The Biologic Rejection Problem

However, the problem of avoiding rejection of the larynx also exists. Rejection is a normal biological process in which cells in the recipient actually invade a living graft transplanted into their midst from another individual, choke off its microcirculation, and cause its destruction. There are two approaches at present that have proved themselves in other transplantation fields. One is donor selection—the attempt to match the donor and the recipient. National tissue typing and donor matching programs represent a complicated and expensive undertaking. Hypothetically, every time a cadaver larynx became available, that donor's tissues could be typed, recorded, and matched with potential recipients through the same national registry that currently serves our liver transplant program. Unused transplants would have to be preserved until a recipient whose tissue types were a close match was identified. The specificity of transplantation antigens is such that it is rare to get a favorable match between cadaver and recipient. The chance of achieving *perfect* donor selection is nil for practical purposes. Nevertheless, by getting as close a match as possible, the patient's lymphocytes would have the least stimulus toward the act of rejection.

The second antirejection approach is immunosuppression. Immunosuppression mechanisms are used to turn off the patient's lymphocytes so that they fail to react against the transplant. The entire blood volume can be circulated outside the body temporarily and then returned after the lymphocytes have been removed. This is an expensive and temporary process. The patient makes new lymphocytes rapidly from sources outside the bloodstream. Another approach has been to reroute the thoracic duct into the esophagus, so that all the body's lymph passes into the gastrointestinal tract. The cellular materials in the lymph, which include almost all the lymphocytes, eventually would be broken down and destroyed. This might reduce a patient's lymphocyte count effectively while allowing resorption through the gut of the fluids and protein that would have been lost. Attempts to explore this intriguing idea in dogs have failed. Gastrointestinal microorganisms spread retrograde up into the thoracic duct, and the resulting infection eventually blocks off the flow.

The only practical immunosuppression achieved in humans has been that produced by immunosuppressive drugs; however, pharmacological immunosuppression is nonspecific. It impairs the ability to reject many undesirable agents, such as bacteria, viruses, fungi, and, worst of all, cancer itself. Patients receiving a kidney transplant are probably not at great risk for developing cancer; their original trouble was renal inflammatory disease. But someone who has already had one cancer is highly at risk (12 per cent) for a second one, and this is the situation in laryngeal cancer survivors. Because of the hazard of encouraging new cancer, immunosuppression of the laryngectomee is not considered an acceptable practice.

THE REINNERVATION PROBLEM

Suppose the problem of immunosuppression were solved tomorrow, and the technology for vascular anastomosis were readily available: A cadaver larynx could be placed in a patient and nourished with a blood supply. Would the larynx work? It is not much use to the patient unless it can open to breathe, partially close to talk, and close tight to swallow. These functions depend on appropriate reinnervation; the larynx must respond to the commands of the recipient's brain. Sensation is important; if the patients cannot feel food sliding over their epiglottis and false vocal cords, they may aspirate. Active abduction of the vocal cords is very important; movement of the vocal cords away from the midline is essential to resist the negative pressure that encourages the glottis to collapse and obstruct on inspiration. Adduction must be finely controlled for voice yet be responsive to the more forceful and generalized constriction necessary for the exclusion of swallowed materials.

Leaving aside the question of sensation, attention must be turned to motor functions of the larynx. What happens when surgeons try to encourage motor nerves to grow back into a denervated muscle? First of all, where the live proximal nerve stump and the dead distal nerve graft are united, a wound must heal. This is associated with fibrosis. Fibrous repair tissue can and often does block up many of the little channels in the graft that the growing nerve fibers need to guide their regrowth into the muscle. Fibrosis is a much quicker and more active process biologically than is neural growth. If a nerve is cut, there is a long delay, measured in weeks, before that nerve can produce axon filaments robust enough to enter a distal graft. (No donor axons survive in the graft; they have been separated from their sustaining cell bodies, which were left back in the brain stem of the donor.)

Even if fibrosis might be offset with clean surgical technique, protection of the anastomosis site, and drugs to inhibit fibrosis, most of the nerve fibers that sprout out the cut end of the patient's recurrent nerve will never make it into the transplant. They do not find their tube; they exit at the neurorrhaphy site or they turn back on themselves and go up their own tubes again. Others coil on themselves and turn around and around and never find an opening. Quantitatively, the number of nerve axons reaching the transplant is reduced.

Some nerve fibers may get out to the new larynx. They will not have quite the normal ability to induce their own insulating material (myelin), and their thresholds of stimulation and refractory periods and so on—all the physiological aspects of a nerve fiber that can be measured—are not up to the capability of the original nerve fibers. Qualitatively, they are not as good at conducting an impulse and transmitting it into new muscle as the original equipment.

Assuming a perfect anastomosis and the best growth of nerve fibers and none of the shortcomings already mentioned, the biggest problem remains that of misdirected reinnervation. The cut stump of the recurrent laryngeal nerve has some fibers that are destined to reach the abducting muscles. If adductor-destined fibers reach abductor muscles, when they fire, the larynx will open instead of close, and vice versa. This is repeated on a random basis for thousands of axons. The donor and the recipient are two different people, and there is no way of matching the two cut nerve ends exactly, even with the finest of microsurgical techniques. In experimental animals in which reinnervation has been achieved, investigators observe "mass action" of the larynx; that is, the whole larynx just quivers, whether the brain says "open" or "close."

Of course, papers can be published to show tracings of tremendous electrical activity of the larynx, proving that nerve fibers did reach the larynx, innervate muscle, and stimulate contraction. But these tracings do not tell whether or not the larynx was under control of the brain in terms of adduction and abduction. In fact, dogs with reinnervated larynxes were not able to lose their tracheotomies. The cords did not firmly sit together and they did not clearly open apart. Thus, even the fully vascularized, living, and immunocompatible reinnervated larynx fails to function. Such a result would surely be of little use to the patient.

Perhaps one innovative approach to the reinnervation problem should be mentioned. The recurrent laryngeal nerve can be traced into the larynx, and the muscle group it supplies can be dissected out of the diseased larynx as a block, pedicled on the nerve. The larynx is then removed and the transplant brought in. The preserved muscle-nerve pedicle is put into the transplanted larynx. Misdirected reinnervation is defeated because the nerves still go to the muscles they were supposed to, and there is no time delay because no nerve fibers have been killed. The muscles will have innervation and tonus right away. Unfortunately, such an approach would be feasible only for a medium-sized cancer, one that would allow preservation of such a pedicle without leaving any of the original cancer in the patient. Most patients who come to laryngectomy have larger tumors. Furthermore, the problem of attaching the muscles in the pedicle to the appropriate points in the donor larynx without inducing so much fibrosis that the larynx is immobilized is unsolved.

CONCLUSIONS

At present, although several excellent investigators have worked diligently on transplanting and reinnervating and revascularizing larynxes to replace the one the cancer patient loses, the end to such research is nowhere near in sight. It seems more likely that success will depend on the reconstructive efforts of laryngeal surgeons who attempt rebuild with the patient's own tissues than on further attempts at transplantation and reinnervation. When these efforts fall short of the goal, it seems likely that patients and physicians alike will continue to rely on the energy, sympathy, and competence of speech pathologists to guide each individual patient to the best rehabilitation possible.

QUESTIONS

1. What is the main lesson to be learned from the one reported attempt to transplant a larynx? Why do you think that if the patient had a reason for laryngectomy other than cancer the outcome would have been or would not have been worth the effort?
2. Disregarding all factors other than neurological problems, why is it that transplanted larynxes probably would not be functional?

Chapter 19

Office Examination of the Laryngectomee

Bruce W. Pearson

This chapter tries to answer the questions posed by a speech pathologist: "How do you examine the laryngectomee? What do you look for at follow-up examinations?"

In the first 6 to 8 weeks after surgery, interest is focused on the three sites of wound healing: the pharynx, the neck, and the tracheal stoma. From then on (and for the next 5 years), the overriding interest is to detect residual or recurrent cancer in the pharynx or neck, if it should arise. If cancer recurs, the only way to avert the patient's death is to detect it early enough that secondary radiation or surgery can still contain the disease.

RADIOGRAPHIC STUDIES

Recent advances in laboratory, radiographic, and endoscopic technology have not helped us meet these obligations in any meaningful way. The detection of recurrent cancer is still almost entirely dependent on the clinical office examination. Radiographs show us little of the internal pharyngeal anatomy once the larynx has been removed. The air contrast, present when the hyoid and thyroid cartilages braced the pharynx open, is gone. The pharynx *can* be visualized with a barium swallow, but irregularities and narrowings are commonplace and are due to aspects of wound healing that vary from person to person and overshadow the subtle manifestations of recurrent cancer.

Tomography is a technique in which the body is radiologically divided into thin slices, like a loaf of bread. It permits detailed assessments of bone and air shadows, but does not distinguish tumor from nontumor in the neck. Xerography, a method that enhances minor differences in tissue density, is unhelpful too because cancer and scar tissues are equally dense. Lymphangiography, a technique whereby the lymph nodes of the neck are demonstrated by introducing radiopaque dye into the lymphatic system, remains a research technique. If a lymph node is full of cancer, the dye fails to enter it, but the position of lymph nodes is highly variable and the clinician cannot ascribe an area with no dye uptake to cancer. There may just be no node at that site. Computed tomography (the CT scan) is the first imaging technique that does distinguish soft tissues of varying density and allows the clinician to differentiate between fat, water density soft tissues, blood vessels, air, and bone. It fails to detect cancer. It is used to demonstrate distortions of normal anatomy, which are important to a surgeon who is called upon to operate when cancer is already known by other methods. The most recent imaging device is the magnetic resonance imaging (MRI) scanner. The physics are complicated but no x-ray radiation is used. Certain tissues like blood vessels can be brilliantly defined but, once again, recurrent cancer is not especially well seen. At the present time, there is little reason to believe that the great promise of this new technique will help much with the specific problem of laryngectomee follow-up.

Endoscopic Diagnosis

Endoscopic techniques to detect tumor recurrence include direct laryngoscopy, the technique by which the original cancer was examined and biopsied. This has been refined in recent years by the addition of brighter fiberoptic illumination, suspension devices that leave the examiner's hands free to manipulate the larynx and instruments simultaneously, along with the operating microscope, which permits magnified highly illuminated direct binocular vision. By means of optical extensions more people than the operator can watch the endoscopist's view. These refinements have improved medical educators' abilities to teach residents and should result in more sophisticated topographical diagnoses, which should permit more subtotal laryngectomies. Perhaps this will reduce the proportion of patients with laryngeal cancer who will receive total laryngectomy in the future. However, direct laryngoscopy is of little use in the postoperative laryngectomee. Recurrent cancer tends to grow in the deep tissues of the neck, often beneath normal-looking epithelium, and in the cervical lymph nodes, which are outside the area observable by rigid endoscopic techniques.

Fiberoptic endoscopy has grown from an uncommon operating room procedure to a widely used office technique in recent years with the introduction of the flexible nasopharyngolaryngoscope. Its principal role in the laryngectomee is to help in the detection of second primary tumors. It offers no special advantages in the discovery of local recurrences, and the "multidot" wide angle image obtained is not quite as clear as an office examination with the mirror.

Mediastinoscopy, an endoscopic technique developed for the assessment and removal of lymph nodes of the upper mediastinum, has proved valuable in the assessment of lung cancer patients, as it helps identify those who are inoperable. However, the detection of mediastinal lymph nodes in laryngeal cancer remains of little use, since secondary procedures or radiotherapy for cure in this area (an area to which subglottic cancers or stomal recurrences spread) generally fail to result in cure.

In the final analysis, office assessment of the laryngectomee depends on careful physical examination, by visual observation and manual palpation. If recurrent cancer is suspected by a lump in the neck or in the stoma, a surgical biopsy for microscopic interpretation is of urgent importance. It should never be forgotten that the two most important factors in the success of a follow-up program are a well-motivated and courageous patient and a careful and responsible physician, each of whom understands his obligations to the relationship.

CLINICAL EXAMINATION OF THE STOMA

Small projections of extra tissue around the tracheal stoma are not likely to represent recurrent cancer within the first few months of surgery. Granulation tissue is more likely. During the first few weeks, granulation tissue is inevitable. Its persistence, however, is usually a sign of the presence of foreign material in the wound, such as a suture or a piece of exposed dead tracheal cartilage. Occasionally it stems from poor hygiene, from inadequate cleaning of the skin around the tracheostomy tube. The patient may still be wearing one because of the granulations, and a vicious cycle of tube irritation and stomal inflammation and granulation is established. Removal of the granulations and a foreign body, if one is present, or reinforcement of the procedures for local hygiene can usually solve the problem.

The appearance of new tissue at a stoma that has previously completely healed is much more worrisome and may represent cancer. Stomal recurrence is particularly prone to develop in a patient who presented with advanced obstructive disease, one who may have required emergency tracheotomy prior to laryngectomy. Some of these will have had such a large lesion that extension to the subglottic region and upper trachea was present at the initial surgery. Early recognition of stomal recurrence is vital if corrective measures are to be successful. The only effective treatment is a major operation, performed before the recurrence has become adherent to blood vessels or metastatic to the lung.

Stomal Appliances

Perhaps a few remarks are in order about appliances worn on the neck. Metal tracheostomy tubes are usually used in the first 6 weeks postoperatively. They are very thin walled and therefore add little obstruction to the airway. They have an inner cannula, which is easily removable for cleaning. Patients generate quite a lot of tracheobronchial secretions in the first month after surgery and the ability to remove the inner cannula and wash it easily greatly facilitates hygiene.

Until the tracheal lining (epithelium) is completely healed to skin, there is a tendency for the tracheal stoma region to contract. Beyond 6 weeks this tendency is usually absent and a tracheostoma tube is no longer required. Decisions must always be individualized, however, as premature tube removal in an unstable stoma will lead to the potentially serious problem of stomal stenosis.

Other appliances may be encountered in the office from time to time. Some patients never completely lose the tendency to stenosis at the stoma, so they wear a small plastic button or "collar" in this opening. It is usually fixed to a string around their neck so that it is not lost if coughed out.

One method of vocal rehabilitation used to add quite a bit of hardware to the neck; namely, the Taub vocal rehabilitation apparatus. The patient wore a tracheotomy tube all the time. A further tube hung down from this and had an inferior opening that remained patent during quiet breathing but closed with a stronger exhalation such as might occur during attempts to talk. When it closed, air was forced laterally and upward through the rest of the apparatus, which consisted of a series of tubes ultimately connected to a fistula into the pharynx. By this means air was shunted on demand into the esophagus, just below the cricopharyngeus. In successful cases, the resulting intrapharyngeal vibrations could be articulated by the patient into a respectable voice.

Newer methods of fistula speech have been introduced by Singer and Blom, and by Panje, that place a much smaller Silastic prosthesis within the stoma itself. The prosthesis consists of a tiny tube, about the size of a golf tee, that keeps a pencil-sized tracheoesophageal connection open. It must not be removed for long or the connection will close. A one-way valve prevents food from entering the trachea, but it permits air to enter the esophagus when the patient covers his or her stoma and exhales. Some patients are, in addition, able to wear a large, basketlike valve over their stoma, held on the skin with an adhesive washer. The basket valve, which can slip out of the adhesive housing for cleaning, closes much like the Taub valve and permits the patient to talk without occluding the stoma manually.

RECURRENT CANCER

What does cancer look like when it recurs? It usually recurs as a firm, painless lump in the neck, but if it involves the tracheal stoma or breaks through the skin surface externally or the mucosal surface internally it has features typical of primary squamous cell carcinoma anywhere. Its central portions are ulcerated and may bleed easily. The active margins are firm, irregular, and fleshy. Because the epithelial barrier to topographical microorganisms is broken, the tumor ulcer may be surrounded by inflamed tissue. It may not be particularly painful, and it tends to look much worse than it feels. Squamous cell malignancies tend to appear in the throat or the neck before they metastasize elsewhere.

During office visits, a routine examination of the throat, nose, ear, and neck is carried out. The incidence of second cancers in patients cured of laryngeal cancers is around 12 per cent, and as these are usually aerodigestive system or lung cancers, early diagnosis may reward the careful examiner and the cautious patient with a second cure. Early symptoms may be difficulty swallowing, a pain in the ear or the chest, persistent bleeding and cough, or a change in the patient's ability to speak.

The cause of a patient's difficulty in swallowing can sometimes be diagnosed by mirror examination of the throat. Occasionally a web forms near the base of the tongue, depending on the manner in which the pharynx was closed or healed after laryngectomy. Stenosis of the pharynx can occur if a large cancer required removal of a good deal of pharyngeal tissue as well as the larynx. This can usually be suspected from the nature of the original surgery. Division of the web or dilatation of the stenosis is often all that is required to restore deglutition.

Examination of the trachea and even the main brochi is becoming more frequent in the office now that flexible fiberoptic viewers are widely available. When the trachea is sprayed with lidocaine the coughing that would normally result from the introduction of an instrument into the stoma is eliminated. Although traces of blood are not unusual in the exhaled secretions from a dry or irradiated trachea, unusual or persistent bleeding demands this examination to rule out or discover a second primary endobrochial carcinoma.

Examination of the nose usually reveals a characteristic change in the laryngectomee. The turbinates become pale and shrunken. Neither air nor cigarette smoke is being drawn through this chamber any more and the result seems to be a recovery from the beefy red chronic rhinitis usually observed in the patient prior to laryngectomy.

The examiner should look at the ears; patients with recurrent cancer may complain of pain in the ear. Both the ninth and tenth cranial nerves (which innervate the base of tongue and the pharynx respectively) receive small sensory branches from the ear, and not infrequently a patient with a lesion in the oropharyngeal region feels as if pain is coming from the ear. If examination reveals that the ear is normal, the pharynx must be looked at more critically.

SURGICAL SCARS

Perhaps a few words on the incisions an examiner will encounter on the necks of laryngectomy patients are in order. In the past, many laryngectomies were carried out through a vertical T incision. Nowadays, a shallow transverse U incision is common. The fact is, the structures of the neck are accessible through a whole alphabet of incisions, and the surgeon's preference has much to do with the particular one the examiner sees.

Over 70 percent of the patients seen and treated by this author for laryngeal cancer do not require a total laryngectomy. Total laryngectomy is usually restricted to patients with very large laryngeal cancers, cancers that also often involve the pharynx, and cancers that have invaded lymphatic channels. Any or all of these may have spread to the lymph glands in the neck. Elaborate neck scars usually indicate the patient has had a laryngopharyngectomy, a reconstruction of the pharynx, or a unilateral or bilateral neck dissection. The complexity of any individual patient's situation may be increased by subsequent wound infection or tissue necrosis, problems frequently encountered in debilitated or postirradiated patients. The result may be a defect for which there is insufficient tissue available locally for reconstruction. In this case the surgeon may have had to mobilize tissue from other areas, such as the chest, shoulder, or back of the neck and bring these into the area. Usually such tissues have been outside the field of radiation, so their potential for healing is preserved.

The problem with using irradiated tissues for reconstruction is that their ability to heal and resist infection is severely impaired. Nonirradiated tissue from somewhere else is usually required before a gullet can be repaired or a defect in the neck can be resurfaced. Needless to say, the chances of someone being able to achieve esophageal voice whose pharynx has been made out of a skin tube from the chest, which lacks the pliability, wetness, and innervation of the normal pharynx and esophagus, are considerably reduced. The same may be said when the stomach has been used to reconstruct the pharynx or when a freely transplanted segment of small bowel serves as the PE segment.

NECK LUMPS

The appearance of a lump in the neck demands prompt evaluation. However, not all the lumps and bumps that appear in the neck of the laryngectomy patient represent residual or recurrent cancer. After the more extensive neck procedures, subcutaneous fat and the sternomastoid muscle are gone. Therefore, one may easily feel the carotid artery, the tail of the parotid gland, or a thyroid lobe remnant in the neck. In the case of the thyroid remnant, actual enlargement of the lump may even occur. This may mean simply that the pituitary gland has detected the need for more thyroid hormone. The residual thyroid lobe can hypertrophy in response to thyroid-stimulating hormone, secreted by the pituitary. The surgeon who performed the operation and knows the patient is in a far better position to assess the significance of lumps in the neck than any other physician. The practice of relegating follow-up examinations to different individuals substantially increases the chance for error. The examiner must appreciate that every case is individual, and to enunciate standard expectations for the various times in the postoperative period for all laryngectomees is unrealistic.

RADIOTHERAPY EFFECTS

As mentioned previously, many patients presently undergoing laryngectomy have previously undergone radiotherapy. Like surgery, radiation produces findings observable in the follow-ups. Visible evidence in the skin may be loss of hair and vascular telangiectases. Deeper in the neck, radiofibrosis may cause normally pliable tissues to become woody and stiff. Examination of the throat will reveal desiccation of the mucosal surface and edema of the underlying tissues. After surgery alone, any persistent or progressive deterioration can be considered to represent cancer until proved otherwise. After radiation, however, it is quite difficult to judge whether it is cancer or radiation necrosis. Patients are at their worst immediately after surgery and tend to improve with time. After radiation, on the other hand, patients are soon at their best; the radiation wound tends to worsen with time. Deterioration in any manner becomes much more difficult to assess. Dysphagia may represent postirradiation desiccation or stricture or tumor. Pain may represent tumor or radionecrosis. Fistula formation may represent tumor or radionecrosis. Tissue swelling and distortion is expected, and severe induration of tissues locally renders the ability to search for recurrence by palpation quite futile. Deterioration of the radiation wound with time is partly due to endarteritis obliterans, a process by which walls of small blood vessels are thickened and eventually occluded, resulting in atrophy and fibrosis of the tissues supplied by these vessels. If this process is mistaken for tumor recurrence and an operation is applied, a severe wound necrosis ensues.

CONCLUSIONS

These remarks should make it apparent that the laryngologist and speech pathologist are co-partners in rehabilitating the laryngectomee. It should also be apparent that although surgical methods may seem primitive or mechanical, they are so only out of necessity. The voice is important, but life is more important. Follow-up management must be individualized for each laryngectomee and have as its object the healing of wounds and the early detection and eradication of recurrent or residual cancer. Efforts at speech rehabilitation can then be applied to a patient with a normal life expectancy.

QUESTIONS

1. In the introductory comments, Pearson relates the rationale for routine office examinations. State this rationale in your own words using two or three sentences.
2. Why is radiographic examination of the pharynx of limited value in discovering small cancers?
3. Why is looking directly at the pharynx of limited value in detecting postlaryngectomy cancers of the neck?
4. Of what significance is the duration following laryngectomy in determining whether new tissue is or is not cancer?
5. How many out of 10,000 laryngectomees might develop second cancers?
6. What significance might be attached to a laryngectomee's complaint of an earache?

7. How many in 10,000 new patients with laryngeal cancer might receive a laryngectomy?
8. Make a list of potential complaints postlaryngectomy patients might relate to you that would warrant your referral of the person to his laryngologist for evaluation.
9. Some laryngectomees wear "new adornments" in their stomas. Why?

Chapter 20

The Feminine Viewpoint on Being a Laryngectomee

Frances Stack

THE FEMININE VIEWPOINT: A FEMALE LARYNGECTOMEE'S SURVEY

In reviewing the problems of female laryngectomees, I decided that my own experiences as a laryngectomee were inadequate to describe their viewpoint. I prepared a survey to determine what problems other women encountered. Some of the questions had been asked before in a larger survey by Gardner (1966), but there have been many changes in our society with regard to women, and most of the women I surveyed had their surgery after Gardner's paper was published. This survey recognizes the total person, and the questions asked were of a social and personal nature.

Thirty-four women were sent a questionnaire with a cover letter. These women were chosen from lists of local New Voice Clubs. Twenty-nine responses (an astonishing 91 per cent) were received. Three of these came from the southwestern part of the country from newly laryngectomized women who included letters with their questionnaires. One questionnaire was not completed properly in all categories, and two letters came back marked "Addressee Unknown."

Table 20–1 summarizes the information obtained from these questionnaires. As shown in Table 20–1, four respondents (14 per cent) were under the age of 50 years; the youngest was 35 years of age. Ten respondents (34 per cent) were between the ages of 51 and 60. Twelve (41 per cent) were between the ages of 61 and 70, and three (10 per cent) were over 70 years of age.

Table 20–1.   Age and Marital Status of 29 Female Laryngectomees Surveyed

Age Range	Married	Single	Total
31–40	1	1	2
41–50	1	1	2
51–60	7	3	10
61–70	6	6	12
71–80	2	1	3
Total	17	12	29

Table 20–2 shows that one respondent had had surgery 27 years ago, and five respondents had had surgery less than 1 year ago. One response did not include this information. Fifty-one per cent of the women reported that they had received radiation therapy.

The question of smoking brought what was expected: 27 of the 29 women (93 per cent) smoked prior to surgery. Two of the respondents reported that they still smoked because they were "too nervous" to quit. The comments on smoking were varied: Some reported that they were too scared to smoke any more, some said they could not inhale, and some said they simply did not enjoy it any more.

When asked what method of speech they used, 22 respondents (76 per cent) reported that they used esophageal speech, and 7 respondents (24 per cent) used an electrolarynx. Six of the instrument users had had surgery in the last 2 years and reported that they were working on acquiring esophageal speech. The other instrument user reported that she "just could not do it."

Table 20–3 records the length of time it took the respondents to acquire esophageal speech. Of the 22 esophageal speakers, 17 (77 per cent) learned to use esophageal speech in less than 6 months. Of the two who gave no response, one was the woman who had been laryngectomized 27 years ago; she has probably forgotten how long it took her. One respondent said it took her 7 months, and two respondents reported that it took them 1 year to acquire esophageal speech.

Table 20–2.   Date of Surgery of 28 Female Laryngectomees Surveyed

Date of Surgery	Number	Date of Surgery	Number
1978	5	1969	2
1976	1	1968	3
1975	3	1966	1
1974	1	1964	2
1973	2	1963	1
1972	2	1961	1
1970	3	1952	1
Total			28

Table 20–3. Time Required by 22 Female Laryngectomees to Develop Esophageal Speech

Time	Number	Time	Number
2 weeks	1	5 months	1
1 month	3	6 months	3
2 months	5	7 months	1
3 months	2	1 year	2
3½ months	1	No response	2
4 months	1		
Total			22

A question concerning the acceptance of esophageal speech by family and friends brought forth extremely positive responses from most of the women. They reported that their family and friends accepted their speech with no reservations. Only two women indicated negative response to their speech.

The survey asked the questions, "Are you employed? If so, in what capacity?" Twenty-three respondents (79 per cent) were not employed. Many of these women were of retirement age, which may account for the high number. Six of the women were employed in the following jobs or areas: sales, dietary, printer, typist, waitress, and mental health aide. One answered, "Although my doctor gave me a clean bill of health, my boss would not take me back."

Another question asked was, "Do you feel surgery has affected your work situation?" Eleven women (38 per cent) answered "no," and 11 answered "yes," with 7 women (24 per cent) not responding to this question. However, the age range of the nonrespondents to this question was from 60 to 80 years of age, and some reported that they were retired.

In responding to a question about whether they had had difficulty coping with being a laryngectomee, seven women (24 per cent) answered "yes." Thirteen (45 per cent) answered "no," four (14 per cent) said "sometimes," and two (7 per cent) answered "yes and no." One woman said "only in the beginning," and two women did not respond. One newly laryngectomized woman responded with, "This has been hard to cope with! I have always worked with people in a profession in which communication is a very important part. I have been coping well with family, friends, my own emotions, and a changed life style—but not feeling useful or able to work is lonely and a blow to one's self-esteem. I miss laughing, singing, humming, and playing my harmonica."

Responses concerning marital status were as follows: 17 women were married, 4 were divorced, 7 were widows, and 1 had never married.

Women today are less reticent about revealing their thoughts and feelings than ever before and are moving into a new era (for these women especially) of "letting it all hang out." The younger newly laryngectomized women were more open about the changes that were difficult for them to handle. For many of them, it has taken about a year to adjust physiologically and emotionally to their altered state.

"Has being laryngectomized had an effect on your marital status?" brought forth some interesting replies. Twenty-four women (82 per cent) answered "no." Three respondents (10 per cent) said "yes" with no clarification, and two did not respond. One woman felt that her surgery hastened her husband's death because of his worry about her. Not one mentioned any negative reactions about her status as a laryngectomee in a marital situation. Many of these women are known to me, and I feel that their responses were honest.

The respondents were asked whether they led an active or an inactive life. Twenty-one women (72 per cent) acknowledged an active social life, seven said they were inactive, and one woman responded with "so-so." The youngest respondent, age 35 years, wrote that her spouse left her because he could not cope with her tracheostomy. When she meets prospective suitors, they promise to call her but never do. "It's a nice way of saying, 'I'll see you around,' so I just stay home," she said.

Responses to a question concerning membership in a New Voice Club indicated that 20 women (69 per cent) were members, whereas 9 women (31 per cent) did not belong to any clubs. Comments that were made about being uneasy around other people or being shy may account for the noninvolvement. The younger women thought there were too many older people in the clubs.

Asked if they were interested in educational programs for laryngectomees, 23 women (79 per cent) responded "yes" and 5 women (17 per cent) said "no." Many wrote little notes of encouragement on the questionnaires concerning this project.

Another question asked whether the person had any hobbies and if so, what kind? Twenty women (69 per cent) reported that they had hobbies, whereas 8 women said "no." The hobbies included hand crafts, theater, tennis, bowling, cooking, dancing, art work, golf, plants, bridge, and helping others. The majority preferred hand crafts and bowling.

In answer to the question, preference of neck covering? eleven women preferred high-neck blouses, seven women chose scarves, eight women used a combination of both, and two women reported that they prefer jewelry. Most women are creative in their choices of neck covering, but one woman surprisingly chose the crocheted stoma cover.

A question was asked about adaptability to weather changes. Fifteen women (52 per cent) reported they had no difficulty in adjusting to weather changes, 11 (38 per cent) said yes they did, and three women (10 per cent) reported that they had difficulty sometimes.

THE AUTHOR'S PERSPECTIVE AS A FEMALE LARYNGECTOMEE

I can remember undergoing many of the same problems that these women reported in this survey. I was younger than the average laryngectomee (26 years of age). I was a smoker who went through "withdrawal symptoms," and it took me from 4 to 6 months to acquire functional esophageal speech. But, in 24 years, here are some of the ways I have been able to overcome some of my problems.

I recognized my limitations with regard to noisy, smoky places and I avoided them as much as possible. I became determined to be involved and to excel in my work. I found people who were willing to work for me in a business I started 10 months before surgery. I was able to do volunteer work as a speech aide 1 day a week at the hospital where I had received speech therapy. What started out as therapy sessions became volunteer work to assist others in achieving esophageal speech.

I have traveled extensively and achieved a measure of success in my former profession that enabled me to continue my volunteer work in the speech clinic with laryngectomees. I was encouraged to return to school to acquire the necessary expertise and credentials, that is, Bachelor's and Master's degrees in speech pathology. Going back to school was a traumatic experience for me, and learning to study again after a 25 year absence was a whole new scene. I was encouraged by my former teacher, who became my mentor.

During that time I became more active socially. I started dating, and I was married for a short time, but I found that I preferred my independence too much. I relate this only because it may be of some value to younger women laryngectomees who feel that these doors in life may be closed to them because of their surgery.

At this time I am a practicing speech and language pathologist in a large suburban hospital's rehabilitation department, working not only with laryngectomees but with other communicatively impaired adults—aphasic, dysarthric, and trauma patients.

There are many things that most people deem impossible, but my own experience is that nothing is impossible. With faith and determination and a large measure of hard work, all things are possible.

QUESTIONS

1. What would tend to make Ms. Stack's survey more believable than Gardner's?

2. How do the women surveyed fit the national average for laryngectomees in terms of successfully rehabilitated voice?
3. How acceptable is speech with esophageal voice produced by women
   laryngectomees?
4. What evidence is reported in this chapter that suggests the effect of
   a laryngectomy on a woman would vary as a function of the person's age?
5. What issues related to being a female laryngectomee might have
   been raised that were not?
6. In what ways might the results of the survey have been different if
   male laryngectomees were surveyed?

REFERENCE

Gardner, W. H. (1966). Adjustment problems of laryngectomized women. *Arch. Otolaryngol., 83,* 31–42.

Chapter **21**

Development of the Feminine Voice and Refinement of Esophageal Voice

James C. Shanks

Laryngectomees frequently report that the use of esophageal voice is met by the public with what appears to be rejection. This may take the form of a female esophageal speaker being identified on the telephone as a male speaker. It may take the form of a listener hanging up on the laryngectomee on the assumption that children are playing a trick on him. In either case, the evidence is that alaryngeal voice sounds somewhat unnatural and, when the listener uses auditory cues alone, may lead to the perception of masculinity. Thus the problem is the low, coarse voice of alaryngeal communication. That there is some objective support for this perception is revealed in the fact that whereas the average prelaryngectomy fundamental frequency is approximately 230 hertz (Hz) for the female and 125 Hz for the male, several studies have indicated the average esophageal fundamental frequency to be around 65 Hz for both sexes. Moreover, the quality of this low-pitched utterance is impaired with aperiodic noise, as indicated by the studies of Shipp (1967) and Weinberg and Bennett (1972).

The question then is whether the assumption may be made, on the basis of auditory perception of phonation or of connected speech, that listeners will identify a female speaker as male in the absence of visual or other identifying features. A study was conducted by Weinberg and Bennett (1971) using 33 esophageal speakers, 15 of whom were female. Thirty-three speech samples were presented, each a reading of the second

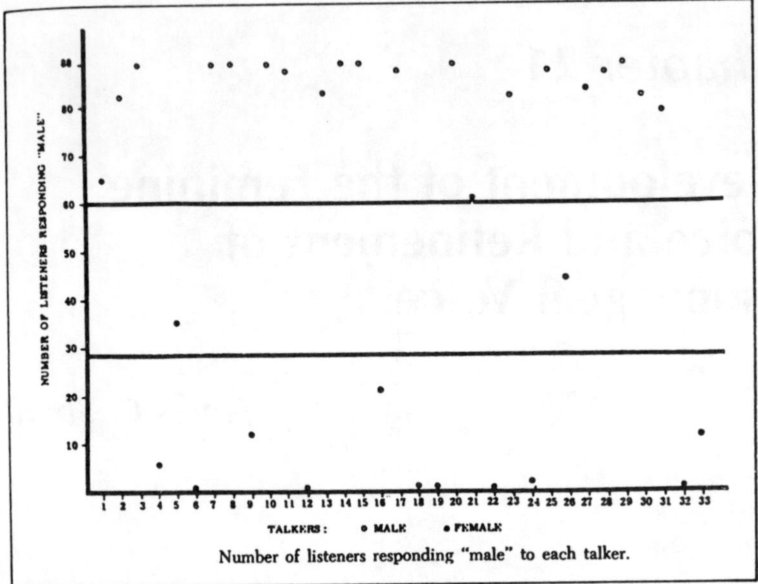

Figure 21–1. Perceived sex of esophageal speakers.

sentence of the ''Rainbow'' passage,* to 88 young adults, who were asked, on a forced choice basis, to identify the speaker as male or female. These judges identified the sex of the male speakers with 98 per cent accuracy but with only 80 per cent accuracy for the female speakers. It should be noted that this procedure combines 88 listeners and all speakers, that is, over 1,500 judgments of men and almost 1,300 judgments of women. Viewed graphically (Fig. 21–1) on a subject-by-subject basis, it may be seen that the men were uniformly identified as male speakers, but there was considerable scatter in the identification of the female speakers. Some, those six or seven at the very bottom of the scale, were almost never identified as male. Another four women had occasional identification as male speakers; two were more likely to be identified as male than as female.

Despite the previous report that both male and female esophageal talkers have an average fundamental frequency (F_O) in the neighborhood of 65 Hz, there is evidence that some individuals have a considerably higher fundamental frequency. For example, Snidecor (1968) found some

---

*From Fairbanks, G. (1960). *Voice and articulation drillbook,* 2nd ed. New York: Harper and Row, p. 127.

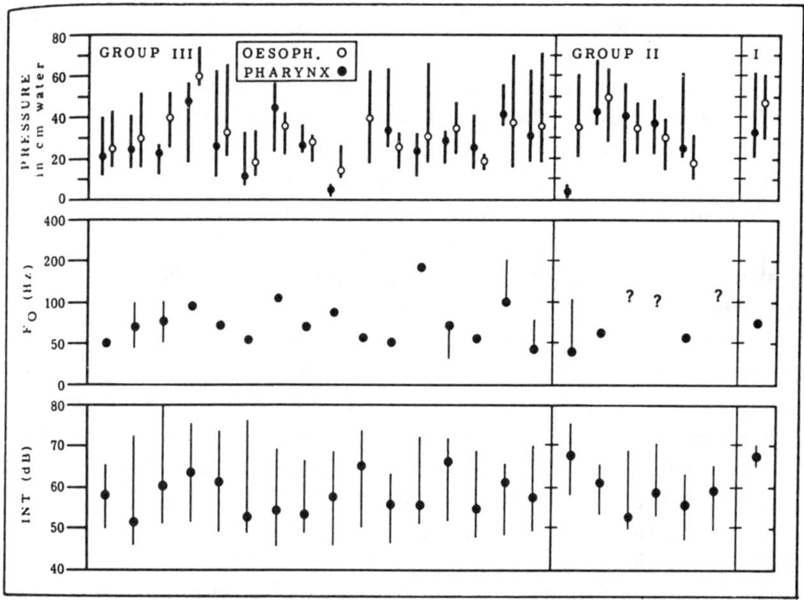

Figure 21–2. Pressure, voice characteristics of esophageal voice.

male speakers to reach 130 Hz. Shipp (1967) reported that one of his speakers reached 200 Hz, and in the data of Damsté (1958) (Fig. 21-2), again an individual F_O in the neighborhood of 200 Hz is seen. In another study, Weinberg and Bennett (1972) ascertained the fundamental frequency for females and males. Females had a mean of 28.87 semitones above 16.35 Hz. The males had a mean of only 21.74 semitones above base. The mean difference between sexes was significant at the 1 per cent level. This kind of evidence suggests that the female laryngectomee, if not the male, can be admonished to raise the fundamental frequency of her esophageal phonation. Parenthetically, the same admonition could be given to a speaker using an artificial larynx.

One of the subjects used in the Shipp study was a lady who had been a school teacher, was laryngectomized, and then obtained a new teaching position after laryngectomy. Her voice is, indeed, one of those identifiable as feminine in the series. As indicated in this woman's observation, the raising of her own fundamental frequency appeared to be related to an increase of tension in the area of the neoglottis. Such increased tension may be accompanied by a vertical elevation of the vibrator as seen radiographically from the side. Such an elevation was noted, for example, in the classic film *Oesophageal Speech* produced in the Netherlands in 1955 by van den Berg, Moolenaar-Bijl, and Damsté. Concomitantly, the voice will likely have a better quality if the intensity is reduced. Raising the pitch and lowering the loudness constitute a neat maneuver that often eludes the laryngeal speaker but is feasible.

However, just as mutational falsetto or effeminate voice is often not completely corrected by the mere act of lowering the fundamental frequency but requires some quality changes as well, so it is necessary to supplement work on pitch and loudness with additional maneuvers designed to compensate, to enable the listener better to perceive the speaker as being feminine in voice and in toto. What kinds of compensatory efforts may be of help?

It is first suggested that the female laryngectomee study herself not only in the initial stages of voice acquisition but regularly and periodically throughout the use of alaryngeal voice. This may be accomplished by self-study alone; however, it may well involve periodic therapy with a clinician. In addition to periodic assessment and ongoing monitoring, there is a need for one more ingredient. That ingredient is illustrated in a story told by the late motion picture actor Bill Gargan about the musician who got off the bus in New York City with a violin case under his arm and asked a nearby beatnik, "Can you tell me how to get to Carnegie Hall?" The young man's reply was simple: "Practice, man, practice." Too often laryngectomees deem the use of esophageal speech in everyday situations as tantamount to practice. The problem is that day-to-day communication does not involve an objective assessment of the individual parameters that go into making that communication most effective. Specifically, a female laryngectomee ought to think, act, and dress in a feminine manner. This extends from the use of attractive jewelry for stoma cover to the way her hair is done, and to recognizing that she, by her mere presence, can command attention as a woman. These nonverbal aspects of the person contribute to the overall impression of acceptability in identification of the femininity of the speaker (Gilmore, 1974).

Another focus for improved voice should be development of a significant change in pitch in the form of inflection and step change. This may take the form of conscious practice on producing an isolated vowel "o" with rising or falling inflection. (Tape) It may include stress changes accomplished by emphasizing specific words within a phrase such as, "I like it." It may include specific practice in singing up the scale. The number of laryngectomees who have cultivated the capacity to sing is far too limited. Notice the specific pitch changes in the following tape samples. (Tape) Not only is a song an appropriate vehicle; even a jingle or a three-word phrase (e.g., Bev loves Bob) may suffice (Gandour, Weinberg, and Garzione, 1983).

Related to the matter of inflection and stress is the use of phrasing and rate. There is good evidence from the studies by Hoops and Noll (1969) and others that rate is highly correlated with acceptability of esophageal speech. Not only should the laryngectomee assess the rate at which she, or he, speaks, but she or he should make this assessment periodically to measure progress. In assessing rate, some significant variables are noted. Many laryngectomees have a greater than average proportion of speaking time devoted to silence, presumably related to air intake. For example, as a person who exhibited slower rate than average (about 100 words per minute [wpm]) and longer than average pauses, Bill Gargan did not have superior speech. However, his long pausetime was offset by Mr. Gargan's stage presence, his lack of being flustered or bothered by that pause, and, indeed, his apparent intent to use that long pause for dramatic effect. (Tape) In the totality of the time domain, not only time spent in silence, or pausing, but the duration of individual phrases and the duration of vowels matters. The speaker who is able to give sufficient duration to vowels will appear to be speaking at an acceptable rate, even when the word-per-minute data indicate otherwise.

Yet another area for the laryngectomee to study as a means of compensating has to do with perfecting articulation skills. Without belaboring the issue, it should be noted that the laryngectomee may have errors of omission, surd-sonant confusion (Connor, 1982), and certainly /h/ difficulty. Drills on specific consonants and vowels should be pursued assiduously and not discontinued too soon. Note the following example of a very feminine lady who does the impossible, producing not only /h/ in connected esophageal speech but in isolation. (Tape)

Another dimension of assistance to the laryngectomee may simply be to provide more than a visual clue to the listener. To look like a woman is one thing; it is another to be able to give a hint to the listener, particularly in a taped message or on the telephone. In answering the telephone, the speaker may well preface her remarks by saying, "Hello, this is Mrs. Smith." In working on quality, the speaker should attempt to find that combination of pitch level and loudness level that is comfortable and provides the greatest clarity. This may involve not only digital pressure, but a slight turn of the head to one side, a posture that can be carried off without being obstrusive to the observer. Finally, it should be noted that acceptability, intelligibility, and the approximation of normality of the female alaryngeal voice must be accompanied by freedom from distracting auditory and visual mannerisms such as stoma noise, undue thump of air intake, visual grimace, and shoulder heaving.

In discussing procedures for improving voice and speech it should be acknowledged that the speaker would hope to avoid certain physical obstacles. Foremost among these is significant hearing loss. If the speaker has a substantial hearing impairment, the entire process of self-improvement is impeded. It is just more difficult for the speaker to monitor and to modify output. Second, it is to be hoped that the speaker would be free of the physical stigmata of a pharyngeal pouch, noted by Damsté (1958) to be associated with poor quality, with a long tortuous fibrotic pharyngoesophageal junction often resulting from extensive radiation. It is to be hoped that the person would be free of significant added surgery involving the removal of significant portions of the tongue, palate, or pharynx. To say that it is to be hoped that these obstacles can be avoided is merely to acknowledge that they may occur, as well as to acknowledge their possible interference with the attainment of voice improvement.

After having pursued a number of avenues in an effort to compensate for lower than average pitch, a female laryngectomee needs to consider two other changes: changing the environment to reduce the penalty and changing the speaker's attitude. Under the heading of environmental changes would be to draw from a listener's feedback how understandable and acceptable alaryngeal speech is. When the female speaker talks to someone, she should not accept the social nod, implying that her speech was understood. She should ask questions such as, ''What did I say?'' and even throw in questions that might be out of context and misleading, such as, ''What color is the sky?'' By employing the listener, the speaker not only improves her ability to monitor her speech but helps the listener to understand better.

Another suggestion is to have a phone amplifier installed to permit reduced loudness of speech production without sacrificing perceived loudness or intelligibility. For many laryngectomees this will not be needed because the instrument already will eliminate the need for louder speech. Further, female laryngectomized speakers should avoid situations involving considerable noise, if at all possible. If a large noisy group is in a room, a listener should be steered to a relatively quiet corner. If need be, the speaker must try to overarticulate so that she may even be lip-read in lieu of being heard. And, finally, if need be, an artificial larynx or written communication can substitute for an attempt to talk loudly with esophageal voice. The female laryngectomee must not succumb to the urge to override the ambient noise level. Another possibility is the exploration of the use of a hearing aid for a hard-of-hearing spouse or relative. A female laryngectomee may be penalized by her husband's hearing loss. However, that is *his* problem. For example, the father of one laryngectomee was so hard of hearing that the laryngectomee felt compelled to speak loudly, to the detriment of his own voice and speech.

Virtually every suggestion given to a woman to make her esophageal voice sound more feminine could be heeded by a man to improve the quality of his voice and speech. Indeed, many of the suggestions made are applicable to the individual male or female who is using an artificial larynx. Finally, time is necessary in which to accomplish all of the refinements and development hoped for.

As the female laryngectomee accepts herself as a person, as a speaker, and as one who is in process of improving her esophageal voice and speech, she gains convictions and behavior that others perceive as femininity, with or without low pitch. Even a "Tallulah" (Lanpher, 1965) can be feminine.

QUESTIONS

1. Comment on the likelihood of a male laryngectomee being confused for a female and of a female laryngectomee being confused for a male on the basis of the sound of the speaker's voice.
2. Shanks recommends at least two factors related to pitch that might contribute to more accurate identification of female speakers. What are these factors?
3. Articulation development is encouraged by Shanks. Do you think female speakers should give more attention to this factor of excellence than male speakers?
4. What advice does Shanks give regarding cuing the listener on the telephone as to the sex of the speaker?

REFERENCES

Connor, N. P. (1982). *Physiological correlates of consonant confusions in esophageal speech: Clinical applications.* Unpublished thesis, University of Maryland, College Park, MD.

Damsté, P. D. (1958). *Oesophageal speech after laryngectomy.* Gronigen: Hoistema.

Gandour, J., Weinberg, B., and Garzione, B. (1983). Perception of lexical stress in alaryngeal speech. *J. Speech Hearing Res., 26,* 418–424.

Gilmore, S. I. (1974). Social and vocational acceptability of esophageal speakers compared to normal speakers. *J. Speech Hearing Res., 17,* 599–607.

Hoops, H. R., and Noll, J. D. (1969). Relationship of selected acoustic variables to judgments of esophageal speech. *J. Comm. Dis., 2,* 1–13.

Lanpher, A. G. (1965). "Hello Tallulah" in *The Climate is Hope* (pp. 34–50). Englewood Cliffs, NJ: Prentice-Hall.

Shipp, T. (1967). Frequency, duration, and perceptual measures in relation to judgments of alaryngeal speech acceptability. *J. Speech Hearing Res., 10,* 417–427.

Snidecor, J. C. (1968). *Speech rehabilitation of the laryngectomized* (2nd ed.). Springfield, IL: Charles C Thomas.

Weinberg, B., and Bennett, S. (1971). A study of talker sex recognition of esophageal voices. *J. Speech Hearing Res., 14,* 391–395.

Weinberg, B., and Bennett, S. (1972). Selected acoustic characteristics of esophageal speech produced by female laryngectomees. *J. Speech Hearing Res., 15,* 211–216.

Chapter 22

Pre- and Postoperative Conferences with the Laryngectomized and Their Spouses

Shirley J. Salmon

When surveying the literature associated with the topic, "Counseling of the Laryngectomee," it is possible to read 30 to 40 articles written by medical doctors, nurses, psychologists, laryngectomees, and speech pathologists. The thoughts expressed in such articles typically reflect a professional or personal bias, or both. Consequently, opinions differ regarding what should be said and who should say it. This author used to believe these opinions were important but is not so convinced any more. It is of little concern whether most of the information is provided pre- or postoperatively and even of less concern who has the right to provide special segments of it. The only matter of importance is that the laryngectomee and spouse receive information that is as accurate and complete as they wish it to be.

This change in thinking occurred about 4 years ago after the author evaluated responses to a questionnaire survey of laryngectomees and their spouses. The questionnaire was designed to determine what their personal experiences had been with pre- and postoperative counseling and how they felt about them. Some of the information obtained from their responses follows.

Sixty-six of the 100 laryngectomees who received the questionnaires completed and returned them; this is considered a high percentage of response. Respondents were from 17 states. The number of spouses of laryngectomees who returned questionnaires was 53 and represented 15 states.

The average age of the laryngectomees, 12 females and 54 males, was 59 years, whereas the average age of the spouses, 7 males and 46 females, was 57 years.

Eight of the laryngectomees were single, whereas 58 were married. The average length of time the couples had lived together since laryngectomy was 5 years.

Forty-two per cent (22) of the spouses reported they had children still living at home when the laryngectomy was performed. In such homes, the average number of children was two. The ages of these children ranged from 3 to 25 years, with an average age of 13 years. Sixty per cent of the spouses were working full- or part-time prior to the laryngectomy. However, at the time of the survey, only 47 per cent were working. This decrease in employment of spouses is interesting to consider. Remember that the average age of the spouses was 57 years, so it may be related to factors other than retirement age.

When removal of the larynx was first recommended by the surgeon, 72 per cent (38) of the spouses were present. As you might expect, several of the spouses (11, or 21 per cent) reacted to the news with "sheer fright."

Their most immediate concerns were (1) whether their spouses would live through surgery (16, or 28 per cent) and (2) whether they would be cured of cancer (10, or 17 per cent). After having a little time to think about the upcoming surgery, they worried about whether their spouses would learn to talk (9, or 16 per cent), how they would react to surgery, and what effect it would have on their morale (7, or 13 per cent). Some, who apparently had *no* information about methods of alaryngeal speech, wondered how their laryngectomized spouses would adjust to not having a voice (8, or 14 per cent).

PREOPERATIVE CONTACTS

All but one of the laryngectomees had at least one preoperative hospital contact with their doctor. Some, perhaps those receiving cobalt prior to surgery, had as many as 30. The average number of contacts was 4 and the average number of minutes per contact was 17. Seventy-seven per cent (41) of the spouses were present during an average of three such conferences.

Forty-five per cent (30) of the laryngectomees reported preoperative contacts with nurses. The mean number of such contacts was ten, each of which lasted an average of 5 minutes. Thus, it would seem that those scheduled for laryngectomy see nurses more frequently than their surgeons but for briefer periods of time. Regrettably, 83 per cent of the spouses reported not being present during such contacts.

Only about one third of the laryngectomees (21, or 32 per cent) reported preoperative contacts with speech pathologists, esophageal speakers, artificial larynx speakers, or spouses of other laryngectomees. They saw speech pathologists (19, or 29 per cent), esophageal speakers (21, or 32 percent) or both much more often than they saw artificial larynx speakers (5, or 8 per cent) or spouses of laryngectomees (8, or 12 per cent). More than 80 per cent of the spouses were not present during any of these contacts, so again, as with nursing contacts, spouses are evidently being neglected preoperatively by the rehabilitation team.

The inference is that doctors and, to a lesser extent, nurses are providing most of the information preoperatively; consideration of what they reportedly are saying follows.

PREOPERATIVE INFORMATION

More than half of the patients (45, or 68 per cent) indicated that their doctors discussed *only* the surgical procedure. Thirty-six per cent (24) were told about the pathologic condition, were told that the surgery was a lifesaving procedure, were given information related to prognosis, or any of these. Fewer than one third of the patients (19, or 29 per cent) were provided additional information by their doctor or the nurses.

The patients who saw an esophageal speaker or a speech pathologist—and remember that they represent fewer than one third of the laryngectomees surveyed—most frequently were told that they would have to communicate at first by writing and later learn to use an artificial larynx or esophageal speech. Less frequently they were given information pamphlets such as those published by the American Cancer Society (ACS).

Are you becoming uncomfortable with the idea that these patients reported having received such a dearth of information? Spouses received even less information. *Almost* half (25, or 47 per cent) were given information from doctors about the surgical procedure, the prognosis, and the likelihood of the patient's being able to resume most activities. Only 25 per cent (13) of the spouses were given any other information from surgeons or nurses prior to surgery.

PREPARATION FOR SURGERY

In view of the information they received, you may be interested in how the laryngectomees and spouses felt about their preparation for the surgery.

Thirty-three per cent (22) of the laryngectomees felt "well prepared," whereas only 13 per cent (7) of the spouses did so. Twenty-three per cent (15) of the laryngectomees felt "adequately prepared," whereas 15 per cent (8) of the spouses felt that way. Forty-four per cent (29) of the laryngectomees felt "poorly prepared," felt "not prepared at all," or refused to comment. Almost the same percentage (45 per cent, or 24) of the spouses felt "poorly prepared" or "not at all prepared." Seven spouses (13 per cent) suggested that, "You don't miss what you don't know about," four (8 per cent) indicated that they "avoided talking or thinking about the surgery," and three (6 per cent) wrote that they felt all right about surgery "because they trusted in the Lord."

WHOM WOULD YOU LIKE TO SEE?

When these respondents were asked whom they would like to have seen prior to surgery, the laryngectomees listed in order of preference a laryngectomee, an esophageal speaker, a counselor, a speech pathologist, a member of the New Voice Club, and an ACS representative.

Spouses listed in order of preference a spouse of a laryngectomee, a laryngectomee, the surgeon, an esophageal speaker, a speech pathologist, and a minister.

WHAT PREOPERATIVE INFORMATION SHOULD BE GIVEN?

When they were asked what information they believe others should have prior to surgery, the laryngectomees listed numerous items.

The most frequently occurring was "information about the different ways to communicate after surgery." Next, listed in order of frequency, were (1) the surgical procedure, (2) the prognosis, and (3) the anatomical and physiological changes associated with such functions as laughing and coughing, the feeding tube, the swallowing problems, the stoma, the mucus, the impaired sense of taste and smell, the inability to blow the nose or to sneeze, and the altered physical appearance. Many also listed encouragement such as the following: (1) being visited by a laryngectomee, (2) being told that an artificial larynx can be used, (3) hearing that it is possible to resume a normal life with few exceptions, (4) being told that there are various avenues open for financial assistance, (5) learning that most can return to work, (6) being reassured that the surgery is virtually painless, (7) being told that they must be patient with themselves following the surgery, and (8) being assured that they will in some way learn to cope with the aftereffects of it.

Two unique suggestions were (1) to provide the laryngectomee and the spouse with an opportunity to attend a meeting with members of the rehabilitation team that includes a laryngectomee and, then, let them ask their questions, and (2) to prepare a written abstract to be left with the patient and spouse that outlines the most important information typically mentioned during conversations with each contact person on the rehabilitation team.

Spouses believed that the most important preoperative information other spouses should receive is that associated with physical aspects: (1) details of the operation, its urgency, and the seriousness of it; (2) the anticipated outcome and prognosis; (3) what to expect the laryngectomee to look like in the intensive care unit (ICU); and (4) how to care for him or her during the immediate postoperative period when nurses are not available. They wanted to be told about the feeding tube, the stoma, the mucus, the breathing difficulties, that the coughing sound was "normal," and, particularly, about how to use the suction machine. Other information they thought important to receive was how to cope with the patient's immediate reactions, change in outlook, depression, need for support, and their own mental strain and tendency to encourage dependency. Finally, they believed that spouses should be told about the various ways to communicate after a laryngectomy and should be given some estimate of the length of time it might take to acquire esophageal speech. They also stressed the desire for a visit from a laryngectomee and from the spouse of a laryngectomee.

When spouses were asked to list the information they would impart privately to another spouse whose mate was about to undergo laryngectomy, they offered advice instead: (1) be patient, loving, and kind; (2) pray a lot; (3) seek religious counseling; (4) stress the chance for cure; (5) take one day at a time; (6) assure the laryngectomee that it will not change your relationship; and (7) be optimistic about alaryngeal speech. The only information that they would impart is that concerning the physical appearance of the laryngectomee immediately following surgery.

By far the most difficult time for spouses to endure is waiting through the surgery without having information about prognosis and without receiving any information about how the surgery is going or the outcome of the surgery until late in the afternoon or into the evening. Other items mentioned less frequently were (1) not knowing how to help the laryngectomee when he or she was emotionally upset preoperatively and when he or she was expressing the desire to die, (2) not knowing how to cope with feeling so alone in the waiting room and nobody seeming to care, and (3) being shocked at all of the tubes in the ICU and feeling that their very presence meant for certain that their spouse was going to die.

A summary of the information obtained from this survey can be begun by stating that the information given to laryngectomees and their spouses most frequently is being provided by surgeons. It would seem from the reports that surgeons focus almost entirely on the surgical procedure. Nurses represent the professional group seen next most frequently by laryngectomees and their spouses. Preoperatively, they also seem to discuss only aspects associated with the surgical procedure itself. Apparently speech pathologists are seeing fewer than half of the laryngectomees and their spouses preoperatively.

The laryngectomees from this survey indicated that, preoperatively, they would have liked to have been given much more information than was provided. They believe laryngectomees should understand the surgical procedure and the associated anatomical and physiological changes associated with it. In addition, they believe laryngectomees should be told about the survival rate, the fact that there are ways to communicate after surgery *including* use of an artificial larynx, that many laryngectomees can return to their former employment, and that various kinds of financial assistance are available to them. They want to be encouraged by having someone tell them they will experience very little pain from the surgery itself, that they must be patient with themselves, that they will learn to cope with the aftereffects of surgery, and that it is possible to resume a near-normal life. They believe it is desirable to receive a visit from a well-rehabilitated laryngectomee. Finally, they recommend that preoperative information, which is usually given orally during face-to-face conferences, be supplemented with printed material that can be studied and shared with their families at a later time.

Spouses from this survey indicated they wanted most for someone to talk to them preoperatively. They think spouses should be told about the surgical procedure, the seriousness of the operation, and the necessity for it. They, like their mates, believe it is important to have information about survival rates. They recommend that spouses be warned about the appearance of their mates immediately following surgery in ICU. They think spouses should be advised how to cope with the depression and other psychological reactions demonstrated by their mates prior to surgery. They also believe spouses should be told about ways to communicate postoperatively and about how they might help with immediate postoperative care.

The introduction of the topic of postoperative counseling leads to a discussion of what these patients and spouses thought about the adequacy of the postoperative information they received.

All but two of the laryngectomees reported postoperative visits with their surgeons. In general their contacts with the doctor postoperatively were more numerous but averaged shorter time periods. The number of contacts ranged from 0 to 150 with a mean of 17 contacts, compared with four contacts preoperatively. The average number of minutes per contact was reduced from 17 minutes preoperatively to 13 minutes postoperatively. Seventy-five per cent (40) of the spouses reported postoperative contacts with the surgeon. The average number of their contacts was six, compared with the average of three contacts postoperatively.

As would be expected, most of the laryngectomees (57, or 86 per cent) reported more contacts with their nurses. Contacts ranged from 1 to 300, with a mean of 23, compared with the average of 10 reported preoperatively. Also, the average number of minutes per contact increased from 5 minutes preoperatively to about 8 minutes postoperatively. The average number of contacts that spouses reported having preoperatively was 9, compared with 10 (10.06) postoperatively.

More than half of the laryngectomees and almost half of their spouses reported *postoperative* contacts with speech pathologists, esophageal speakers, artificial larynx speakers, or spouses of rehabilitated laryngectomees. More than three times as many contacts were with speech pathologists or esophageal speakers than with the other two groups. The average number of contacts with speech pathologists was six and with esophageal speakers, two. The average number of minutes taken for each of the conferences was 17 minutes with esophageal speakers and 16 minutes with speech pathologists.

POSTOPERATIVE INFORMATION

The postoperative information most frequently received by laryngectomees was that "they could learn to speak again." The next most frequent information provided was that concerning a general description of current physical status and self-care, particularly of the stoma. Only four laryngectomees were provided information about New Voice Clubs and the same number, four, were assured they could lead an essentially normal life.

Three were given an estimate about when they could return to work. One or two laryngectomees were assured that the surgeon removed all of the cancer, were told how to obtain emergency help at home if necessary, were advised not to become constipated, and were warned to avoid use of aerosol sprays. Only one laryngectomee was presented with a written schedule of upcoming appointments with both the surgeon and the speech pathologist.

Thirteen of the fifty-three spouses (25 per cent) indicated they did not receive *any* postoperative information. The most frequent type of information provided to those spouses who *did* receive some was about the various types of alaryngeal speech. Several spouses expressed disappointment in not being advised about how to help care for their spouses at home. Some suggested that one reason for their not being provided with this type of information was that the nurses themselves did not seem to know.

WHAT POSTOPERATIVE INFORMATION SHOULD BE GIVEN?

When laryngectomees were asked to list the information they would like to have been given or that they would impart to other laryngectomees, they showed high agreement on three items. First, they suggested that it is important for the newly laryngectomized to hear that it is possible to learn to talk again; second, that there is a good chance of cure; and third, that the recovery from surgery is or is not progressing at a normal rate. Other items mentioned frequently were (1) a visit from a laryngectomee and spouse (one fellow mentioned he wanted to see a well-healed stoma); (2) an explanation of how esophageal speech is produced; (3) an estimate of the length of time it takes to acquire esophageal speech; (4) where therapy can be obtained and the approximate cost; (5) a written explanation of self-care and what to expect as normal, such as bloody mucus, impaired taste and smell, less stamina and less strength; and *finally,* (6) a demonstration for the family showing procedures to follow for mouth-to-stoma resuscitation.

Spouses believe other spouses should be told how to take care of their mates' stoma problems, how to cope with their mates' depression, and how to make communication easier between the two of them. One spouse indicated that she would suggest having an extension phone installed in the home so that when the laryngectomee first arrived home he could listen in on phone conversations with friends and relatives.

When asked to list some of the more difficult situations for them after the surgery but before hospital discharge, spouses agreed that "attempts to communicate" were the most difficult. The second most frequently mentioned item was "not knowing what to expect in terms of coughing and suctioning" and so not knowing how to help care for the patient when he or she was in distress and the nurses were not available. One spouse mentioned feeling so lonely because of the imposed silence, and another mentioned that she was frightened by her husband's sudden dependency on her.

ADVICE ON WHAT TO DO AT HOME

When spouses were asked to indicate some things they thought should be mentioned to a spouse after hospital discharge when the laryngectomee is at home, numerous items were mentioned. Some of the most frequent were (1) be patient; (2) resist the urge to "baby" him or her, (3) provide lots of love and encouragement; (4) help him or her to practice his speech lessons and encourage him or her to use speech as much as possible; (5) maintain social life as previously; (6) continue as before as much as possible; (7) help the laryngectomee stay busy; (8) try to understand how each other feels; (9) pay closer attention during attempts to communicate; (10) expect flare-ups and depression; (11) phrase conversation for "yes" and "no" answers; (12) try not to panic when he or she cannot swallow or is having trouble breathing; (13) be as cheerful as possible; (14) remember that no matter what people say, your spouse will no longer be able to do some of the things he did before, for example, swim, blow his nose, laugh, sip his coffee, and drink through a straw; (15) obtain a humidifier because it is essential; and (16) look forward to better days ahead.

PROBLEM AREAS

When spouses were asked to look at a list of potential problem areas and to indicate which, if any, they thought were problems for them and their mate as a direct result of the laryngectomy, they rank-ordered the areas, from greatest problem to least, as follows:

Speech communication
Social
Psychological
Employment
Sexual
Alcohol
Financial
Family
Marital

None of the spouses indicated religious problems.

A summary of the main points from these responses indicates that laryngectomees believe patients should be told their chance for cure and whether their recovery is or is not progressing at a normal rate. They believe laryngectomees should be given information about the different methods of alaryngeal speech, how to acquire an artificial larynx, how esophageal speech is produced, where they can obtain speech therapy, and how much it costs. They suggest a visit from a laryngectomee and a spouse, and finally, they recommend that printed materials be prepared to remind laryngectomees of self-care procedures when they go home and to warn them about the everyday occurrences at home, such as swallowing difficulties, stoma crusting, and choking sensations about which they need not become overly alarmed.

Spouses recommended postoperative information be provided about the feeding tube, the suction machine, and the humidifier. They suggested preparing spouses for the unusual coughing sound and excess mucus. They proposed that spouses receive advice about how to cope with their mates' and their own psychological reactions to the effects of surgery. Finally, they recommend that spouses receive instructions about ways to make communication easier with their mates.

Data such as these that have been obtained from a questionnaire survey must be interpreted with some degree of caution. Admittedly, laryngectomees whose names are available on mailing lists such as for the International Association of Laryngectomees (I.A.L.) probably represent a biased sample. Use of averages cancels out extremes and factors such as memory, individual experiences, learning difficulties, and time lapse. Consequently, it seems that specific numbers or percentages from this questionnarie should not be quoted to justify one or another position, but that they should instead be examined for indications of general trends. When used in this broader sense, the responses can help identify the topics speech clinicians might want to emphasize during pre- and postoperative conferences.

If you accept my interpretation of the survey responses, you may find useful the "Check List" (Fig. 22–1) handout developed by Barbara Cady and me. It helps us provide consistent service from one patient to another. If you will refer to it now, I would like to make some specific comments about a few of the items noted. Space prevents a discussion of all of them.

When I review the patient's medical chart, I am interested in pinpointing factors that may influence my interactions with the patient postoperatively. For instance, if radiation or cobalt was administered prior to surgery, it is likely that the neck tissue will take longer to heal and that sutures may more easily pull loose following surgery. Consequently, there is greater likelihood of a fistula or hard necrotic tissue postoperatively that may necessitate cheek placement of an electronic neck-type artificial larynx or use of an intraoral device. A history of pulmonary disorders such as emphysema or asthma may significantly reduce pulmonary function or cause excessive accumulation of mucus. In such an instance use of a pneumatic-type artificial larynx would be contraindicated, and the likelihood of excess stoma noise during esopha-

CHECKLIST FOR PRE- AND POSTOPERATIVE
LARYNGECTOMEE CONSULTATIONS

Barbara B. Cady, M.A., and Shirley J. Salmon, Ph.D.
Veterans Administration Hospital
Kansas City, Missouri

Patient's Name: ____

	Date Completed	*By Whom*
I. Preoperative Consultation with Patient		
A. Review medical chart	__________	______
B. The patient and spouse	__________	______
C. Facts the couple can relate about the upcoming surgery	__________	______
D. Alternatives for postoperative communication	__________	______
E. Services provided by speech-language pathologist and Karam and Gray's handout	__________	______
F. Postoperative appointment	__________	______
G. Referral to counselor	__________	______
H. Consultation report written and placed in medical chart	__________	______
I. If needed, investigate referral sources for alaryngeal speech therapy	__________	______
II. Postoperative Consultation with Patient		
A. First Visit		
1. Selected literature from American Cancer Society given to patient	__________	______
2. Various types of stoma shield shown to patient	__________	______
3. Stoma shield literature given to patient	__________	______
4. Letter written to IAL and to New Voice Club to place patient's name on newsletter mailing lists	__________	______
5. Medic Alert information discussed: "Neck breather" to be engraved on back of bracelet and printed on billfold card	__________	______
6. Visit recorded in medical chart	__________	______
B. Second Visit		
1. Discuss literature provided at first visit	__________	______
2. Film, *To Speak Again,* and Mark 4 projector to patient's room	__________	______

      3. Alaryngeal speaker and spouse visits scheduled   __________   __________

      4. Head nurse notified of visits   __________   __________

      5. Visit recorded in medical chart   __________   __________

  C. Third Visit

      1. Pick up projector and film; answer questions   __________   __________

      2. Show the patient a videotape, demonstrate artificial larynx devices, or both   __________   __________

      3. Visit recorded in medical chart   __________   __________

  D. Other Visits

      1. Discuss visits from alaryngeal speakers and spouses   __________   __________

      2. Begin instructions in the use of an artificial larynx   __________   __________

      3. Recommend and, when possible, issue an artificial larynx device   __________   __________

      4. Loan patient "Self Help for Laryngectomees," "Looking Forward," and "Hello, Tallulah"   __________   __________

      5. Refer for physial therapy   __________   __________

      6. Schedule patient as an outpatient   __________   __________

      7. Record each visit in medical chart   __________   __________

Figure 22–1. Checklist for pre- and postoperative consultations created by Barbara B. Cady and Shirley J. Salmon, Veterans Administration Hospital, Kansas City, Missouri.

geal speech is increased. Ulcers or hiatal hernia may be irritated with attempts to acquire esophageal speech or may impede the ability to do so. Those who are alcohol- and drug-dependent may demonstrate less motivation or ability to carry out the instructions and drills necessary for acquiring good alaryngeal speech.

When I first visit with the patient and spouse, I try to observe whether their speech discrimination is adequate. I am interested in whether children are an integral part of their life, since many patients report that children are easier to communicate with first via alaryngeal speech. I ask whether the patient intends to return to work and about his work environment. I try to discern whether he is a "big talker" or a "man of few words" and whether he has heard alaryngeal speech. Finally, I must ascertain whether he is literate and, if so, provide him with a communication booklet.

To determine what information the patient and spouse can relate about the surgery, I begin by asking them questions such as, "What has your doctor told you about the surgery?'' *and* ''What have the nurses told you?'' If they seem to understand some of the concepts but have misconceptions about others, I try to reinforce their correct ideas and to explain why the others are not correct. I use layman's terminology, lots of imagery, and sometimes, *simple* diagrams. In most instances I am probably reiterating what has already been said at least twice before, but I believe that each time it is said the patient and spouse have an opportunity to understand a little bit more of what they are about to undergo.

My *primary* purpose is fourfold. I believe the patient and spouse should understand that (1) the voice box will be removed and the patient will breathe through a permanent hole in the neck; consequently, it will be necessary to learn a new way to produce voice; (2) while the patient is recovering from laryngectomy he will be swollen around the neck and face areas, probably will be bandaged about the neck, will have a nasogastric tube in place, and will require suctioning from his new airway, the stoma; (3) there are alternate methods of alaryngeal communication with which the patient can soon become familiar; and (4) the speech clinic staff will be available as soon after surgery as the surgeon deems advisable and will return for the first postoperative visit on the fifth day following surgery.

Generally I terminate the conference by writing down my name and extension number and inviting them to notify me if they think of unanswered questions. Then I leave a handout prepared by Farid Karam, an otolaryngologist, and Eugene Gray, a speech pathologist (Karam and Gray, 1979). It was developed to communicate with patients about the medical, nursing, and alaryngeal speech aspects associated with laryngectomy and can be reviewed by them and family members at their leisure.

Most of the items under the Postoperative Consultation section are self-explanatory. I wish to make only two comments. The ''selected literature'' that we use from the American Cancer Society (ACS) includes *Helping Words for the Laryngectomee* (American Cancer Society, 1964), *Your New Voice* (Waldrop and Gould, 1969), and *First Aid for (Neck-Breathers) Laryngectomees* (American Cancer Society, 1971). Although some of the information in these pamphlets is outdated or biased in favor of esophageal speech, we believe the good information outweighs the bad. These pamphlets are free from ACS and even now are being revised by the International Association of Laryngectomees (I.A.L.) to reflect more accurately current attitudes.

I began this presentation by saying that my primary concern is that laryngectomees and their spouses receive information that is as accurate and complete as they wish it to be. There is an abundance of information that we need to provide them in incremented steps over time. In this chapter I have focused only on that which should be given priority during the pre- and immediate postoperative period. I hope you will find my suggestions helpful.

QUESTIONS

1. What percent of laryngectomees have preoperative contact with individuals knowledgeable about postoperative speech methods?
2. According to Salmon's survey, what areas of information might you raise with spouses in order to allay their concerns?
3. What information seems important to the laryngectomees before their operation that might be contributed by specialists in speech rehabilitation?
4. Draft an outline of the content of a postoperative visit that you might be called on to make.
5. What changes would you make to the "Check List"?

REFERENCES

First aid for (neck-breathers) laryngectomees. (1971). New York: American Cancer Society.
Helping words for the laryngectomee. (1964). New York: American Cancer Society.
Karam, F., and Gray, E. (1979). *Total laryngectomy: Patient information.* Bay Pines, FL: VA Medical Center.
Keith, R. L., Shane, H. C., Coates, H. L. C., and Devine, K. D. (1977). *Looking forward—A guidebook for the laryngectomee.* Rochester, MN: Mayo Foundation.
Lanpher, A. (1967). "Hello Tallulah," in *The Climate Is Hope,* by W. Ross. Reproduced by New York: American Cancer Society.
Lauder, E. (1978). *Self-help for the laryngectomee.* Antonio, TX: Author.
To Speak Again [Film]. (1967). New York: American Cancer Society.
Waldrop, W., and Gould, M. (1969). *Your new voice.* New York: American Cancer Society.

Chapter 23

Factors in the Choice of Treatment of Patients with Laryngeal Cancer

H. Bryan Neel, III, and Lawrence W. DeSanto

Squamous cell carcinoma of the larynx is the most frequent cancer involving the upper air and food passages. Glottic cancers—those arising on the true vocal folds—constitute about 75 per cent of all laryngeal cancers. Hoarseness almost invariably occurs with the development of glottic cancer; therefore, glottic cancer often can be diagnosed while the tumor is still small and confined to the vocal folds. Because the diagnosis can be made early, treatment can be expected to be successful.

Cancers that arise in other regions of the larynx, the supraglottis, and the subglottis—that is, above or below the true vocal folds—often give no early warning. Symptoms develop after the tumors have become large. Such patients complain of a vague sore throat, referred ear pain, a lump in the neck due to metastasis, difficulty in swallowing, or hoarseness if the tumor has enlarged to the extent that it has spread to the vocal folds.

More than 80 per cent of the patients in whom squamous cell carcinoma of the larynx develops are or have been cigarette smokers. Such patients are at a higher risk than a comparable nonsmoking population for the development of other primary cancers that can be related to smoking, namely carcinoma of the lung, mouth, tongue, lip, bladder, pancreas, and esophagus.

DIAGNOSIS AND STAGING

Indirect (mirror) laryngoscopy in the office is the usual method of diagnosis and the principal source of information used in planning treatment. A complete head and neck (otorhinolaryngological) examination is done after a thorough history has been elicited from the patient. Direct laryngoscopy is required for biopsy and histopathological confirmation by a pathologist; at the same time, the extent of the tumor can be determined in more detail. Clearly, vocal cord mobility is best assessed in the office. Rarely are tomographic roentgenograms or contrast laryngography needed. The authors cannot recall a single instance in which a primary cancer of the larynx was discovered by a roentgenographic examination.

The clinical staging of cancer of the larynx—the system developed by the American Joint Committee for Cancer Staging and End-Results Reporting—provides a basis for predicting the effectiveness of various forms of treatment and comparing results from various medical centers. It incorporates the surgeon's clinical appraisal of the size and site of the primary tumor, the presence or absence of metastases to the neck, a rough estimate of the amount of disease in the neck, and the presence or absence of distant spread. The system does *not* take into account several other important considerations used in determining an approach to treatment, namely the patient's general health, age, sex, occupation, reliability, motivation, and preference; nor does it incorporate the skill and experience of the surgeon, radiotherapist, surgical pathologist, speech pathologist, and associated personnel.

TYPES OF TREATMENT

Conservation surgery—that surgery designed to spare a functional portion of the larynx—is carried out in carefully selected patients who have either glottic or supraglottic tumors. However, it is important to emphasize that in many patients it is not safe to carry out partial laryngectomy. Preservation of a functional larynx (or part of it) is important, but life itself is more important. Total laryngectomy is necessary for the eradication of cancer in more that 30 per cent of all patients the authors see, and it is the "gold standard" in patients with laryngeal cancer that is too far advanced for partial laryngectomy. In many centers, radiation therapy is employed for almost all patients, but it has been found that for most tumors surgery in the form of partial or total laryngectomy, with or without neck dissection, leads to better survival and is more "cost effective." In some instances, combinations of surgery, irradiation, and chemotherapy lead to a better outcome.

SELECTION OF TREATMENT

Selection of treatment of patients with laryngeal cancer is influenced by different attitudes. Each attitude has its advocates, and each advocate is armed with supporting statistics, some of which are often difficult to interpret. To summarize, the following are the various positions and treatment options:

1. Cancer of the larynx is a surgical disease and the only therapeutic decision is the choice of the operation.
2. Early cancers should be treated by external irradiation for cure, intermediate cancers should be dealt with surgically, and advanced cancers should be treated by a combination of irradiation and surgery.
3. Early and intermediate cancers should be irradiated, and surgery is employed only when the tumor cannot be controlled by radiation therapy. This is the "radiate and watch" method.
4. Treatment should be *individualized*. Selection of treatment is influenced largely by the type, location, and size of the primary tumor; the presence or absence of regional metastases (or the likelihood of regional metastases); and the general health of the patient. The availability of a surgical pathologist skilled in frozen-section diagnosis, the distance between treatment facilities and the patient's home, the likelihood of follow-up, the patient's occupation, and the patient's preference also influence the selection of treatment. With individualization of treatment, any forms of conventional treatment (radiation, conservation surgery, laryngectomy, and chemotherapy) may be used, and the form of treatment recommended for a given patient is based on an estimate of the probability of success and an analysis of the many factors that have been noted above. (This is the approach the authors' group takes.)

QUESTIONS

1. What portion of laryngeal cancers do not reveal themselves by hoarseness?
2. What method does the physician use to investigate whether a patient might have laryngeal cancer?
3. Why does the American Joint Committee for Cancer Staging and End-Results Reporting recommend a staging of laryngeal cancer?
4. What does "conservation surgery" mean?
5. Treatment by surgery and radiation therapy combined is given under what condition compared with radiation therapy alone?

Chapter 24

Physical and Occupational Therapy for the Patient With Laryngectomy: Why and What For?

Ann H. Schutt

In patients who have had radical neck resection in conjunction with laryngectomy, the disability that results from the resection, rather than the laryngectomy itself, necessitates physical and occupational therapy. With radical neck resection, the loss of important structures—the spinal accessory nerve as well as other motor nerves, sensory nerves, and muscles—leads to disability.

The neurological deficit may be due to neurapraxia, incomplete nerve lesions, or complete nerve lesions (Villanueva and Ajmani, 1977). These three forms of nerve lesions result in the same kind of shoulder dysfunction during the early postoperative course. With neurapraxia, full motor function of the trapezius muscle cannot be expected until approximately 6 to 9 months postoperatively. With incomplete nerve lesions, part of the nerve has lost its ability to transmit electrical activity, and denervation of a portion of a muscle or loss of the activity can result. The regrowth of the nerve may take months, and the weakness of the trapezius muscle can persist for as long as 18 months. The muscles of these patients need to be protected until there is little or no shoulder disability; this period usually lasts from 9 to 12 months. In the patient with incomplete nerve lesions, total muscle reinnervation will not take place before 18 to 24 months. Because of this denervation, there can be a loss of muscle mass and a resultant loss of muscular function. Stress placed on the muscle will cause overstretching and pronounced dysfunc-

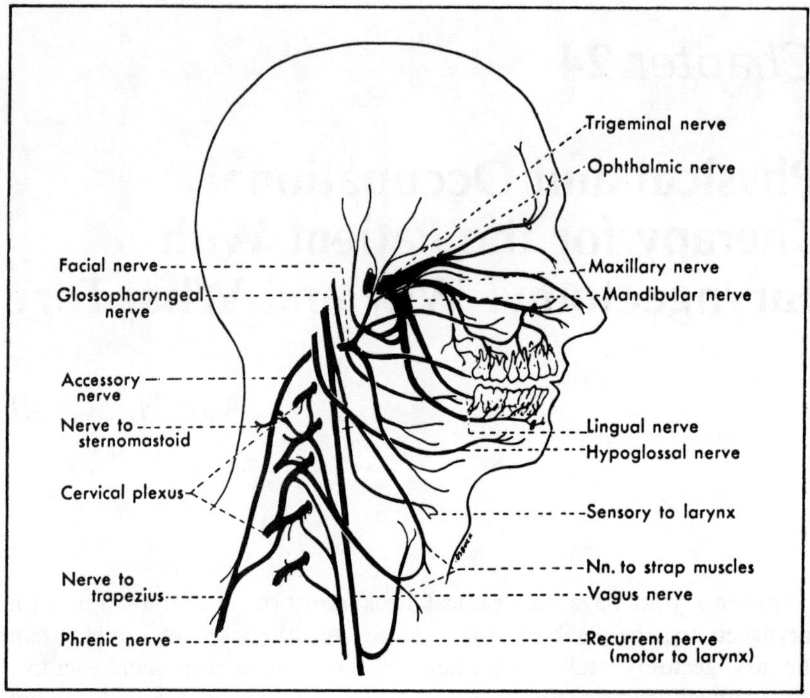

Figure 24–1. Nerves of the neck and face. (From Hollinshead, W. H. [1976]. *Functional anatomy of the limbs and back* [4th ed.] [p. 383]. Philadelphia: W. B. Saunders. By permission.)

tion. When the nerve and the muscle are completely sacrificed, education of the patient and strengthening of remaining structures to assume the role of the lost function are necessary.

The spinal accessory nerve innervates the trapezius muscle and is extremely important to shoulder function (Hollinshead, 1956) (Fig. 24-1). Its loss causes a great deal of disability. The spinal accessory nerve also innervates the sternocleidomastoid muscle. In a radical neck resection, the sternocleidomastoid muscle is sacrificed and the deeper neck muscles must be taught to rotate the neck (Fig. 24-2). The greater auricular and greater occipital nerves are responsible for the sensation in the lower scalp area, the posterosuperior part of the shoulder, the lateral and posterolateral cervical area, and the skin over the parotid gland and the auricle. Because these nerves are sacrificed with radical neck resection,

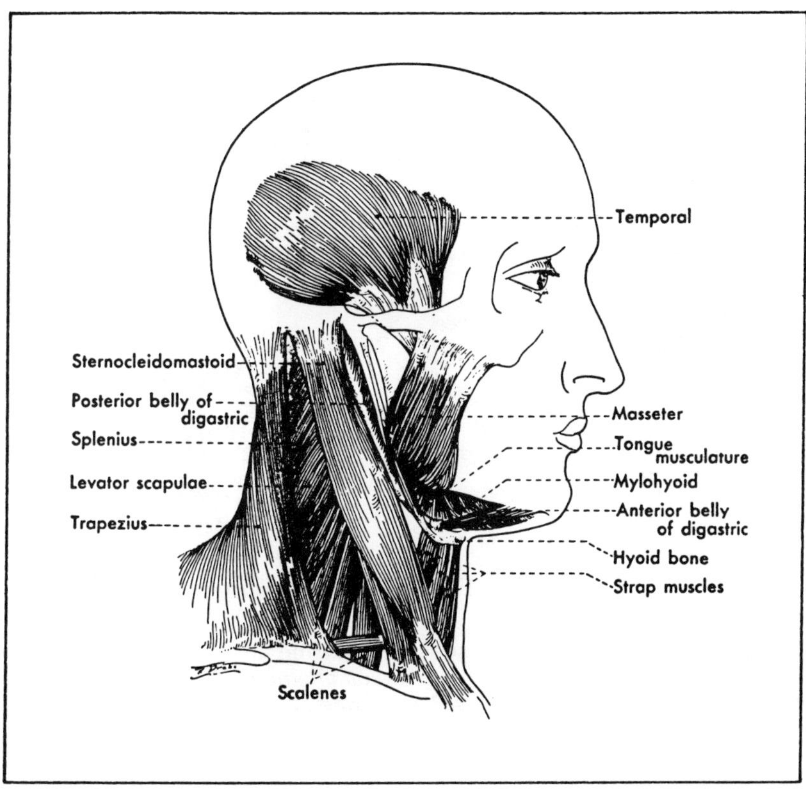

Figure 24–2. Muscles of the neck and head. (From Hollinshead, W. H. [1976]. *Functional anatomy of the limbs and back* [4th ed.] [p. 376]. Philadelphia: W. B. Saunders. By permission.)

sensation is lost in these areas and patients should be cautioned concerning the increased risk of burning, cutting, or injuring the remaining skin. Rarely there is damage to the phrenic or vagus nerve or to the brachial plexus at surgery. Usually the phrenic or vagus nerve is resected only when there is extensive involvement of the nerves by tumor.

Functional losses result from these anatomical losses. The trapezius muscle is responsible for stabilizing and smoothly rotating the scapula. This muscle has an important role in positioning the humerus optimally for abduction and flexion of the upper extremity. The loss of the spinal accessory nerve causes permanent paralysis of the trapezius muscle, resulting in a drooping, sagging shoulder. This muscle imbalance can cause overstretching of the remaining muscles (Fig. 24–3), mainly the levator scapulae and the rhomboids, with decreased range of motion of the shoul-

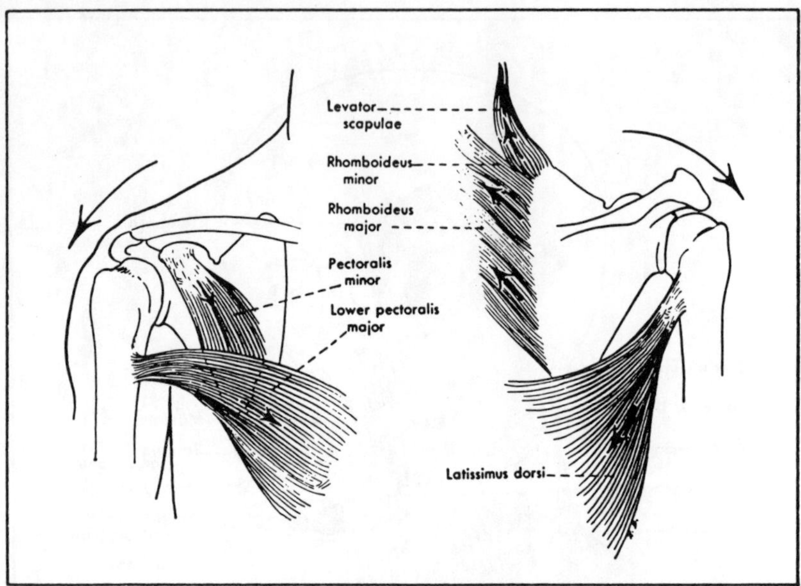

Figure 24–3. Muscles that can substitute for the absent trapezius muscle. (From Hollinshead, W. H. [1976]. *Functional anatomy of the limbs and back* [4th ed.] [p. 112]. Philadelphia: W. B. Saunders. By permission.)

der, decreased strength of the shoulder girdle, stretching of the posterior muscles, and inability to perform effectively some of the activities of daily living and self-care. This muscle imbalance can also lead to tightness of the anterior muscles, such as the pectoralis major (Fig. 24–4).

The degree of disability varies greatly from one patient to another. Disability can be more evident in patients who have osteoarthritis of the neck and shoulder. Usually the median age of patients who undergo radical neck resection is 55 to 60 years. At this age preoperative osteoarthritis or degenerative changes in the shoulder can intensify the postoperative disability. Although both flexion and abduction motions of the shoulder are affected, the loss of the motion of abduction causes more disability than does that of flexion. The loss of the sternocleidomastoid

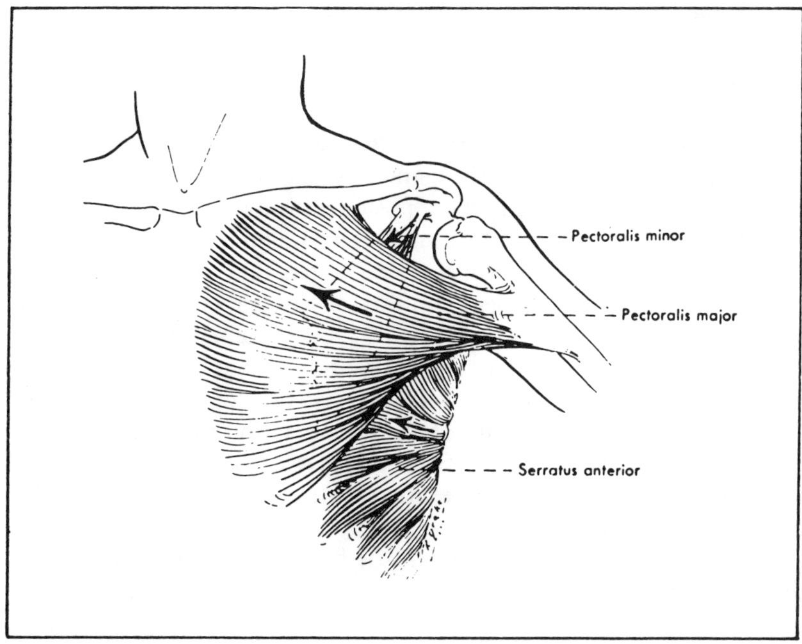

Figure 24–4. Location of pectoral muscles. These muscles often tighten when the trapezius muscle has been sacrificed. (From Hollinshead, W. H. [1958]. *Anatomy for surgeons,* Vol 3 [p. 33]. New York: Hoeber. By permission.)

muscle can lead to dysfunction in the neck and can cause pain and tightness, since only small weak muscles deep in the neck structures remain as substitutes. Bilaterally the sternocleidomastoid muscles assist in flexion and extension of the neck; unilaterally this muscle acts as a flexor and rotator of the neck to the opposite side. Patients with radical neck resection have sternocleidomastoid and trapezius loss as a result of spinal accessory nerve loss, and the circulation of the arm and brachial plexus can be compromised from drooping of the shoulder. Drooping of the shoulder can result in cold hands and tingling fingers. The remaining muscles—the levator scapulae, the rhomboids, the serratus anterior, and the deep muscles of the neck—must assume the function of the lost muscles. Tightening of the pectoral muscles must be avoided.

If possible, physical therapy for the patient who is to undergo radical neck resection should begin preoperatively (Johnson, Casper, and Lesswing, 1979; Gates et al., 1982). The patient can learn what type of exercises are to be done and why these exercises will be necessary (Appendices 24–A and 24–B). Furthermore, the patient can be informed that other muscles can be used to substitute for those that have lost function and that the patient must work to overcome the loss of muscles by the substitution of other muscle groups.

Early pain in these patients is often a result of the neck-extended posture during surgery, which aggravates degenerative arthritis of the neck. Swelling can also cause pain postoperatively. The necessary drainage tubes can lead to discomfort, incisional swelling, and soreness. Early during therapy the patient must be reassured that no damage will be done if the neck and shoulder are moved. These patients are often reluctant to move because of either fear of pain or actual discomfort. The patient should begin assistive range of motion exercises on the second or third day postoperatively. The patient is usually supine, and therapists assist in flexion and abduction of the shoulder while the scapula is supported. Re-education of the muscles to take over lost function is started. It is important to encourage relaxation with movements to avoid guarding, muscle misuse, and pain.

Late pain may be due to loss of the nerves or of muscle function in the area or to scarring. When irradiation is used preoperatively or postoperatively, fibrosis and scarring can lead to shoulder and neck dysfunction. The scarring, loss of muscle, and weakened remaining muscle result in pain.

Postoperatively, the scapula will wing. There will be downward and forward movement of the scapula, and it will swing laterally. There can be pectoral tightness. All these conditions can lead to compromised circulation of the arm if they are not corrected with substitution of the muscles that remain after surgery. Early use of a sling is often necessary to correct the drooping shoulder. The sling should not be worn longer than 1 month because shoulder immobility in itself can lead to stiffness and discomfort. If the arm is not supported by a sling, the patient should hold the arm up at the elbow.

For the first 1 to 2 weeks the exercises should be done with the patient supine (Appendix 24–C). Assisted flexion, abduction, and rotation motions of the shoulder should be done on a mat or bed (see Appendix 24–A). Mild back extension exercises and mild stretching can be done while the patient is supine. After 2 weeks these exercises can be done with the patient in a sitting position (see Appendix 24–B). In this position mild back extension exercises such as pulling the shoulder blades together are begun. In addition, re-education of the muscles for neck flexion, rotation, and lateral bending can be started. Because of the usual presence of degenerative arthritis of the cervical spine, neck extension exercises, which can lead to increased tightening of the posterior cervical muscles, are not advocated. Shoulder stabilization in a relaxed position can be important. To avoid overstretching of the remaining muscles, the patient should ensure that his arm is supported while he is walking or sitting.

One to 2 months (see Appendix 24–C) after surgery moderate pectoral stretching can be accomplished. Exercises for strengthening the upper back area should be done at this time. If the rhomboid muscles are of antigravity strength, they can be strengthened by weight lifting. The levator scapulae muscle, which raises the scapula, can also be strengthened. Caution is necessary in the strengthening program so that the muscles are not overworked. Special positions of the shoulder to support the humerus in the glenoid fossa of the scapula are usually helpful. To relieve some of the strain on the levator scapulae and the supraspinatus muscle, a small Orthoplast sling attached to the belt can be constructed to support the arm. The hand can be placed in the pants pocket, or the fingers can be supported in the belt loops. These positions are helpful for resting the shoulder. Placing the hand on the hip can relieve the pull and strain of the weight of the arm on these muscles.

Preoperatively, a magic slate should always accompany the patient to surgery. A word board or picture board should be available for the first day postoperatively. One to 2 weeks postoperatively it is important to begin occupational therapy. Just getting the patient out of the hospital room and around people who are training him to be comfortable with his new type of communication is important. Being in settings with understanding people who are not speech pathologists may also help alleviate some of the frustrations of these patients. Therapy is additionally beneficial, occupying the patient's time while he is recuperating from surgery and providing a supportive atmosphere while he is adapting to his disability.

A few "do's" and "don'ts" have been used in many cancer centers (Villanueva and Ajmani, 1977) (Appendix 24–D). These are important for achieving maximal recuperation. The patient should use good posture at all times and should pull the shoulders back frequently to prevent tightness of chest muscles and excessive strain on the weakened muscles over the scapula. In the early postoperative period the patient should avoid sitting for long periods to prevent tiring of the scapular muscles. It is best to sit in a chair with a straight back and arms so that the affected arm can be supported on the arm of the chair; otherwise, the involved hand can be placed on the hip to relieve downward pressure. To protect the involved arm, the patient should place the uninvolved arm under the involved elbow and should push it up to elevate the shoulder. When sleeping, the patient should lie on his back as much as possible. If he must lie on his side, he should lie on only the uninvolved side and should place the involved arm over the side of the body with the elbow bent and the arm supported on a pillow. It is important to emphasize that the arm must be supported so that the posterior musculature is not stretched until these muscles become strong enough to assume their new functions. In addition, the patient should not carry or lift objects weighing more than 3 pounds (1.4 kilograms) with the involved arm. Shoulder purses or shoulder bags should not be worn or carried on the involved arm, as heavy objects can cause damage or increase pain in the shoulder. Early postoperatively strenuous activities such as moving furniture and vigorous exercises should be avoided. The patient should also avoid injuries such as burns, pressure, lacerations, and insect bites. Because of the loss of sensation, direct application of heat to the involved skin area should be avoided. Men should be cautious while shaving the involved area.

Exercise programs for home use are prescribed. These exercises should be done daily, and the correct position for doing them should be emphasized. The patient should be cautioned to increase his strength and endurance gradually. Range of motion exercises, endurance exercises, and strengthening exercises are important. Re-education for suitable and proper substitution patterns is necessary. Late strengthening of the rhomboid, levator scapulae, and serratus anterior muscles may be necessary but can be done only if the arm is pain free. Strengthening exercises must not be done if they cause pain. A sling should not be worn all the time, as it can cause stiffness and loss of motion in the shoulder, and loss of motion causes pain. Shoulder shrugging, pushing against a wall, and shoulder retraction can help to strengthen the remaining muscles. Isometric exercises should be done slowly and with no more repetitions than are helpful. Overexercising should be avoided. Failure to exercise or incorrect exercises can lead to decreased range of motion and further tightening of the anterior shoulder muscles. Biofeedback has occasionally been useful in relaxation of tense, tight muscles and in re-education of the remaining muscles to take over new muscle action. As the nerve reinnervates, biofeedback can also be helpful for re-education of the reinnervated muscle.

In summary, patients who have had laryngectomy with neck dissection may need and benefit from physical and occupational therapy. Loss of the spinal accessory nerve results in shoulder dysfunction and can cause pain. Early treatment with range of motion exercises, strengthening of the musculature of the posterior shoulder girdle, and stretching rather than strengthening of the anterior shoulder musculature are important. The goal is to train muscles to substitute for trapezius action so that the patient will be able to stablize the scapula and raise the arm for use in a higher plane. It is important to teach the patient to protect the areas of sensory loss. Education, understanding, and participation of the patient and family are vital in any program of physical and occupational therapy.

QUESTIONS

1. How long should a patient work toward gaining return of function from a shoulder that has been affected by radical neck resection?
2. Why does return of function take so long?
3. Physical therapy often concentrates on helping the patient learn to rotate his neck after neck resection. Why does the patient have problems and what does therapy attempt to do for the patient?
4. If a patient has had a left radical neck resection, would rotation to the left or to the right most likely be a problem?
5. How soon after surgery should physical exercise of the neck and shoulder begin?
6. Discuss the relationship between pain of the shoulder and the "hand on the hip" position.

APPENDIX 24–A. SHOULDER MOBILIZATION EXERCISES

(These directions are intended for home treatment and **not** as a prescription for use by a professional physical therapist.)

Repeat required number of times as indicated by the therapist.
1. **Pendulum exercise is done while standing and leaning forward.**
   a. Swing affected arm forward and backward like a pendulum.
   b. Swing affected arm in and out like a pendulum.
   c. Extend affected arm toward the floor and swing it like a pendulum in gradually increasing circles. Then gradually decrease size of circles and let arm come to a complete stop.
   d. To increase comfort and relaxation, a two-pound weight (sandbag) may be held in the hand on the affected side while doing this exercise.
2. **Range of motion exercises may be done while sitting, standing, or lying down.**
   a. With arm straight at your side, raise it forward and upward so your elbow is near your ear. Keep trunk straight.
   b. With arm straight at side, raise it sideways and upward overhead so your elbow is near your ear. Keep trunk straight.
   c. Put palm of hand on or near back of neck; then rotate arm downward and place hand in small of back. Place hand on hip, if lying down.
3. **Wall creeping exercises with the finger tips are done while standing.**
   a. Stand erect, face the wall, and extend affected arm directly in front of your body so that finger tips touch the wall. Creep up the wall with the finger tips. Walk toward the wall as you reach higher and higher. Avoid arching your back. Repeat with finger tips going down the wall; walk backwards this time.
   b. Repeat above, only this time do the exercise with the affected arm extended sideward. Keep body erect. Do not lean toward the wall or shrug shoulders. A mark or a piece of tape may be placed on the wall each week to evaluate your progress.
4. **Range of motion exercises with the use of an overhead pulley may be done in an erect position, sitting or standing. Attempt to keep the shoulders level at all times. Do not hunch the shoulders.**
   a. Holding the rope in each hand, begin with your good arm over your head and the affected arm at your side. Raise the affected arm actively forward and upward overhead and assist this motion by gently pulling downward with your good arm in front of you. Then gently return to initial position.
   b. Holding the rope in each hand, begin with your good arm up over your head and the affected arm at your side as before. This time raise your affected arm actively sideways and upward overhead. Assist this motion by gently pulling downward with your good arm. Then return to initial position.

APPENDIX 24–B. NECK AND UPPER BACK EXERCISES

Good Posture Principles:

1. Tuck chin in slightly (make a double chin).
2. Stretch the top of head toward ceiling.
3. Keep upper back and neck comfortably straight.
4. Keep shoulders relaxed and down.

To Avoid Poor Posture:

1. Try not to look up.
2. Try not to let chin protrude.
3. Try not to slump.
4. Try not to shrug shoulders up.

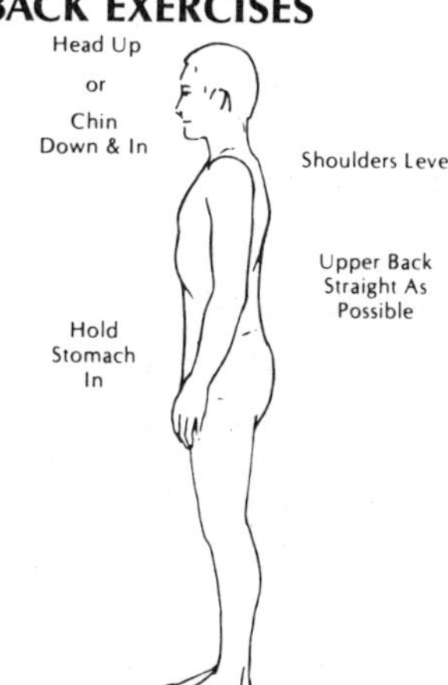

MAKE GOOD POSTURE A HABIT. BEGIN BY SETTING ASIDE A SPECIAL TIME DURING THE DAY TO PRACTICE GOOD NECK POSTURE. BE AWARE OF HAVING GOOD NECK POSTURE IN ALL YOUR DAILY ACTIVITIES.

Relaxation Exercises of Upper Back and Neck:

1. Sit in a comfortable chair in a quiet room with head well-balanced and arms hanging loosely at both sides, or on the lap.
2. Inhale slowly through the nose while drawing shoulders slowly up and backward. Keep chin down and in (double chin).
3. Hold position until tightness is felt in the muscles of the neck and upper back. AVOID PAIN!
4. Exhale slowly through the mouth as you return to the original position by gradually relaxing muscles of the neck and upper back.
5. Rest between repetitions.
6. Repeat ___________ times. DO EXERCISES SLOWLY!

Hints for Avoidance of Neck Pain:

1. Avoid prolonged activity with the head raised or hanging.
2. Avoid holding your neck and head in any one position for a long period of time.
3. Use a drafting board, or lectern, while reading or writing.

Exercises for Normal Range of Movement:

1. Bring head and neck down until chin is touching chest.
2. Turn face to left side and then to right side. Keep neck, shoulders and trunk straight. Keep chin down and in.
3. Tilt head and neck toward left shoulder; avoid raising shoulder toward head.
4. Tilt head and neck toward right shoulder; avoid raising shoulder toward head.
5. Bend head and neck back.

Pectoral Stretch in Lying Position

The pectoral muscles are the large muscles on the front of your chest from breastbone to your shoulders.

Lie on your back with knees bent and with feet flat on the floor. Do not put a pillow under your head, but place a folded towel between your shoulder blades. For a stronger stretch, clasp your hands behind your neck and let your elbows fall toward the floor. Remain in this position for _____________.

Isometric Strengthening of the Neck Muscles

1. Neck Flexion—With your neck bent slightly forward, place your hand under your chin. Attempt to bend your head and neck down, but resist the motion with your hand. Hold _____________ seconds.
2. Lateral Tilt—With your chin level and your head straight, place your hand on the left side of your head. Attempt to tilt your head to the left, but resist this motion with your hand. Hold _____________ seconds. Repeat this to the right side.
3. Rotation—With your chin level and your head turned slightly to the left, place your hand on the left side of your head. Attempt to turn your head to the left, but resist the motion with your hand. Hold _____________ seconds. Repeat this to the right side.
4. Neck Extension—With your head and neck straight, place your hands at the back of your head. Attempt to move your head backward, but resist in the motion with your hands. Hold _____________ seconds.

Courtesy of Mayo Clinic Department of Physical Medicine and Rehabilitation.

APPENDIX 24–C. MAYO CLINIC DEPARTMENT OF PHYSICAL MEDICINE AND REHABILITATION: EXERCISE PROGRAM FOR PATIENTS AFTER HEAD AND NECK SURGERY

1. Second to fifth postoperative day
   A. To be done passively by the therapist while the patients are supine.
      Shoulder flexion, abduction and rotation.
      Avoid cocontraction and guarding of the muscles.
      Avoid pectoral muscle guarding.
      Stress shoulder retraction.
2. Sixth to fifteenth postoperative day: Keep the neck in a neutral position.
   A. To be done supine on a firm surface, with the hips and knees flexed and feet flat on the mat to avoid substitution.
      Shoulder elevation with levator scapula and with the mat supporting scapula.
      Keep the pectoral muscles relaxed.
      Active assistive range of motion of the shoulder. Teach patient to assist motion with the other arm.
      Active pectoral stretching in supine position.
   B. To be done sitting on a straight backed chair.
      With hands on hips, do active shoulder rotation.
3. Beginning fifteenth postoperative day
   A. To be done sitting on a straight-backed chair while maintaining good posture.
      Active neck flexion, extension to neutral, lateral bending and rotation.
      Watch for sternocleidomastoid tightness on the nonoperated side.
4. Beginning twenty-second postoperative day
      Active pectoral stretching
5. Beginning thirtieth postoperative day
   A. To be done lying on the abdomen on a mat.
      With arms at sides, have the patient raise the head and then the shoulders. When this exercise can be performed with ease, substitute the following exercise in its place.
      With the hands clasped behind the neck, raise the head and then the shoulders off the mat, keeping the elbows pulled toward the back.

PRECAUTIONS
Skin over dissection is anesthetic.
Carotid arteries are very superficial.
Avoid pressure on anterior surface of the neck.
Note sternocleidomastoid muscle is resected.
Avoid Codman's exercises, as they tighten pectorals and cause neurovascular compression.

APPENDIX 24–D.   MAYO CLINIC DEPARTMENT OF PHYSICAL MEDICINE AND REHABILITATION: INSTRUCTIONS FOR HEAD AND NECK PATIENTS

1. *DO* maintain good posture at all times. Pull back your shoulders frequently. Good posture is essential to prevent the chest muscles from tightening and pulling against the weaker muscles on the back of the shoulder and to prevent excessive pressure and minimize discomfort when you are wearing the brace.
2. *DO* avoid sitting for long periods to prevent tiring the muscles that maintain good posture. It is best to sit in a chair with a straight back. If this is not possible, place a pillow behind your back for support.
3. *DO* exercise only in the position indicated.
4. *DO* wear your arm support at all times when you are sitting, standing, or walking. If it is not possible to wear the support, protect the affected arm by placing your _______________ hand under your _______________ elbow and gently pushing the elbow upward.
5. *DO* lie on your back as much as possible when you are sleeping. When lying on your back, place the back pillow under your spine between your shoulder blades and the neck pillow under your neck. If you must lie on your side, lie only on your _______________ side and place your _______________ arm over the side of your body with your elbow bent and your hand supported on a pillow.
6. *DO NOT* use your _______________ arm (unless it is absolutely necessary) until advised to do so.
7. *DO NOT* lift or carry objects weighing more than 3 pounds with your _______________ arm. Heavier items can cause damage and increased pain in your shoulder.
8. *DO NOT* lie on your _______________ side.
9. *DO* place your _______________ hand on your hip to relieve pressure under the arm, whenever necessary, when wearing the brace.

REFERENCES

Gates, G. A., Ryan, W., Cooper, J. C., Lawlis, G. F., Cantu, E., Hayashi, T., Lauder, E., Welch, R. W., and Hearne, E. (1982). Current status of laryngectomee rehabilitation: I. Results of therapy. *Amer. J. Otolaryngol., 3,* 1–7.

Hollinshead, W. H. (1976). *Functional anatomy of the limbs and back* (4th ed.). Philadelphia: W. B. Saunders.

Johnson, F. T., Casper, J., and Lesswing, N. J. (1979). Toward the total rehabilitation of the alaryngeal patient. *The Laryngoscope, 89,* 1813–1819.

Villanueva, R., and Ajmani, C. (1977). The role of rehabilitation medicine in physical restoration of patients with head and neck cancer. *Cancer Bull., 29,* 46–54.

Chapter 25

Special Problems of the Alaryngeal Speaker

Marshall Duguay

This chapter specifies "special" and "alaryngeal." The speech clinician must never forget that each laryngectomized individual is an individual. His problems are his special problems, individual and unique. Although most of the comments in this chapter will be directed toward problems in developing esophageal voice, many comments also have relevance to artificial larynx users and to those who have surgically and surgically-prosthetically restored voice. They apply generally to the alaryngeal speaker.

Problems can be categorized into four areas. The laryngectomee may experience a problem in learning to communicate orally because of (1) anatomical and physiological reasons, (2) physiological and sociological reasons, (3) teaching and learning reasons, and (4) a category that can be called OGK's, that is, "Only God Knows." Designation of this fourth group, the OGK's, is not meant to be flippant. There will always remain a few individuals who do not learn to speak and clinicians will never be able to determine exactly why. Fortunately, however, the reasons for failure by the majority (of failures) can usually be determined.

The speech clinician's major concern is generally problems in acquiring esophageal speech. Very simply, patients who cannot or do not learn esophageal speech (1) lack the ability or facility to force air into the esophagus, (2) lack the ability or facility to retain air briefly in the esophagus, (3) lack of ability or facility to return the air from the esophagus, or (4) lack ability or facility in the function of the pharyngoesophageal (PE) sphincter. These four areas are not mutually exclusive.

Why do these patients fail to learn? Obviously some do not want to learn. They are too depressed; they cannot accept the operation or the voice; they cannot cooperate or concentrate because they are alcoholic; they are feebleminded or senile, or they fail to practice. They fail because some clinicians are poor teachers or they are poor learners or both. They live alone and have no reason to talk: there is no one to talk to. The areas of psychological-sociological reasons and teaching-learning reasons are extremely important and undoubtedly account for large numbers of our clinical failures.

A consideration of those individuals who lack the ability or facility to force air into the esophagus and a review of some of the hypothesized problems in this area follow. As is well known, a total laryngectomy does not involve any of the cranial nerves. However, if an accompanying neck dissection is performed (and it often is to excise metastatic disease), it does involve Cranial Nerve XI, the accessory nerve. A more extensive radical neck dissection can involve Cranial Nerve X (vagus), Cranial Nerve XII (hypoglossal), and the lingual branch of Cranial Nerve V (trigeminal). These disruptions hamper oral sensations and tongue movements. It can be speculated that the result is a reduction in both the oral tactile and the kinesthetic feedback systems. Perhaps air injection (or at least some types of injection) is hampered.

In order to break through the closed PE barrier via injection, an oral-pharyngeal pressure build-up must be accomplished. To do this, two of the exits from the oral-pharyngeal cavity, the oral port and the nasal port, must be closed off. The oral port can be closed with a lip seal or a tongue seal. Lingual problems may necessitate teaching a lip seal, and individuals who have labial problems need to use a tongue seal. Nasal port closure requires velopharyngeal (VP) adequacy. Consequently, a patient with a cleft palate or palatal paresis would be a poor candidate for an injection technique; but he may experience little trouble with an inhalation method of air intake, since VP adequacy is not required. (In inhalation higher intraoral pressure is not generated but rather lower [negative] esophageal pressure is increased.)

Simpson, Smith, and Gordon (1972) looked at several anatomical factors related to the speech skills of proficient versus poor esophageal speakers. They wrote, "Almost all the proficient speakers show a smooth conical hypopharynx without evidence of permanent constrictions, bulging of the wall or irregular indentations posteriorly. The pharynx shows fully controlled mobility, relaxing to a wide space and contracting under muscle control, almost to the extent of obliterating the air space when required" (p. 971). They reported a relationship between speech proficiency and radiological abnormalities. The relationship is not absolute, but there is a close association. They stated, "Certain individuals showing x-ray changes achieved a high grade of speech indicating their capability of overcoming a basic mechanical inefficiency, but, in general, the greater the radiological abnormality, the poorer the resulting voice'' (p. 988).

Simpson and co-workers (1972) went on to say, "Healthy, well-motivated patients will overcome deficiencies in their vocal mechanism and by application and effort acquire useful voice though they may never be able to acquire superior voice. Patients who are poorly motivated, elderly, or in ill health may be totally unable to compensate for deficiencies in the vocal mechanism caused by a functionally poor reconstruction after laryngectomy and fail to acquire any useful speech.'' Just what kinds of abnormalities are they talking about? They found instances of double constriction, an area of narrowing located between the esophagus and the oropharynx in addition to the narrowing at the PE junction. They describe three types:

Type A: a permanent organic stricture above the PE junction. This is a constant area of narrowing that does not distend even upon swallowing and is likely related to loss of excised mucosa or fibrosis secondary to delayed healing.

Type B: pseudostrictures. These constrictions are due to bulging of the posterior pharyngeal wall into the lumen of the hypopharynx.

Type C: voluntary contraction. They identified two patients who showed normal pictures at rest, on injection, and on barium swallow. However, during phonation the hyoid bone was pulled backward to produce a second narrowing. The effect was to create a small resonating chamber that influenced the pitch of the resulting esophageal voice.

In addition to abnormal constrictions, Simpson and colleagues (1972) described pouches, defined as localized forward bulging of the anterior pharyngeal wall beyond what is considered to be the normal configuration. These pouches occurred at two levels: high pouches situated just below the base of the tongue at the level of the hyoid bone and low pouches located between the PE junction and the hyoid bone.

The functional effect of these constrictions and pouches superior to the neoglottic PE segment can only be speculated upon. Do they increase the effort needed to move air in? Is more oral-pharyngeal pressure needed to override the constrictions as well as the closed PE segment? Does air or mucus and saliva get trapped in the pouches, affecting the quality of voice as well as the effort needed to drive the increased mass? The anatomy, the physiology, and the coordination of suprapharyngoesophageal PE segment strictures need to be considered when looking for reasons to account for esophageal speech failures, for they can negatively affect the ability to force air into the esophagus.

Now let us drop down from the supraesophageal structures to the esophagus itself. Unlike normal vocal folds, which are longer in the male than in the female, the length of the esophagus is similar in males and females, about 25 centimeters (cm) (9 inches). At its superior end can be found the upper (proximal, cricopharyngeal, PE) sphincter. This sphincter is approximately ½ inch long and ½ inch in diameter. This sphincter is in a closed state except for esophageal air intake and expulsion and during swallowing, belching, gagging, and regurgitation. It is this upper sphincter, or PE segment, that functions as the neoglottis in esophageal speech. Part of this musculature is composed of striated muscle, hence the possibility of some degree of voluntary control. There is a lack of agreement among surgeons ranging from the point of view that great care should be taken during surgery to spare the fibers of the cricopharyngeal muscle and, if possible, the integrity of its innervation, to an attitude of "Do not worry about it because almost any remnant of tissue or muscle can serve as the basis for the development of a neoglottis." In addition, there is obviously great variability in terms of PE segment location. Diedrich and Youngstrom (1966) showed it ranging from as high as C4 all the way to down to C7; most often it was located around C5 or C6 in their subjects. Since the PE segment is longer than the width of the cricopharyngeus muscle, it is believed that fibers from the inferior pharyngeal constrictors also help to compose the neoglottis.

Dey and Kirchner (1961) found no apparent constriction at the level of the cricopharyngeus and suggested that its control for esophageal voice is irrelevant. In contrast, Damsté (1975) wrote, "Before sound can be produced by the esophageal opening, air must be passed into the esophagus. This requires a relaxed sphincter of the pharyngoesophageal segment" (p. 650). He felt that "the patient must now learn to relax the esophageal opening voluntarily (usually it is closed and relaxes only reflexly after the constrictive phase of the second stage of swallowing) at the precise moment when the pumping action of the floor of the mouth raises the pressure of the air in the pharynx" (p. 650). He also stated, "It has been our experience that the habit of pseudo-whisper and pharyngeal voice enhance the reflex closure of the esophageal mouth" (p. 657). Therefore, these must be discouraged.

The ability voluntarily to relax the PE segment in order to get air in for speech suggests the need for at least some neural intactness in this region. Shipp (1970) using electromyographic (EMG) equipment found that poor esophageal speakers (as opposed to good ones) displayed either extremely weak or uncoordinated or inconsistent EMG patterns of the cricopharyngeus muscle during phonation, suggesting interruption of neural innervation.

Bagshaw (1967) in her experience with 123 laryngectomized patients found six patients with too tight a sphincter who were unable to obtain voice easily or at all. She said, "The cricopharyngeus sphincter was so tightly closed in the swallowing phase that it was difficult for the patient to make it function voluntarily . . . it required great air pressure from the esophagus and made smooth control difficult" (p. 62).

Mountcastle (1974) stated that results of radiographs and manometrical studies on normal subjects indicate that the greatest movement of a bolus occurs when the pressure gradients are low. Winans, Reichbach, and Waldrop (1974) found that their good esophageal speakers had significantly *lower* cricopharyngeal pressures than their poor speakers. To be exact, the good speakers had pressure readings averaging only 13 mm Hg, whereas the poor speakers had readings around 30 mm Hg.

Hurst (1943) indicated that a tight, spastic cricopharyngeal sphincter may have to be treated mechanically with dilators such as a gastric tube or muscle-relaxing drugs. Levin (1952) and van den Berg and Moolenaar-Bijl (1959) were also of the opinion that a tight PE segment may be a barrier to esophageal speech.

Ingelfinger (1958) in his classic article entitled "Esophageal Motility" commented on the mechanism of sphincteric opening. "Three possibilities exist: (1) The sphincter opens passively in response to oropharyngeal pressure; (2) it is pulled apart by other muscles; or (3) its intrinsic tonicity is inhibited" (p. 538). After discussing 1 and 2, he wrote, "By a process of exclusion, it would appear that intrinsic muscular relaxation in the sine qua non of sphincteric opening: it may to some extent be forced or pulled apart, but first of all the sphincter has to relax" (p. 539). A word of caution is in order: he is writing about its physiology in normals during swallowing.

Evidence from a study by Kirchner, Scatliff, Dey, and Shedd (1963) suggests that "the absence of a functioning sphincter at the esophageal inlet does not, of itself, promote regurgitation or produce dysphagia" (p. 12). The authors also mention that neither does it interfere with good esophageal voice.

The importance of the function of the PE segment has become quite apparent through the ever-increasing knowledge generated by work with tracheoesophageal shunts and surgical-prosthetic speech restoration (Panje, 1981; Shapiro and Ramanathan, 1982; Singer and Blom, 1980).

An especially significant article (Singer and Blom, 1981) reported on patients who failed to acquire fluent speech subsequent to tracheoesophageal puncture. The authors used the term "pharyngoesophageal spasm" to identify the reason for the failure. They concluded that ". . . air-flow-induced spasm of the cricopharyngeus and pharyngeal constrictor muscles seems to be an important factor in failure of some patients to acquire fluent speech, with both tracheoesophageal puncture and conventional esophageal voice therapy'' (p. 673). They solved the problem of these failures by the technique of selective myotomy, reporting that "all 14 patients eventually achieved fluency after myotomy." (p. 671).

McGarvey and Weinberg (1984), in discussing the Singer and Blom work regarding pharyngoesophageal spasm, stated, "The implication of this characterization is that airtight closure represents an abnormal response which merits treatment in the form of selective myotomy" (p. 275). Their study of 15 nonlaryngectomized adults indicated that airtight closure and the absence of the ability to produce voice continuously are not unusual (abnormal) characteristics of the normal (nonlaryngectomized) human esophagus in response to air insufflation testing. They wrote, "Laryngectomized patients exhibiting airtight closure of the PE segment or failure to produce voice continuously during insufflation testing exhibit responses that correspond to those exhibited by each of the non-laryngectomized subjects. In contrast, we believe that laryngectomized patients who fail to exhibit airtight closure and who consistently produce voice continuously during air insufflation exhibit unusual response characteristics and altered (compromised) function" (p. 275).

It is obvious that PE segment function is critical to phonatory success. It is also obvious that there is a great need for additional research of the PE area in order to optimize surgical reconstruction after total laryngectomy and hence facilitate both conventional esophageal speech and tracheoesophageal speech restoration.

Speech clinicians have all seen patients struggle and strain to force air past a very tight and unyielding upper sphincter and struggle and strain to get that air (once in) back out past this same tight, unyielding upper sphincter. If this is indeed a problem in a given patient, perhaps relaxation and control can be taught, especially in those who have good "striated" segments and good neural innervation. Faulkner (1940) and Greene (1947) both indicated that spasms of the esophagus can be increased and the lumen narrowed by suggestions that arouse emotions of anger, grief, anxiety, apprehension, and fear. They also report that suggestions that arouse pleasant emotions such as elation, happiness, enthusiasm, security, and contentment actually caused relaxation of the spasms and a widening of the esophageal lumen.

Thus, teaching relaxation, reduction of anxiety and tension, and even the use of biofeedback techniques can be useful. Other patients may require muscle relaxants and tranquilizers; others with less than optimal physical abilities may need to be considered for pharyngoesophageal dilation via bouginage or, even more drastically, a myotomy.

The other end of the continuum is a too loose or too flaccid PE segment or pharyngeal wall at the level of the neoglottis. This situation can be helped by the use of digital pressure, neck bands, prosthetic devices, or even surgical procedures such as a sternomastoid muscle swing operation as described by Montgomery and Lavelle (1974).

It may be perplexing to the reader that the subject of addressing the problem of getting air in changes to a discussion of the flaccid segment that distends or bulges to cause a lack of maximal vibrating function upon phonation. This is mentioned here because clinically problems may be induced by the use of neck bands and digital pressure that is too forceful. If digital pressure is too hard, the segment will be tightened and the resistance to air intake increased. Digital pressure, for example, should be applied *after* air intake and not *prior to* air intake. This author also has a strong clinical hunch that digital pressure and bands prevent bulging or ballooning by introducing resistance anterior to the neoglottis and is not really pushing the segment closer together, at least in most patients. So much for area (1), the ability or facility to get air in.

The next two hypothesized areas, namely, the ability or facility to retain the air and then to force it out (return it) tend to overlap. In constructing a "four-problem model," the fact that esophageal phonation is a process that really should not and cannot be fractionated has been ignored; models should be flirted with and not married.

Another area of concern for hypothesized problems is the distal or cardiac sphincter. This is the area believed to separate the gastric (stomach) and esophageal lumens. It should theoretically remain closed except when it is physiologically advantageous for the organism to have something (food, liquids, air) flow one way or the other.

Wolfe, Olson, and Goldenberg (1971) used radiographic and pressure instrumentation to look at this site in 13 laryngectomees. They found that seven patients, who had failed to develop esophageal speech, demonstrated hiatus hernia or gastroesophageal reflux or regurgitation with varying degrees of esophagitis present. To quote Wolfe and colleagues (1971), "A cause and effect relationship is suggested" (p. 1977). All seven complained of one of the following symptoms: heartburn, regurgitation, chest pain (all of these increased by bending over or lying down), a sensation of food sticking in the throat, a watery voice quality, and difficulty or failure in acquiring esophageal speech. The other six patients, who had developed good to excellent esophageal speech, were shown to have ". . . competent distal esophageal sphincters" (p. 1977).

Another interesting point made in Wolfe and co-workers' (1971) article was that when the Asai procedure as well as other air-directing prostheses were used with unsuccessful conventional esophageal speakers, they developed good voice without any further change in the condition of the upper esophagus. Wolfe and co-workers (1971) suggested that the failure, prior to the Asai procedure, was in the esophagus as an air reservoir: "It is our contention that the trapping of a usable supply of air in the esophagus is dependent upon a competent distal esophageal sphincter" (p. 1976).

They also speculated that hernia and reflux were likely present prior to the laryngectomy in many of the patients and that perhaps attempts to learn esophageal speech aggravated the gastric problem. They urged that when complaints warrant, the possibility of hiatus hernia be considered and investigated. Then, if the presence of hiatus hernia is confirmed, they recommended the use of an artificial larynx or an anti-reflex hernia-plasty procedure.

Wolfe and co-workers (1971) also refer to a postoperative fluoroscopic study of 30 laryngectomees reported by Doubravsky and Prasil (1969). Among their 30 subjects they found eight patients with "retrograde aerophagia," six with gastroesophageal reflux, and five with hiatus hernia. These investigators felt that re-education of voice via esophageal speech created an undue strain on this sphincter and that a potential danger of peptic esophagitis was thus created. They did not report the quality of esophageal speech.

Another problem, rather serious, can occur in this lower esophageal area: a condition called achalasia. In achalasia the lower esophageal region does not relax, with resultant obstruction in the passage of the bolus into the stomach. Basically, this "disease" is one of incoordination between the muscles of the esophageal wall and those of the sphincteric lower area. The anatomical cause is not known. However, most believe that it is of a neural character, since on postmortem examination there is a degeneration of terminal nerves between two muscle layers of the esophagus, specifically in the region of Auerbach's plexus. The disease affects all ages. It is the most frequent cause of dysphagia in women and the second most frequent in men (Shapiro, 1974). It is generally chronic, and progressive deterioration occurs. There is much difficulty in swallowing, weight loss occurs because of the difficulty, and pain and regurgitation may occur. In early cases barium studies indicate delayed emptying of the esophagus, and in more advanced cases the characteristic appearance of stenosis is seen. There are no less than 35 different operative procedures to relieve esophageal achalasia. The best results, it seems, come from a type of esophagocardiomyotomy.

Two additional comments can be made. Winans and associates (1974) found that although both their "fluent" and their "poor" esophageal subjects had nearly identical lower esophageal sphincter pressures, the good ones had significantly higher gastric pressures (high gastric–low cricopharyngeal pressure). They stated, "Although air reaching the stomach probably is of no use in speech production, the fact that some air does pass into the stomach of good speakers is attested to by the difficulties they experience with bloating and flatulence" (p. 13).

Finally, since there appears to be so much concern and focus on the upper (proximal) esophageal sphincter in the recent literature (McGarvey and Weinberg, 1984; Panje, 1981; Shapiro and Ramanathan, 1982; Singer and Blom, 1981), speech clinicians may lose sight of the importance of this lower (distal) esophageal sphincter. Undoubtedly, its intactness contributes to speech success as well as to physical comfort. A number of laryngectomees who use conventional esophageal speech and are a number of years postoperative complain of stomach distress, discomfort, and gas. What effect does long-term esophageal loading of air have on the distal sphincter? As more and more patients receive tracheoesophageal procedures and continue to pump huge volumes of air into the esophagus, will an increase of complaints and symptoms consistent with reflux, distention, hiatal hernia, and serious stomach and gastric disturbances be seen? Clinicians should have a very real and serious concern about these problems and should hope that they are carefully monitored by those who are quick to "puncture." It may prove not to be an innocuous and harmless procedure with passage of time.

A brief look at the body of the esophagus is warranted. The capacity of the esophagus has been estimated to approximately 80 cubic centimeters (cc) of air (2½ ounces or five tablespoons). Moreover, the esophageal speaker uses only about the upper one third for storage and release, and this is a very rapid air–air out phenomenon. Diedrich and Youngstrom (1966) found that their better speakers seemingly had a more widely dilated esophagus. Good speech depends to a degree, then, on trapping sufficient air in the esophagus. Exactly what constitutes "sufficient" is not easy to specify.

In normals and in esophageal speakers the esophagus is usually collapsed during a resting state, although small amounts of air or food or liquid can be present as long as they are not sufficient to trigger a peristaltic reaction. Intraesophageal pressures have been measured in several studies. However, instrumentation differs from study to study, so it is hard to compare findings. There is some agreement about the average pressures in the esophagus during phonation. Positive pressures averaging 20 to 50 cm H_2O have been measured in good speakers, whereas in poor speakers positive pressures averaged 40 to 80 cm H_2O.

Such investigators as Damsté (1958), Salmon (1965), Bozymski and Pharr (1972), and Crouch (1974) have studied the relationships between pressures in the pharynx, the PE segment, and the esophagus in good versus poor esophageal speakers but have failed to find any significant correlations. Such variables as the presence of a foreign object within the PE segment affecting voicing, positioning of the pressure-sensing device, or PE segment movement during intake and phonation may affect results. In addition, Zinner and Fleshler (1972) remind us that the phonation task under study may contribute to esophageal pressure variance. For maximal duration tasks requiring sustained effort they found that pressure rises uniformly throughout the esophagus. On the other hand, for a brief yet forceful effort, mean pressures at the medial and distal levels are greater than at the proximal level. This finding also implies a degree of voluntary control over the esophageal speech apparatus and the concept that intrinsic esophageal activity may play a role in esophageal speech rather than simply behaving as a passive tube having the air squeezed out of it.

Another consideration regarding the body of the esophagus is interesting in view of data relating age to failure to develop esophageal voice. Ingelfinger (1958), in his review of esophageal motility, wrote, ". . . In all people beyond the age of 50 an increasing incidence of abnormal esophageal motor phenomena may be detected" (p. 557).

The last study related to problems in learning is one by Samuel and Adams (1976). They examined esophageal and diaphragmatic movements in 19 patients. (To the best of this author's knowledge, few investigators have studied the diaphragm as a problem site in esophageal speech failures.) After reviewing their video recordings, they reported the emergence of a consistent basic pattern consisting of the following stages:

(1) Commencing from rest, the neoglottis relaxes and the diaphragm begins its descent.
(2) At some point, usually near the end of the descent of the diaphragm, the oesophagus suddenly dilates throughout most of its length.
(3) With complete descent of the diaphragm all the oesophagus except the lower-most 2–3 cms. is dilated. The sequence of events so far can be likened to inflating a "sausage type" balloon.
(4) In preparation for speech, the neoglottis closes and the diaphragm begins its ascent.
(5) As the diaphragm ascends, a variable segment of the lower oesophagus collapses and the remainder increases slightly in diameter. This is the maximum width attained and simulates squeezing the end of an inflated balloon.
(6) The neoglottis opens and during speech the oesophagus collapses as the diaphragm completes its ascent. The neck of the balloon has undergone a controlled release. (p. 1107)

When Samuel and Adams (1976) compared the patterns of their poor speakers with this series of events, they found "non-dilation of the oesophagus presumably due to failure of relaxation of neoglottis during expansion of thoracic volume" (p. 1108).

If diaphragmatic ascent is not coordinated with movements of the neoglottis, further problems arise even in those patients who manage a good air intake. The neoglottis must remain closed during diaphragmatic ascent to allow a sufficient build-up of pressure. Premature neoglottic opening results in quiet or absent speech. If neoglottic opening is delayed, the diaphragm heaves up and down and the patient appears to be suffering from acute indigestion.

Although the preceding observations are subjective, it is tentatively suggested that the following conclusions are valid:

1. No patient whose diaphragmatic movements are poor or incoordinated will have good speech.
2. Patients with good speech tend to have coordinated neoglottic and diaphragmatic movements.
3. Varying degrees of incoordination between the neoglottis and the diaphragm result in varying percentages of intelligible syllables.

To summarize, this chapter has tried to show how problems can occur in the process of esophageal speech acquisition. These problems can occur with air intake, air retention, and air return. The problem area may be superior, anterior, posterior, or inferior to the PE segment. It also may be in more than one area, or the problem may be a result of improper coordination between areas. The clinician must not think just "physical." The patient's attitude, drive, and motivation; his anxiety and fear; his level of understanding; what he practices and how often he practices; and what he is asked to do and how he is asked (i.e., psychological-sociological-teaching-learning variables) can and will affect his physical assets and liabilities.

Any speech clinician can help the great esophageal speakers. They will learn (sometimes in spite of the clinician); they really need little help. The real challenge, the real joy of clinical work is helping and succeeding with the difficult cases. The speech clinician must get out there and help the tough ones: They are the ones who really need the help.

QUESTIONS

1. Outline some of the anatomical and physiological reasons for esophageal voice failure.
2. If a patient has a palatal paresis, what air charge method would you advocate?
3. Supraesophageal abnormalities may account for some liabilities in speaking with esophageal voice. Which abnormalities are indicated by Duguay and how may they influence speech?

4. What specific problems of the esophagus may limit esophageal voice development?

5. Do you agree with Damsté (1975) that pseudo-whisper may trigger reflexive closure of the esophagus? Why might this be so? How could one teach a pseudo-whisper without risk of this problem?

6. How well trained are you to carry out Duguay's recommendation on the teaching of relaxation? What might you do to effect such a state in your clients?

7. When a person is failing esophageal voice, to what potential problem might you first attend?

8. What might be the major indications that a patient injects air but cannot (does not) store it in the esophagus?

9. What evidence would suggest that in teaching a glossal or glossopharyngeal press method of air intake you should also consider respiratory action of the diaphragm?

REFERENCES

Bagshaw, M. J. (1967). Rehabilitation of post-laryngectomy patients. *Brit. J. Dis. Commun. 2,* 54–63.

van den Berg, J., and Moolenaar-Bijl, A. J. (1959). Cricopharyngeal sphincter, pitch, intensity, and fluency in oesophageal speech. *Pract. Oto-Rhino-Laryngol., 21,* 298–315.

Bozymski, R. M., and Pharr, S. Y. (1972). Esophageal manometry and speech proficiency in post-laryngectomy patients (abstract). *Gastroenterology, 62,* 726.

Crouch, Z. B. (1974). *The relationship of intraluminal swallowing, resting, and phonation pressures to esophageal phonation "goodness" and maximum duration of phonation.* Unpublished doctoral dissertation, University of Kansas, Lawrence, KS.

Damsté, P. H. (1958). *Oesophageal speech after laryngectomy.* Groninger: Boekdrukkerij Voorheen Gebroeders Hoitsema.

Damsté, P. H. (1975). Methods of restoring the voice after laryngectomy. *Laryngoscope, 85,* 649–655.

Dey, F. L., and Kirchner, J. A. (1961). The upper esophageal sphincter after laryngectomy. *Laryngoscope, 71,* 99–115.

Diedrich, W., and Youngstrom, K. (1966). *Alaryngeal speech.* Springfield, IL: Charles C Thomas.

Doubravsky, J., and Prasil, J. (1969). X-ray picture of the esophagus and the esophagogastric junction in laryngectomized patients. *Cesk Radiol., 23,* 111–116.

Faulkner, W. B. (1940). Objective esophageal changes due to psychic factors. *Amer. J. Med. Sciences, 200,* 796–803.

Greene, J. S. (1947). Laryngectomy and its psychologic implications. *N.Y. State J. Med., 47,* 53–56.

Hurst, A. (1943). Nervous disorders of swallowing. *J. Laryngol. Otol., 58,* 60–71.

Ingelfinger, F. J. (1958). Esophageal mobility. *Physiol. Rev., 38,* 533–584.

Kirchner, J. A., Scatliff, J. H., Dey, F. L., and Shedd, D. P. (1963). The pharynx after laryngectomy. *Laryngoscope, 73,* 18–33.

Levin, M. M. (1952). Speech rehabilitation after total removal of the larynx. *J. Amer. Med. Assoc., 140,* 1281–1286.

McGarvey, S. D., and Weinberg, B. (1984). Esophageal insufflation testing in nonlaryngectomized adults. *J. Speech Hear. Dis., 49,* 272–277.

Montgomery, W. W., and Lavelle, W. G. (1974). A technique for improving esophageal and tracheopharyngeal speech. *Ann. Otol. Rhinol. Laryngol., 83,* 452–461.

Mountcastle, V. B. (1974). *Medical physiology* (13th ed.). St. Louis: C. V. Mosby.

Panje, W. R. (1981). Prosthetic vocal rehabilitation following laryngectomy. The voice button. *Ann. Otol. Rhinol. Laryngol., 90,* 116–120.

Salmon, S. J. (1965). *Pressure variations in the esophagus, pharyngeal-esophageal construction and pharynx associated with esophageal speech production.* Unpublished doctoral dissertation, State University of Iowa, Iowa City, IA.

Samuel, P., and Adams, F. G. (1976). The role of oesophageal and diaphragmatic movement in alaryngeal speech. *J. Laryngol. Otol., 90,* 1105–1111.

Shapiro, M. J., and Ramanathan, V. R. (1982). Trachea stoma vent voice prosthesis. *Laryngoscope, 92,* 1126–1929.

Shapiro, S. L. (1974). Achalasia of the Esophagus. *The Eye, Ear, Nose and Throat Monthly, 53,* 184–188.

Shipp, T. (1970). EMG of pharyngoesophageal musculature during alaryngeal voice production. *J. Speech Hearing Res., 13,* 184–192.

Simpson, I. C., Smith, J. C. S., and Gordon, M. T. (1972). Laryngectomy: The influence of muscle reconstruction on the mechanism of oesophageal voice production. *J. Laryngol. Otol., 86,* 961–990.

Singer, M. I., and Blom, E. D. (1980). An endoscopic technique for restoration of voice after laryngectomy. *Ann. Otol. Rhin. Laryngol., 89,* 529–533.

Singer, M. I., and Blom, E. D. (1981). Selective myotomy for voice restoration after total laryngectomy. *Arch. Otolaryngol., 107,* 670–673.

Winans, C. S., Reichbach, E. J., and Waldrop, W. F. (1974). Esophageal determinants of alaryngeal speech. *Arch. Otolaryngol., 99,* 10–14.

Wolfe, R. D., Olson, J. E., and Goldenberg, D. G. (1971). Rehabilitation of the laryngectomee: The role of the distal esophageal sphincter. *Laryngoscope, 81,* 1971–1978.

Zinner, E. M., and Fleshler, B. (1972). Intraesophageal pressures during phonation in laryngectomized patients. *J. Laryngol. Otol., 86.* 129–140.

Chapter 26

Nursing Care of the Laryngectomee Outside the Hospital Environment

Nancy Morozink

After a patient has undergone a laryngectomy, he or she will find several areas of life affected to such a degree that adjustments are necessary in order to maintain a life style that is comfortable for both patient and family. The changes include management of a tracheostomy tube, adequate humidification of the environment, bathing, personal hygiene, stoma coverings, adjustments in eating, treatment of colds, activity involvement, and awareness of problem signs.

When teaching is begun with a patient, it is emphasized that even though there will be problems, adjustments can be accomplished and life can be enjoyable. Surgery does require some new self-care procedures; if the goal of total rehabilitation is to be achieved, the patient must have the cooperation, understanding, and acceptance of the family. This is why it is preferred that a close relative accompany the patient coming for instruction.

MANAGEMENT OF THE TRACHEOSTOMY TUBE

The patient receives care management instructions while still in the hospital, before returning home wearing a tube. The parts of the tube and their functions are explained. Wearing of the tube should not cause discomfort. If the trachea becomes irritated or if pressure develops at any point, the physician should be notified. Cleanliness of the tube is important both for good hygiene and providing an open airway for easy breathing. This is accomplished by using warm tap water, soap, and brushes. It is important to clean the inner tube as often as necessary for easy and quiet breathing; the number of times each day depends on the amount of mucus present. The outer tube does not have to be cleaned daily, but it is advisable to do so in the interest of good hygiene. Cooking oil functions as a safe, inexpensive, and easily available lubricant to facilitate comfortable reinsertion of the tracheostomy tube. A small, preferably unbreakable dropper bottle can be used to dispense the oil directly onto the tube. The amount required per time is usually 1 drop on the tube part being reinserted. The oil is evenly distributed on the tube surface using a clean finger. Excessive amounts of oil will cause increased coughing and discomfort and will not promote easier reinsertion. Olive oil is not recommended because of its strong odor and its tendency to become rancid. The gauze bib worn behind the tube should be changed when it becomes wet or soiled. Brushes should be cleansed thoroughly with soap and water and allowed to dry.

The laryngectomee is no longer breathing through his nose. A new opening for breathing purposes has been made into his neck by surgical means and leads directly into his windpipe, or trachea. This new opening is called a stoma. The primary purpose of the tube is to keep the stoma from closing while healing is taking place and thus provide an adequate airway at all times.

If the stoma is of sufficient size, approximately 6 weeks following surgery the weaning process from the tube may begin. It is necessary to do this gradually to prevent the stoma from shrinking in size. The tube is usually left out for an hour the first time. If it can be replaced easily, the next time another hour may be added. As long as the tube can be easily reinserted and no shrinking of the stoma is noted, the time interval for leaving out the tube may be increased daily until eventually the patient will be without it all day. It is advisable to wear the tube during the night until it can be left out all day for at least 2 weeks without any change in stoma size. If difficulty in replacing the tube arises at any time, the amount of time it is being left out should be decreased for a few days; then the patient can gradually increase the time interval again, carefully observing whether the stoma is becoming smaller. At the time of the first check-up following surgery, which is usually after 3 months, a "stoma button" may replace the original tube if the stoma is not staying open sufficiently by itself. This is a small, pliable device, resembling a spool, worn only to keep the stoma from becoming too small. It is more convenient to clean and wear than a tube.

ADEQUATE HUMIDIFICATION OF ENVIRONMENT

Before surgery, the nose acted as a humidifier and moisturized the air before it reached the trachea. Following surgery air is taken directly into the trachea without the benefit of moisture from the nose and upper respiratory tract. The tissues of the trachea attempt to compensate for this dryness by producing excessive secretions, which tend to produce more coughing. This combination of excessive secretions and coughing can present potential health hazards for the patient. Without sufficient humidification, these secretions may become dried, forming crusts and mucus plugs that greatly impair breathing. As months pass, the lining of the trachea adapts to dryness, undergoing a change in the cells that makes them more compatible with dryness. This change will assist in decreasing the excessive secretions and their effects.

However, during the winter months when dryness in the air is increased, proper humidity is most important in promoting an airway free of thick, sticky secretions and crusts. Adequate humidity will keep the secretions sufficiently thin so that they can easily be coughed up and removed. There will always be some necessary secretions present in healthy tissues; these can usually be managed with little difficulty. A vaporizer is essential in the bedroom during the winter months, as is keeping the windows closed. Having adequate humidification for several hours during sleep will help carry the patient through the day, when it may not be possible to run a vaporizer. A humidifier is mandatory in promoting adequate humidity throughout the entire house; a 40 per cent level is usually sufficient.

Wearing a foam bib over the stoma will help keep more humidity in the trachea. If crusts form in the trachea and the air seems too dry, sometimes it is necessary to use a medicine dropper to instill saline directly into the trachea. It has been found beneficial to use a dropper or two of saline routinely morning and evening to prevent dryness complications. (Saline may be made by dissolving ⅛ teaspoon of salt in one cup of water.)

In a hotel room without sufficient humidity, it is helpful to turn on the shower or bathtub faucet. For optimal results, the laryngectomee can close the bathroom door and remain inside until there is some relief from thickened secretions. If increased humidity is desired for the sleeping area as well, the laryngectomee may leave the water running with the door open or wear a dampened bib over the stoma.

Car air can be found to be quite dry to a laryngectomee traveling for several hours. Again, wetting a gauze bib and wearing it over the stoma will usually provide adequate moisture.

Some signs of excessive dryness are increased, unproductive coughing; noisy breathing; bloody mucus; expelled crusts; and thick, sticky mucus. When these symptoms occur, the amount of humidity should be increased immediately. Usually air conditioning can be used successfully in summer if the laryngectomee remains aware of the signs of dryness and the conditioner is used accordingly. During summer months, no extra humidification is usually required.

BATHING AND PERSONAL HYGIENE

There is usually great concern about keeping water from entering the trachea. Excessive water can be dangerous, but water splashed in from bathing or shampooing is not of serious consequence and can be removed easily by coughing. Mucus collecting around the stoma is more of a problem in the beginning and lessens in time. Regular bathing, including the area up to the edge of the stoma, is essential for proper cleanliness and prevention of odors. The laryngectomee can use a regular wash cloth, soap and water, and bathe as usual, but should *not* use perfumed soaps, which tend to be more irritating in this area. Sometimes the use of a small amount of petroleum jelly around the stoma will help to prevent crusts from adhering to the skin. Tub bathers need no special protection from water. Those who shower may find that equipment having a coil and handle that can be regulated directly by the user is satisfactory for both showering and shampoos. Shampoos not done in a shower are most easily accomplished by leaning over a sink with a towel around the neck to prevent water from entering the stoma. Women should also lean over the shampoo bowel in a beauty salon for the first few weeks following surgery rather than place undue stress on the neck by backward extension of the head.

Those who take showers may be interested in a shower shield, which fits around the neck and offers protection from the spray. If help is needed in a tub or shower, a wet palm slapping a hard surface is more easily heard than a pounding fist.

If shaving presents a problem from falling whiskers, a cloth bib may be worn over the stoma. When using a safety razor, the laryngectomee should shave the chin area first to prevent dripping. Hair cuts should pose no problem as long as a cloth drape is used.

The coughing of mucus should be handled in much the same way as someone blowing and wiping the nose. To mask a cough, the laryngectomee holds a handkerchief to the mouth with one hand, cups the other hand over the stoma to reduce the sound and trap the mucus in the bib, then coughs. A clean handkerchief should always be available to wipe away mucus that collects outside the stoma.

Mouth care is especially important since breathing has been rerouted. Tooth brushing, flossing, and use of mouthwash should never be neglected, and a soft brush should be used for the tongue, cheeks, and gums.

A common question concerns being able to blow the nose. This is not possible as before. Cleaning the nose is usually accomplished with cotton swabs and tissues.

STOMA COVERINGS

Another of the concerns of patients following surgery is their appearance with regard to the stoma. It is important for them to know that they *can* look nice and probably dress in much the same manner as before surgery. The style of clothing preferred previously should be tried again to see if it can be worn comfortably. As long as the clothing permits comfortable air exchange, it is suitable.

Cover bibs made from porous cloth material are available and may be worn in open-neck clothing for casual purposes or worn under better clothing for protection from mucus adherence. There are many handsome "ascot" scarves men can wear with open-neck shirts. The ladies are fortunate to have beautiful scarves in abundance if they choose to wear them. Scarves made of material with body are more comfortable because there is less adherence to the stoma area. Many patients make their own bibs of material selected from fabric stores and find that crocheted bibs may be made from various yarns and threads to give the desired texture. They are very smart when coordinated with the right shirt, sweater, or blouse. Turtle necks may also be worn successfully. When wearing a shirt and tie, men sometimes find that if the second or third button is removed and sewn on top of the button hole, it will be easier to reach inside the shirt to wipe away mucus that may collect.

In addition to masking the stoma, stoma coverings act as a filter, permitting the air to be in acceptable condition when reaching the windpipe, thus reducing irritation and subsequent coughing; they offer protection from excessive air when outside; and they warm the air in winter, which also aids in reducing coughing. If radiation has been necessary, these areas should be protected from direct sunlight by a stoma covering or other suitable clothing. Foam bibs are available and are especially useful in filtering fine dust and in helping to retain moisture in the trachea. Foam products also include an adhesive foam patch that is small, lightweight, and usually quite convenient to wear, either alone or under clothing as a protector from mucus and foam strips for those who would like to make their own coverings. Because some patients cannot tolerate coverings directly against the stoma, both a wire frame and a metal rod are available that fit on a soft bib to lift away the fabric and permit easier breathing. A stoma covering should be worn, particularly in the company of others. For the laryngectomee to do otherwise will only invite unnecessary inconvenience for everyone concerned. Plastic coverings must never be used over the stoma. Breathing is impossible through plastic!

ADJUSTMENTS IN EATING

Since air no longer passes through the nose, the senses of both smell and taste are sometimes diminished. Taste largely depends on smell and thus is affected. These senses are not completely absent because there is still some interchange of air through the nose, and the tongue continues to help promote the sense of taste. Some patients do not notice much difference in these senses, but for those who do, there will usually be improvement with time and speech development.

Eating practices usually do not require permanent alterations or restrictions, but certain measures must be clearly understood and closely followed to facilitate pleasant eating experiences and reduce the probability of food's becoming lodged in the esophagus. Please be sure to allow adequate time for eating and chew the food well, taking average size bites. It is suggested that patients refrain from eating popcorn, the white meat of chicken, and steak until swallowing seems normal and comfortable. Swallowing difficulties often relate to the extent and location of the tumor and the extent of the surgical procedure necessary to remove it. The severity of these problems varies, and it is important that the situation be discussed with the physician. Having food return through the nose while eating is a temporary disturbance and will correct itself. If nutritional intake is impaired, it is wise to increase protein intake. Using double-strength milk is an excellent way to do this. It is prepared by adding one cup of dried skim milk to one quart of whole fluid milk. This product may be used for cooking purposes as well as a separate beverage. Cheese may be grated or melted in sauces and served with other foods. Tender meats cut in small pieces adapt well to cream sauces, stews, and soups. Some fruit drinks and nectars are less irritating than others. Dietary supplements such as Instant Breakfast, Meritene, and Ensure may also be used. Several good publications are available on nutrition. Suggestions include "Eating Hints" and "A Guide to Good Nutrition," both available from the National Cancer Society; and excellent booklets from pharmaceutical companies. Information should also be available from your laryngologist's office.

TREATMENT OF COLDS

Fortunately colds do not seem to pose a serious problem. For unknown reasons, patients usually have fewer colds and sinus problems after surgery than before. The nose may "run" or "drip," usually because of lack of air passing through the nose to help absorb the secretions. This condition will improve in time. If a cold does develop, a vaporizer should be used to keep secretions thin and easily removed. If the patient becomes increasingly ill, the physician should be contacted immediately. Cold remedies should not be taken without the physician's permission. These medications may increase dryness of the secretions, making them difficult to remove, therefore causing serious breathing impairment.

ACTIVITY INVOLVEMENT

Most activities need not be restricted, but some pertaining to water sports such as swimming and water skiing require special precautions. Fishing done in a safe boat when wearing a good vest-type life preserver is acceptable. The amount of work and activity allowed should be gauged by the stamina of the participant. It is wise to avoid becoming overtired and to stay active within comfortable limits.

It is helpful for the patient and family members to arrange a "signal system" that can be used by telephone until voice communication is possible. Identification cards regarding some first-aid procedures are available for the patient. Identical information is now also printed on adhesive stickers to be placed in car windows or wherever the patient wishes. Identification bracelets and lockets are available and their use is recommended.

There are laryngectomee clubs located in almost every state and in some foreign countries. These are worthwhile and informative. Information regarding specific clubs and locations may be obtained through your laryngologist's office. The American Cancer Society publishes a free newsletter (I.A.L. News) that carries excellent information of special interest to the laryngectomee. It will be sent to anyone upon request.

AWARENESS OF PROBLEM SIGNS

It is of great importance for the laryngectomee to have follow-up care and to be aware of problems that may arise so that the physician may be alerted between visits to arrange necessary treatment. A lump anywhere in the neck demands the physician's immediate attention. Other important signs include persistent coughing of blood, persistent sore throat and earache, sores around the stoma or in the trachea, difficulty swallowing or breathing, voice changes, unusual and prolonged coughing, or any problems that seem to persist. These signs do not necessarily mean recurrence of cancer, but they should be promptly investigated.

Patients who have had a neck dissection will often experience discomfort and aching in the shoulder on the affected side during the first few months following surgery. To alleviate these symptoms heat and massage are used in tandem with normal activity. These discomforts are normal side effects of this particular surgery and will usually subside in time. Puffiness of the face and neck (usually on the nonsurgical side) often comes and goes. It is more apparent in the morning on arising and usually does not indicate a serious problem.

It has been found to be to the patient's advantage if his or her home physician is aware of findings and treatment in his or her particular case. The preferred procedure is to contact his or her physician, usually by letter, to establish communication for sound follow-up care in the future.

QUESTIONS

1. What is the primary reason for wearing a tracheostomy tube, and how may different types can you list? (Consulting your laryngologist is acceptable in answering this question.)
2. Amplify on the author's comment about the use of cooking oil to insert a tracheostomy tube. (Why, what does the oil do, other instructions that might be given to a client?)
3. List ways of increasing the humidity of air inhaled by a laryngectomee?
4. How many suggestions do you find in the author's discussion of bathing and personal hygiene? Can you rewrite these in the form of 10 Commandments for Activities of Daily Living?
5. Outline a discussion you might have with a client regarding stoma cover-ups.
6. In your circle of laryngectomized acquaintances, have any other adjustments in eating been made that are not discussed in this chapter?

Chapter **27**

Rehabilitation Score-List for the Laryngectomized

P. Helbert Damsté

The 1977 Mayo Laryngectomee Rehabilitation Seminar used Sally Bowman's short speech proficiency check list. This appeared to be a great help for speech pathologists and patients alike in getting started on a therapy program that was adapted to the patient's needs. It suited especially those patients who, 1 or 2 years after their original training period, wanted to check whether there was need for improvement in their speech habits.

Fortunately, there are clubs for the laryngectomized in the Netherlands that stimulate a critical attitude towards the quality of speech. A chance was seen to get the seven Dutch schools of logopedics interested in working with laryngectomized persons. It is practically impossible for most speech therapy students to have live experience with esophageal voice training, because the number of new patients each year about equals the number of students that graduate each year. For this reason 5 years ago the possibility for advanced esophageal speakers to improve their speech habits with the help of speech therapy students, supervised by the voice therapy training staff, was created. This did not always turn out to be a success: the students on the whole did not work in a systematical way; some appeared not to know what to practice with their patients. Often the patients stayed away after one or two sessions. Clearly the parties on both sides did not particularly stimulate each other.

It was thought that an extended score-list for judging the quality of esophageal speaking habits would be helpful to prepare the participants for the voice improvement sessions. A joint committee of one patient, two logopedists, and a phoniatrist worked out the score-list (Fig. 27–1) and manual.

Rehabilitation Score-List for the Laryngectomized

Patient's name:

Examiner:

Examination dates:

1st

2nd

3rd

Needs Treatment

I. Qualities of Voice and Speech

I.1 Type of voice: pseudo-whisper, pharyngeal, esophageal (underline)

I.2 Mode of air intake: inhaling, swallowing, injecting (underline)

1   2   3   4   5

I.3 Elementary Skills

    3.1 Availability of the voice
    3.2 Duration of the sound
    3.3 Number of syllables on one intake
    3.4 Articulation
    3.5 Loudness
    3.6 Tempo

I.4 Supplementary Skills

    4.1 Latency
    4.2 Audible klunk
    4.3 Repeated injections
    4.4 Surplus movements
    4.5 Stoma noise

I.5 Refinements

    5.1 Intensity variation
    5.2 Variation of pitch
    5.3 Variation of tempo

I.6 Intelligibility

II. Social Skills

II.1 Independence

    1.1 Visiting friends
    1.2 Joining clubs, going to meetings or a pub
    1.3 Talking to strangers
    1.4 Going out on errands
    1.5 Using the telephone
    1.6 Job situation

II.2   Assertiveness

    2.1   Eye contact
    2.2   Taking part in discussion
    2.3   Humor

Check II.3   Information
if the

answer   3.1   The clubs for laryngectomees
is no: 3.2   The various means and devices for
          laryngectomees
    3.3   The possibility to swim
    3.4   The possibility to smell

Figure 27–1.   Rehabilitation score-list for judging the quality of esophageal speaking habits.

MANUAL FOR USE OF THE EVALUATION SHEET

The names and the date are entered.

The present performance on each item is judged on a five-point scale and entered by an x:

1.   very poor
2.   poor
3.   medium
4.   good
5.   excellent

This can be done by subjective judgment for rapid screening or by actual counting and measuring and comparing with norm scales. The subjective method is good enough for clinical purposes because there are no hard and fast norms for individual cases. The attainable "norm" is different for each patient, because the outcome of the operation and wound healing vary and the condition of the lungs and other factors related to general health and age are not the same. Therefore an estimate is made of what would be the best attainable score on each item for the patient under examination and this goal-score is entered as ☐. For example, when intonation is very poor, and you expect that by practicing it can be improved to medium, the scale is entered as follows:

☐   pitch modulation   ☒ ▢

The check mark in the left margin means that there is a discrepancy between potential competence and actual performance, so that this item will be a part of the training program. When the screening is repeated from time to time, the different colors of pen or pencil can be used.

1.   The Quality of Voice and Speech
    1.1   Begin by noting what type of voice is being used: when the patient is using pseudo-whispered or pharyngeal voice, it makes no sense to go on with the list, because it is meant for advanced users of esophageal voice. The patient will have to be referred to a phoniatric center in order to learn esophageal voice.

    1.2   The intake of air is recognized by the following features:
- Inhaling is synchronous with an inspiration.
- Swallowing requires a large and slow movement of the hyoid.
- Injecting is rapid and inconspicuous, or it can be heard as audible "klunks."
- Inhaling can be done in an unobtrusive way and is sometimes used in combination with injection.

When an inefficient method of air intake is used, for example, swallowing, a check mark in the left margin will indicate that this will be corrected.

    1.3   Elementary Skills
        3.1   Consistency: Is the voice sound always available? Can it be produced on request ten out of ten times (score 5), eight times (score 4), six times (3), four times (2), two times (1)? Ask the patient to say "pah" in intervals of 5 seconds.

        3.2   Duration: ask the patient to hold an easy syllable (ah, pa, or ta) for at least 2 seconds (score 5), 1.5 seconds (4), 1 second (3), 0.5 second (2).

        3.3   Number of syllables on one intake: ask the patient to repeat quickly wa-wa-wa-wa-wa on one air intake. For five syllables, score 5; for four, 4; and so on. Score the best of three trials.

        3.4   Articulation: Note the overall distinctness and clarity of articulation and mark specific articulation defects.

        3.5   Loudness: Conduct a subjective evaluation of maximal loudness: weak (1), medium (3), loud (5). Objective evaluation with sound-level meter at a distance of 20 centimeters, curve A: for 65 decibels (dB) score (1), 70 dB (2), 75 dB (3), 80 dB (4), and 85 dB (5).

3.6   Tempo: Mark whether the rate of speech is satisfactory without detriment to distinctness and clarity of articulation.

1.4   Supplementary Skills

4.1   Short latency: the duration between the air intake and the utterance. No pause in the midst of words or phrases.

4.2   Silent intake: no audible "klunks" between words and sentences.

4.3   Single intake: no "double pump."

4.4   Simple intake: no accessory movements with the mouth or the head or other parts of the body; no signs of effort.

4.5   Stoma noise: hardly any expiratory thrusts audible during speech and no audible inspiration.

1.5   Refinements

5.1   Intensity modulation: try with accents in two- to five-syllable words and in phrases.

5.2   Pitch modulation: intonation in affirmative and interrogative sentences.

5.3   Variation in the rate of speech: fluent spacing of accentuated parts, intelligible acceleration in casual speech or irrelevant parts of sentences.

1.6   Intelligibility: is it possible to comprehend the details of an extemporaneous story without looking at the patient's face (mouth)?

2.   Social Skills

2.1   Independence

The items are discussed and evaluated by the patient and the speech pathologist together. This gives an opportunity for the patient to recognize problem areas and for the speech pathologist to suggest step-by-step approaches towards solutions. Scoring has to take into account the degree of speech proficiency that is within the patient's reach. When, for instance, the patient still dislikes to enter conversations with strangers, this may be quite justified if his speech is scarcely comprehensible. If, however, his speech is completely understandable to strangers, a practice program would be appropriate in which the patient learns to overcome inhibitions and feelings of inferiority because of an abnormal voice.

2.2   Assertiveness

A discussion of these items is meant to desensitize the patient

> with regard to self-consciousness about his speech handicap.
>
> 2.3   Information
>
> The last series is to be adapted according to the country's customs and needs. There may be countries where information about the possibility of an artificial larynx should be added to the list. In some centers perhaps the hazard of smoking will be on the information check list and the need for a half-yearly radiographic examination of the chest (because this group has a high risk of bronchial carcinoma). In other centers this sort of information will not be given by the persons concerned with rehabilitation.

In this form the evaluation sheet represents a detailed analysis of the qualities of a laryngectomee's speech. More compact forms are conceivable and are in fact being used by several speech pathologists. The merits are obvious. For the speech pathologist it is a helpful instrument: It aids in the discovery of underdeveloped skills and problem areas (diagnosis) and in the assessment of attainable goals for therapy (prognosis). Because he can now "contract" the patient for the amount of time to be spent on the checked items, it helps the speech pathologist to organize his or her work. For the patient it is a motivating device: he can clearly see what can be improved in his speech skills and habits, and he can see the results of his efforts when he has been working on them. It addition, the spouse or other persons in the environment can be informed about the plan of treatment and can be given the task of rewarding the patient when he practices with success the intended speech behaviors.

QUESTIONS

1. Develop a score-list similar to that suggested by Damsté for esophageal voice to enable assessment of the use of an artificial larynx.
2. Do you agree with the heading "Supplementary Skills" for section I.4?
3. For each subsection in Part I of the score-list, develop definitions for the numerical ratings of 1, 2, 3, 4, and 5.
4. Do as directed in Question 3 the same for Part II.

Chapter 28

Essentials for Alaryngeal Speech: Psychology and Physiology

James C. Shanks

The psychological ingredients that a laryngectomee brings to the acquisition of speech after surgery are in great measure determined by his preoperative attitude. It is not facetious to say that it is important to determine whether the person is a pessimist or an optimist. The pessimist will contend that a glass of water is half empty; the optimist will note that the glass is half full.

In an effort to attempt to define the essentials that cause a person to be a pessimist or an optimist, the story is told of twin boys once studied in some detail. One boy was a pessimist of the first order, his brother most optimistic. In the study the pessimistic boy was placed for 3 hours in a room containing many toys, a bicycle, and all kinds of sweet things to eat, including candy and ice cream. Meanwhile, his optimistic brother was placed in a room containing only a small shovel and an enormous pile of horse manure. After the 3 hours had elapsed, the examiners went back to find the pessimistic boy sitting disconsolately. When asked about his feelings about the things around him, he reported that he was afraid that the toys might break, that he might hurt himself on the bicycle, and that the ice cream and candy might make him sick. The examiners then approached the optimistic boy and were somewhat surprised to find him using his small shovel, digging feverishly in the pile of manure. When asked about his activity, the lad replied, "With all of this manure around here, there's got to be a pony somewhere."

Clearly, the laryngectomee who is looking for his pony appears more likely to be successful in acquiring alaryngeal speech. Another scale that can be used in assessing the laryngectomee has to do with introversion and extroversion. Various authors, including Schall (1938), Levin (1952), and Stoll (1958), note the greater likelihood of the outgoing, extroverted person being more successful in the acquisition of speech after laryngectomy.

A third useful scale measures the individual's preoperative dependence versus independence. In this situation many of us are convinced that it is not merely a question of whether the laryngectomee was previously dependent or independent but whether he continued to have the same kind of relationship with his environment after surgery. For example, if an individual, quite independent before surgery, depended after surgery on his spouse to clean the stoma, help with nose blowing, and care for every need, that individual would be expected to make slower progress than one who put up with dependence on others only until the point when he could be independent, not only with regard to work but with regard to care of himself.

A fourth measurement has to do with the general characteristic, motivation. Stoll (1958) is among many authors who have contended, along with individual members of the International Association of Laryngectomees (the IAL), that motivation is the most important single factor in acquisition of speech after laryngectomy. Confirming evidence comes from Goldberg (1975), a researcher and social scientist. He found that motivation or the desire to do is the attribute most highly correlated with successful rehabilitation.

Motivation not only cuts across attitudes of optimism, extroversion, and independence but it also assumes a freedom from special problems. Thus, it should be noted that the individual who lives alone has an added difficulty both as regards amount of practice and justification for practice to improve his speech after laryngectomy. Blake (1974) found that the Minnesota Multiphasic Personality Inventory showed scores on four scales to be related to alaryngeal speech proficiency. The higher the score on these four scales, the lower the speech proficiency. The four scales were (1) schizophrenia; (2) the F scale, relating to eccentricity or carelessness; (3) hypochondriasis, or anxiety about health; and (4) social introversion. Similarly, DeBartolo (1971), using the Tennessee Scale of Self Concept as well as a scale of anxiety, found that in general the better speakers had higher scores on self-concept and body concept. The poorer speakers were more anxious than the better speakers, and the poorer speakers had higher scores on defensive distortion. In other words, concept of self, body image, anxiety level, and defensive distortion were factors differentiating the groups of better versus poorer speakers.

Apart from the entire matter of preoperative attitude is a person's constellation of fears. Stoll (1958) found, for example, that the fears before surgery common to many laryngectomees included fear of the word "cancer" as well as fear of death, fear about operations in general, and fear of the permanent loss of voice, especially as it might affect dealing with other people and the loss of job, money, and security. After surgery the fears noted by Stoll included fear of recurrence of cancer and fear of death. There was also fear of the new ways in which the body would function in lifting, breathing through the neck opening, smelling, and tasting. There was fear of old age, of feeling useless, and of feeling depressed. There was fear of being unable to re-establish old interpersonal relationships. Finally, there was fear that the individual would not be able to learn a new method of speaking.

Another approach in assessing the psychological attitude of the laryngectomee has to do with his reaction to crises. Sanchez-Salazar and Stark (1972) found four specific times at which the laryngectomee might expect a crisis: on being told that an operation is necessary, just after the operation while in the hospital, upon arrival home after discharge from the hospital, and several months later when the individual finds that his environment has settled back into a routine in which he no longer enjoys a favored or special status. Now the significance of these crises is not that they prevent the individual from learning speech after laryngectomy but rather than knowing that such crises may occur enables the others, as well as the laryngectomee, to anticipate them and begin to counteract their negative influence.

Physiological essentials for alaryngeal speech are every bit as important as psychological factors. Gates and coworkers (1982a; Gates, Ryan, Cantu, and Hearne, 1982b) provided a sanguine update on the success and failure of efforts to acquire esophageal speech. Indeed, historically physiological factors have been given greater emphasis in accounting for difficulty in developing *esophageal* speech. Physical factors appear to be less likely to interfere with speech using voice from a mechanical or electrical larynx. This chapter will focus on physical essentials for esophageal speech while implying that the factors are somewhat less essential in instrument speech.

It appears that chronological age correlates with ability to learn speech after laryngectomy. In his book *Laryngectomee Speech and Rehabilitation* Gardner (1971) summarized four studies related to success in acquiring esophageal speech as a function of age. These studies indicated that persons between 20 and 40 years of age have a chance of almost 100 per cent, those between 40 and 60 years have a 56 to 98 per cent chance, and those 60 and over only about a 50 per cent chance of developing good esophageal speech. The factor of age was further investigated by Kahane and Irwin (1975) (Fig. 28–1). Persons older than 60 years had a greater likelihood of requiring a longer time in speech therapy, a greater measure of hearing loss in general and a greater high-

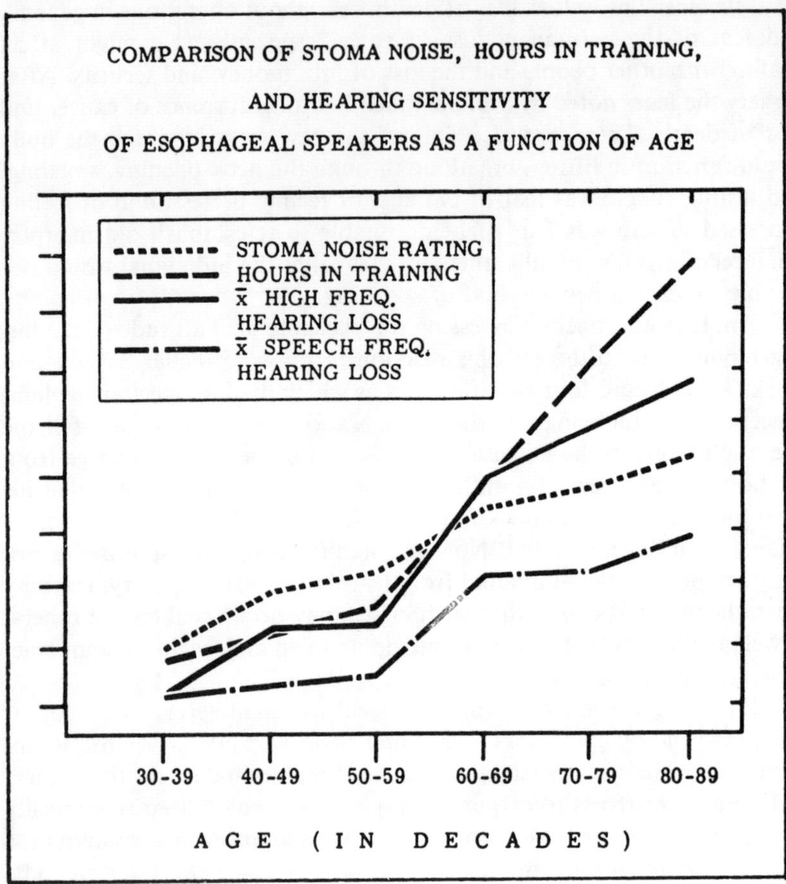

Figure 28–1. Alaryngeal speech and hearing functions by decades of age.

frequency loss specifically, and, finally, a greater amount of perceived or judged stomal noise when speaking.

This finding by Kahane and Irwin (1975) of greater difficulty with hearing and speaking associated with older age may be looked at from another point of view, that is, one having to do with hearing itself. Berlin (1974) and Diedrich and Youngstrom (1966) both found the presence of a hearing loss to be one of the few significant physical factors adversely related to the ability to acquire and develop esophageal speech. Martin (1970) extended the assessment of hearing to include ability to understand esophageal speech. Now it is recognized that when an individual has a hearing loss, expressed in units of intensity called decibels, this does not, by itself, indicate his ability to understand speech of a given loudness. The question of the presumed benefit from a hearing aid or other amplification is related to an additional test of discrimination: Given speech of adequate loudness, is it understandable? In such a test the individual is asked to repeat one-syllable words. With 50 words per test, doubling the number of words correctly repeated gives a discrimination score, expressed in per cent. To have a problem in discriminating average speech from a laryngeal speaker would be a predictable obstacle. Martin's study went beyond that to note that individuals who could understand average esophageal speech were more likely to acquire good esophageal speech themselves after therapy.

The single most important structure needed for articulate speech is the tongue. Many years ago Harrington (1961) indicated that when a person is able to eat average-sized morsels, the mechanism exists to capture air to produce esophageal voice. However, it should be noted that not only does the tongue function for the injection of air into the esophagus for esophageal voice production but it is used also in the articulation of speech, whether voice be produced by the esophagus or an artificial larynx. In the following sample, the lady in question has had much of the back of her tongue removed. She was able to acquire esophageal voice by inhalation. What is more noteworthy is that her connected speech is quite understandable and that she has difficulty only with the back-of-tongue consonants, such as /k/ and /g/. (Tape)

This consideration of the tongue as a mechanism needed for the injection of air for esophageal voice leads us to the next physiological consideration: five areas of pressure (Winans, Reichbach, and Waldrop, 1974) within the alimentary tract important for the production of esophageal voice (Fig. 28–2). Those five areas are (1) the bottom of the throat or hypopharynx; (2) the place where the esophagus and the pharynx meet, identified as the pharyngoesophageal (PE) junction; (3) the body of the esophagus itself; (4) the sphincter at the bottom of the esophagus as it empties into the stomach, designated the gastroesophageal, or GE, junction; and finally, (5) the stomach or gastric area. Taking these five crucial areas in reverse order, it is notable that difficulty in the stomach area is likely to be associated with too much air pressure, leading to discomfort. The unusual circumstance of reduced air pressure in the stomach could occur in the laryngectomee who has also had a colostomy, yet the speaker in the following tape merely had a slightly softer voice after colostomy. (Tape) The area of the GE junction should be tight to retain air in the esophagus. If there is a rupture, such as a hiatal hernia, or if there is undue reflux of stomach contents up into the esophagus, the individual may report discomfort from the distended stomach, too much acidity, and even difficulty in producing voice. One laryngec-

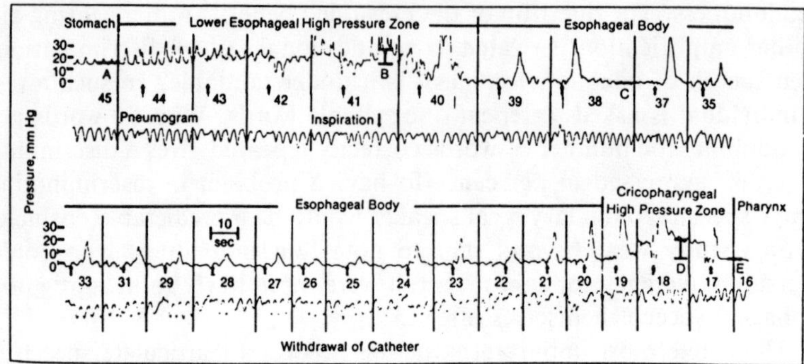

Figure 28–2. Pressure changes through the pharynx, esophagus, and stomach.

tomee had to loosen his belt after 5 minutes of practicing esophageal voice, yet we know of several good speakers with a history of hiatal hernia (Mathis, Lehman, Shanks, Blom, and Brunelle, 1983). Within the body of the esophagus, there should be neither a stricture nor a rupture. Some individuals have an esophageal diverticulum or spasm, which would not assist in the production of esophageal voice.

The most crucial area for the production of esophageal voice is the PE junction. Theoretically, this area could be too loose or too tight. If the PE junction is too loose, a remedy may be had in the form of digital pressure on the neck opposite the PE section or the application of a band, a hand, or a tight collar or tie around that area. In one instance, a patient had both an esophageal diverticulum and a loose PE segment. Even with digital pressure she could produce voice only briefly. The more common and more serious problem is undue tension in the PE area. A study by Winans and co-workers (1974) measured pressures in these different areas in persons with a larynx and in laryngectomized persons. In normals there is pressure in the PE area, pressure at the bottom of the esophagus, and the pressure of an air bubble in the stomach. The laryngectomee differs from the laryngeal speaker (Fig. 28–3) in that he has a bigger bubble of air pressure in the stomach and lower pressure at the PE segment. Moreover, when comparing individuals who were more successful in the acquisition of esophageal voice with those who had difficulty in acquiring it, Winans and colleagues found that those having difficulty acquiring voice (Fig. 28–4) failed to get a larger air bubble in the stomach; that is, they were not getting air down that

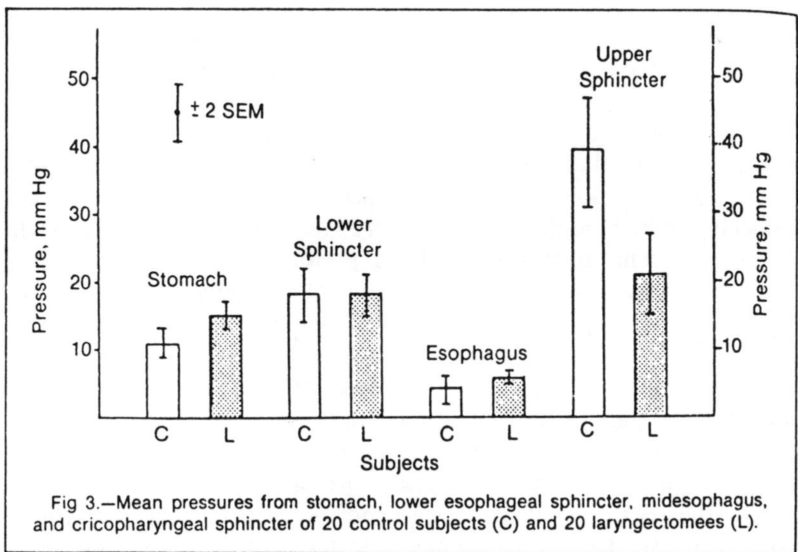

Fig 3.—Mean pressures from stomach, lower esophageal sphincter, midesophagus, and cricopharyngeal sphincter of 20 control subjects (C) and 20 laryngectomees (L).

Figure 28–3. Pressures in laryngeal versus esophageal speakers.

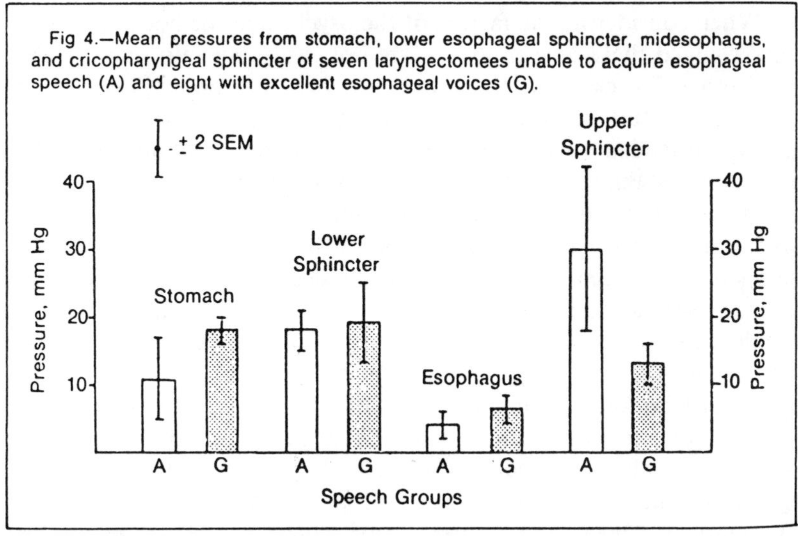
Fig 4.—Mean pressures from stomach, lower esophageal sphincter, midesophagus, and cricopharyngeal sphincter of seven laryngectomees unable to acquire esophageal speech (A) and eight with excellent esophageal voices (G).

Figure 28–4. Pressures in good versus poor esophageal speakers.

far, and, most importantly, they had excessive pressure in the PE segment (see Figs. 28–3 and 28–4). That pressure interfered with the ability to get air into the esophagus and the ability to make that segment vibrate with minimal air forced from the esophagus.

The physical integrity of the vocal tract—the mouth, throat, and nose separated by the palate—is crucial to resonance as well as to the articulation of voice into speech. If the vocal tract is open because the cheek has an opening or because there is a gap in the area under the chin, sound will not have the same quality nor will air pressure be built up within the mouth to articulate the various consonants. This characteristic holds not only for the esophageal speaker but for the individual who uses an artificial larynx or a tracheoesophageal puncture-prosthesis. Notice in the next audiotape sample the poor quality of speech, related to the fact that this gentleman had part of the roof of his mouth cut away by the surgeon. It was difficult to fabricate a prosthetic device to cover that portion of the soft palate that ordinarily moves during speech. (Tape)

Another possible difficulty with the vocal tract has to do with its undue firmness. The laryngectomee who has had heavy radiation may have a firm, fibrotic neck area that interferes with the placement of a neck-type artificial larynx. Although this does not preclude the use of the cheek as a means of delivering sound into the vocal tract or of using an oral device (pneumatic or electric) to put voice into the mouth, it does reduce the speech potential.

When considering the factors of the psyche and the body, it must be acknowledged that some problems are not easily put into one category or the other. For example, if the individual is an alcoholic, his problem affects his attitude as well as his bodily function. This writer recalls a man who attended a workshop 1 year ago who did a commendable job in speaking as well as in relating to other laryngectomees. At the close of the conference he confided that just before his operation a doctor had forced him to make three decisions that affected his life: first, to have the operation for removal of his larynx, a decision about which he was wavering; second, to completely give up the use of alcohol; and third, to completely give up the use of drugs. Only when ordered to do so did this man assent. There was little question in his mind (or the author's) that the doctor who forced him to do these three things literally saved his life.

An indication of the way in which attitude and body interplay is seen in the results of a study by Snidecor (1975), for many years a leading teacher and researcher in Santa Barbara, California. Doctor Snidecor obtained a measure of speech proficiency on a large number of laryngectomees. He also had them answer a number of questions on a three-way multiple choice scale. Of 31 questions presented, 12 turned out to have answers that were highly correlated with speech proficiency

Table 28–1. Questionnaire Answers Given by Better Esophageal Speakers

Number of Item	Subject (Abbreviated)
1.	Eats rapidly when at home in private.
2.	Can swallow food in rather large chunks (steak).
3.	If had a modest retirement income, would work and spend the difference.
4.	Can easily break wind when this will not bother others.
5.	Age: 62 and under.
6.	Relations with family are active and at times scrappy.
7.	Stomach growling (in public) does not bother him or her.
8.	Is more talkative than most in a small group.
9.	Does not fear or hate old age.
10.	Welcomes new learning situations.
11.	Is egocentric or proud of self.
12.	Drinks socially or not at all.

(Table 28–1). The characteristics of individuals who were successful are worthy of study.

The proficient speaker is one who eats rapidly when at home in private. He does not make a fetish of mealtime but realizes that feeding the body is essential. He can swallow food in rather large chunks. It is noteworthy that if he had the chance to retire at a modest income and just get by, he would decline that option and go to work, spending the added money for greater enjoyment in living. His attitude is that he can break wind when this will not bother others. (We sometimes forget that flatus is a common characteristic of the laryngectomee, particularly one who uses esophageal voice. As one laryngectomee said, "I may run out of steam, but I never run out of gas." This might be thought of as an inside joke.) The most important thing is that the laryngectomee looks at his bodily functions as normal and is not upset by them, especially if they do not bother others. That the proficient speaker is aged 62 or under lends further evidence that age is a variable. The finding that relations with the family are "active" or "sometimes scrappy" has two connotations: first, there must be a family with whom to have interactions; second, the person is not a Caspar Milquetoast, does not just accept what comes his way, and has normal, healthy differences of opinion with others in the family. Stomach growling, like flatus, does not bother him. Now note the tendency to talk more than most in a small group, that is, in the absence of undue noise or competition. Notice that the individual does not fear or hate old age and welcomes new learning situations. The fact that he is egocentric or likes himself is a reflection of factors noted by other authors. Finally, the notation that he drinks socially or not at all is in contrast to the problem drinking noted previously.

In summing up the essentials for alaryngeal speech, the conclusion is that the individual must want to talk. If his desire to talk is strong enough and if there is an opportunity to learn, he can learn by one means or another. One of the most frustrating tragedies this author has encountered is the man, declining to try to acquire speech after laryngectomy, who stated, "The Man upstairs doesn't want me to talk." That is sacrilegious. The body must be capable of taking nourishment; even if fed by tube, the body must stay vital. Greater amounts of tongue removal constitute the most important physical obstacle to the conversion of voice into speech. Seldom does an individual with a total laryngectomy and a total glossectomy learn to speak in a satisfactory manner. In some instances people try to learn sign language or resort to writing. But a desire to talk and a body capable of taking nourishment constitute the minimal essentials for speech after laryngectomy.

Finally, it should be noted that in all of the studies reported, including Snidecor's, it has not been said that if someone fails to meet the different criteria that person should be denied the chance to try to speak after laryngectomy. It is a person's right to try to talk. It is a human right to try to sound human. No matter how many strikes there were against a person previously, he or she should be given the opportunity to go to bat to try to learn to speak after total laryngectomy.

The discussion of essentials has proceeded from impressions and reports by observers. The question posed to the laryngectomee may be, "After total laryngectomy, what do you bring for your recovery and rehabilitation?" There are three parts to the answer.

The laryngectomee has gone through a surgical experience that leaves a blend of self-doubt and self-confidence. The doubt springs from lack of awareness of the implications of total laryngectomy for everyday activities, body functions, and the future. How can and will I function? the laryngectomee asks. Some know early on that *they will learn to talk again*. Such people need to be given only a minimum of information about the process of producing esophageal voice, and they proceed to develop communication by combined acquisition of motor skills and self-appraisal. Some excellent speakers are basically self-taught.

Those who teach speech after laryngectomy accept the fact that they are not indispensable. In visualizing their relationship to the recently operated laryngectomee, they see themselves as sharing information gained directly from previous experience and indirectly from the writings of others. For some laryngectomees speech clinicians need do little beyond providing that information. For some laryngectomees clinicians need to do more.

A basic question in the rehabilitation process is what do speech pathologists and other health personnel contribute to rehabilitation? As noted in a study supported by the National Cancer Institute, carried out by Gonnella and co-workers (1978), their role may be (1) identifying and evaluating, (2) informing, (3) instructing, and (4) treating and training. This philosophy of rehabilitation as a process of "I do something for and to you" underlies much of their thinking. However, it need not imply "conditioning" in the cold sense that speech clinicians shape behavior. It may imply being like the minister who saw himself as making the uncomfortable comfortable—and making the comfortable uncomfortable. There is a need to help many laryngectomees become aware of the excellence of speech that can be developed, of flaws that stand in the way, and of means of judging themselves in order to continue to improve as time goes by.

Finally, the process of rehabilitation is not only measured in terms of facts: How fast do you talk, what is your pitch, how clearly do you speak? The end result of rehabilitation should include also the laryngectomee's feelings about himself—as a person and as a speaker. This suggest a qualitative as well as a quantitative side to rehabilitation. Growth as a person may be hard to measure, but it is important. Finally, any assistance speech clinicians provide is with a realization that laryngectomees are entitled to it whether they live for an additional 20 years—or 20 weeks. As long as the laryngectomee lives, he is entitled to use and improve his skills. That conviction is another essential the laryngectomee provides in the act of learning to talk again after laryngectomy.

QUESTIONS

1. List the psychological essentials (which may require some rewriting of Shank's comments) and then indicate that which you think is the most important, the second most important, the third until the rank order is complete. Make your indications by using numerals, 1, representing the most important; 2, the second most important, and so forth.
2. Shanks indicates that age is related to the likelihood of speech reacquisition. Hearing acuity and discrimination are one variable related to age that might account for ease and degree of speech skill development. What are some other factors that might link age to lesser degrees of speech proficiency?
3. What is the difference between hearing acuity and discrimination?
4. What instructional modifications might be needed in order for individuals with partial glossectomies to develop esophageal voice and subsequent speech?

5. Develop a questionnaire that might be used during an initial interview with a prospective client to learn of potential physical limitations for speech acquisition.

REFERENCES

Berlin, C. I. (1974). Hearing loss, palatal function, and other factors in post-laryngectomy rehabilitation. *J. Chronic Dis., 17,* 677–684.

Blake, I. (1974). *Relationship between personality and esophageal speech proficiency.* Paper presented at annual convention of American Speech and Hearing Association, Las Vegas, NV.

DeBartolo, R. (1971). Psychological considerations in the attainment of esophageal speech. *J. Surg. Oncol., 3,* 451–466.

Diedrich, W. M., and Youngstrom, K. (1966). *Alaryngeal speech,* Springfield, IL: Charles C Thomas.

Gardner, W. H. (1971). *Laryngectomee speech and rehabilitation.* Springfield, IL: Charles C Thomas.

Gates, G. A., Ryan, W., Cantu, E., and Hearne, E. (1982b). Current status of laryngectomee rehabilitation: II. Causes of failure. *Am. J. Otolaryngol., 3,* 8–14.

Gates, G. A., Ryan, W., Cooper, J. C., Lawlis, G. F., Cantu, E., Hayashi, T., Lauder, E., Welch, R. W., and Hearne, E. (1982a). Current status of laryngectomee rehabilitation. *Am. J. Otolaryngol., 3,* 1–7.

Goldberg, R. T. (1975). Vocational and social adjustment after laryngectomy. *Scand. J. Rehab. Med., 7,* 1–8.

Gonnella, C., Parker, C., Hollender, J., Lowell, G., Petterson, P., and Miller, S. (1978). *Normative Criteria for Cancer Rehabilitation.* Rehab. Res. Monograph Series No. 1, Atlanta: Emory University.

Harrington, R. (1961). Speech instruction panel. Tenth Annual Meeting, International Association of Laryngectomees, San Francisco.

Kahane, J., and Irwin, J. (1975). *Comparison of hearing sensitivity, stoma noise and speech ratings and duration in therapy in 90 esophageal speakers.* Paper presented at annual convention of American Speech and Hearing Association, Washington, DC.

Levin, N. M. (1952). Speech rehabilitation after total removal of the larynx. *J. Amer. Med. Assoc., 140,* 1281–1286.

Martin, D. E. (1970). *Performance of laryngectomees on selected auditory tests in relation to their esophageal speech proficiency.* Unpublished doctoral dissertation, University of Michigan, Ann Arbor.

Mathis, J. G., Lehman, G. H., Shanks, J. C., Blom, E. D., and Brunelle, R. L. (1983). Effect of gastroesophageal reflux on esophageal speech. *J. Clin. Gastroenterol., 5,* 503–507.

Sanchez-Salazar, V., and Stark, A. (1972). The use of crisis intervention in the rehabilitation of laryngectomees. *J. Speech Hearing Dis., 37,* 323–328.

Schall, L. A. (1938). Psychology of laryngectomized patients. *Arch. Otolaryngol., 23,* 581–584.

Snidecor, J. C. (1975). Some scientific foundations for voice restoration. *Laryngoscope, 85,* 640–648.

Stoll, B. (1958). Psychological factors determining the success or failure of the rehabilitation program of laryngectomized patients. *Ann. Otology, 67,* 550–557.
Winans, C. S., Reichbach, E. J., and Waldrop, W. F. (1974). Esophageal determinants of alaryngeal speech. *Arch. Otolaryngol., 98,* 10–14.

Chapter **29**

Laryngectomee Visitations

Shirley J. Salmon

As you laryngectomees acquire better speech skills, you will probably find yourselves called upon to represent the rehabilitated laryngectomee in a variety of circumstances. Your spouses may also be asked to share this responsibility so that, together, you may be viewed as representatives of a well-rehabilitated couple.

The circumstances in which you and your spouse might find yourself could include

1. Participating in local or state cancer crusades to raise additional funds for the American Cancer Society.
2. Attending New Voice Club meetings at which the two of you will be viewed by the newly laryngectomized patient and spouse as a source of information and inspiration.
3. Visiting laryngectomee patients and spouses in the hospital either preoperatively or postoperatively.

It is for this latter reason that a discussion of hospital visitations is warranted. Because these visits can play such an important role in total rehabilitation it seems advisable to make them as effective as possible. The following are some suggested guidelines that might make your visits more acceptable to patients and to hospital personnel, thereby increasing the chances for your being asked to return in the future. These guidelines are the "do's and don'ts" for hospital visitations.

1. *Do not* risk offending a surgeon by visiting his patient in the hospital until the surgeon has requested it or approved it. Remember that the doctor has the legal right—and the legal responsibility—to decide who will or will not see his patients. All other hospital per-

sonnel (nurses, speech pathologists, and so on) must have his approval before they call you and request a visit. Even the family should mention their desire for a visit to him and solicit his approval before you come.

It is a good idea for you to remember to ask whoever contacts you whether the doctor has approved the visit. In this way you will not offend the doctor and you will not be committing a faux pas.

Such discourtesies occur more frequently than you would believe. Two examples may sound familiar enough to be convincing. Consider the laryngectomees who have acquired speech skills and who return to the hospital for periodic check-ups. Following their check-ups they frequently stop by to visit the nurses on the hospital floor where they recuperated from their own surgery. While there they hear about patients in whom they are interested and, unfortunately, begin visiting with them prior to receiving any official request. A second example may seem even more familiar. It happens when an alaryngeal speaker has received an official request to visit one patient but, while visiting that particular patient, he notices other laryngectomees on the same floor and decides to visit with them also. Unfortunately, he does so without an official request and in so doing commits a discourtesy to the surgeon.

2. *Do not* enter a patient's room without first stopping at the nurses' desk to introduce yourself to the head nurse, to state which patient you would like to see, and to indicate who requested your visit. It is a matter of common courtesy to inform the head nurse of your visit, since she is responsible for all patients on her floor. It also provides her with an opportunity to note your visit in the patient's hospital chart for the benefit of the surgeon and other hospital employees.

    Also, she can be most helpful to you. She knows the condition of the patient and can tell you whether the patient is ready to receive visitors or whether you might wait so as not to interrupt a doctor's visit or a treatment.

3. When you first introduce yourself to the patient, *do* present your name card or write down your name, address, and telephone number so that he can refer to it later. Similarly, if you are a member of a local laryngectomees' club, provide him with written information about it such as the name of it, when and where the meetings are held, and some of the typical activities carried out. At the same time, write down the patient's full name, current address (including zip code), and phone number (including area code). Then, later, when you want to turn the name in to the local New Voice Club or

the International Association of Laryngectomees (I.A.L.) so the patient can begin receiving newsletters and announcements of meetings, you will have all of the necessary information. (By the way, if you do not receive the free newsletters from the I.A.L. just write a letter to them and request that your name be added to their mailing list. The address is International Association of Laryngectomees, 90 Park Avenue, New York, NY 10016.)

4. If the patient's spouse is not present, *do* arrange another appointment that is convenient for you and your spouse to visit with the patient and his or her spouse. Several investigators have found that spouses of laryngectomees often are poorly informed regarding all aspects of laryngectomy. They need to be provided with information and resent being ignored by those interested in rehabilitation.

5. For the sake of the patient and yourself, *do* use your communication skills to your best advantage. The average age of individuals when laryngectomized is about 55 or 60 years and the average person of this age in our country may well have a hearing loss. So, there is a good possibility that either the patient or the patient's spouse will have some degree of hearing loss. With this fact in mind about the listener, consider some other facts known about esophageal speech. The pitch level of esophageal voice makes it more difficult for the human ear to perceive, and most esophageal voices are not as loud as normal voices. Now, considering all three of these factors (the possibility of the patient or spouse having a hearing loss, the lower pitch of esophageal speech, and the lower intensity of esophageal speech), it seems logical to conclude that you as an esophageal speaker must adapt your speaking behavior in order for it to be as effective as possible. What can you do to compensate for these possible communication hazards?

6. *Do* be aware of proximity. Snidecor (1968) and Lanpher (1971) have each reminded us "loudness varies in inverse proportion to the square of the distance." That is, a laryngectomee can be heard four times as well when his listener is 3 feet away as when he is 6 feet away. If you remember this fact, you will apply it by assuring yourself that the seating arrangement between you, the patient, and the spouse assures close proximity.

7. *Do* allow opportunity for speechreading. No matter what the reason may be, if someone is having difficulty hearing a speaker's message, he or she will try to obtain cues by reading lips and by observing facial expressions. Consequently, do not seat yourself directly in front of a window during the day or in front of a table lamp in the

evening. You do not want your listener to have light glaring in his eyes if he is attempting to gain additional information from your lip movements or your facial expressions.

8. *Do* observe the noise level within the hospital room and try to work around it. You may find it advisable to turn off the TV or the radio. You may want to suggest moving to a quieter place if the room is being shared by another patient who has visitors or who is creating competitive noises. You should not visit during the lunch or supper hours, since this is an inconvenient time for hospital personnel. Besides, the clanging of trays in the halls can cause an overriding noise and can also be distracting. Try to observe the regular visiting hours.

9. Gardner (1971) has detailed many fine suggestions as to what might be said to patients. You are encouraged to read what he has to say. Of course, you can never anticipate *all* the questions that might be asked. One word of caution. When you do provide an answer, be honest! If you do not know, say so!

It might be helpful to suggest some topics that should not be discussed. *Do not* try to answer questions about surgery or hospital procedures. *Do not* imply criticism about professional workers involved with the patient by suggesting that something "different" was said or done with you. Statements concerning the length of time before your tracheotomy tube was removed, the length of time before your hospital discharge, or your ideas concerning the disadvantages of using an artificial larynx may be different from information the patient has already received. These differences may only cause uncertainty and doubt in a patient who is already faced with considerable anxiety.

Remember, your purpose in visiting a patient is not to plant seeds of doubt but rather to relieve his mind and to bolster his spirits.

It is desirable to make at least one follow-up contact after the patient leaves the hospital—either in person, by phone, or by card. This will make the patient and spouse feel that someone is truly interested in them.

This presentation is brief yet touches on the more significant points. It is hoped that you will find them helpful.

QUESTION

1. Summarize Dr. Salmon's chapter by composing "Ten Commandments for Visitations."

REFERENCES

Gardner, W. H. (1971). *Laryngectomee speech and rehabilitation.* Springfield, IL: Charles C Thomas.

Lanpher, A. (1971). *Profile of a laryngectomee as related to the clinician's role.* Paper presented at Eleventh I.A.L. Voice Institute, Kansas City, KS.

Snidecor, J. C. (1968). *Speech rehabilitation of the laryngectomized.* (rev. ed.). Springfield, IL: Charles C Thomas.

Chapter 30

Factors That May Interfere With Acquiring Esophageal Speech

Shirley J. Salmon

Many hypotheses have been offered to explain why some laryngectomees fail to acquire esophageal speech. To support these hypotheses, investigations have been designed to acquire information about related topics such as (1) type and extent of surgery, (2) the anatomy and physiology of the esophageal speech mechanism, (3) site and tonicity of the neoglottis, (4) presence of medical problems, and (5) psychological characteristics. Although various facets of each of these topics have been investigated numerous times, there is little agreement about the extent to which each contributes to the failure to learn esophageal speech. Consequently, a review of the findings from related literature is replete with contradictions and, generally, should be considered academic rather than clinically applicable.

The question of how many laryngectomees fail to acquire esophageal speech is basic to the topic. Several investigators (Gardner and Harris, 1961; Heaver, White, and Goldstein, 1955; Kitzing and Toremalm, 1970; Putney, 1958; and Seeman, 1958) have reported percentages ranging from 25 to 45 that represent laryngectomees who do not acquire esophageal speech. The midpoint within such a broad range does not vary greatly from the percentage computed from a questionnaire study conducted by Horn (1962) under the auspices of the American Cancer Society. Findings from this survey seem to be more frequently cited than any other, probably because of the large number of individuals polled. Of the 3,366 laryngectomees who responded, 36 per cent indicated they used esophageal speech only partially or not at all. Thus, despite what some overzealous speech pathologists, physicians, or laryngectomee instructors might say, the evidence strongly suggests that at least one third of the laryngectomized population does not acquire esophageal speech.

It is not surprising that some authorities would suggest that percentages related to failure to acquire esophageal speech must somehow relate to quality of instruction and involvement of various professionals concerned with the total rehabilitation process. Duguay (1979) represented such attitudes in his recent commentary. He stated, "Obviously, some of these failures can be accounted for on the basis of poor teaching. In support of my belief, Dan Martin at the Michigan Cancer Foundation and Walter Amster at a Florida V.A. Hospital have reported less than 20% failure rate. Knowledge, training, equipment, and the availability of ancillary services (psychiatry, dentistry, radiology, gastroenterology, etc.) can and do enhance our success rate" (p. 13).

Speculations, observations, and data suggest there are many factors other than quality of instruction and involvement of ancillary personnel that influence acquisition of esophageal speech. Although this is not intended to be a comprehensive review, some of the factors that are repeatedly mentioned in the literature will be discussed in the following sections.

Type and Extent of Surgery.   Several investigators have been interested in whether adverse effects on esophageal speech skill could be attributed to factors such as pre- or postoperative radiation, total laryngectomy versus total laryngectomy plus radical neck dissection, and presence or absence of the hyoid bone following laryngectomy. Robe, Moore, Andrews, and Holinger (1956), Shames, Font, and Mathews (1963), Hunt (1964), and Diedrich and Youngstrom (1966) all reported no apparent relationship between the first two factors and esophageal speech skill. This consensus of findings is atypical and, thus, must be considered significant despite intuitive feelings of disbelief. A similar concurrence has not been demonstrated regarding the influence of the presence or absence of the hyoid bone following laryngectomy. Diedrich and Youngstrom did not find evidence to indicate that this factor influenced esophageal speech skill. But Vrticka and Svoboda (1961) and Robe and co-workers (1956) reported evidence to suggest that presence of the hyoid bone with intact strap muscles resulted in better esophageal speech.

Anatomy and Physiology of the Esophageal Speech Mechanism.
Several researchers (Damsté, 1958; Diedrich and Youngstrom, 1966; Hodson and Oswald, 1958; Kirchner, Scatliff, Dey, and Shedd, 1963; Seeman, 1958; Vrticka and Svoboda, 1961) have attempted to relate the shape (area and width) of the hypopharynx to esophageal speech skill.

Their findings are inconsistent. Similarly, studies by Schwab (1957), Hobson and Oswald (1958), and Diedrich and Youngstrom (1966) that compared speech skill with differences noted in morphological structure of the pharyngoesophageal (PE) junction have yielded conflicting results.

Site and Tonicity of the Neoglottis. Although there is general agreement that the typical site of the neoglottis is between C4 and C6, the relevance of such agreement is unclear. This is so especially when the discrepancy among results reported by Robe and colleagues (1956), Schwab (1957), Damsté, (1958), Hodson and Oswald (1958), Vrticka and Svoboda (1961), Kirchner and co-workers (1963), and Diedrich and Youngstrom (1966) regarding the relationship between either the length of the PE segment or the width of the esophagus and esophageal speech skill is acknowledged.

Many investigators have been interested in assessing the relationship between proficiency of esophageal speech and pressure measures obtained above, within, or below the PE segment during resting state, swallowing, air intake, or air expulsion. Although swallowing pressures are reported by several (Crouch, 1974; Dey and Kirchner, 1961; Ingelfinger, 1958; and Kirchner et al., 1963) to be lower in laryngectomee subjects than in normal control subjects, the reduced pressures in the laryngectomee group apparently do not relate to speech skill. Similarly, average pressures measured during rest, air intake, and air expulsion as reported by Damsté (1958), Dey and Kirchner (1961), Salmon (1965), Bozymski and Pharr (1972), Crouch (1974), and Winans, Reichbach, and Waldrop (1974) vary between good and poor esophageal speakers. Generally, high pressures are associated with poor speakers and low pressures with good speakers. However, extreme pressure variations within individual speakers during different or identical tasks have caused most of these investigators to doubt the predictive relationship between pressure measures and esophageal speech skill. This seems to be true for the majority of laryngectomees and would differ only when pressures are noted to be exceedingly high or low. Thus, for the average laryngectomee, pressure measurements above, within, or below the PE segment are not predictive of either the ability to acquire esophageal speech or the proficiency that might be developed.

Presence of Medical Problems. Wolfe, Olson, and Goldenberg (1971) are apparently the only investigators who have used radiographic and pressure instrumentation to determine whether a relationship exists between failure of the lower esophageal sphincter and the ability to master esophageal speech. They report that the primary differences between their good speakers and those who either had no speech or poor esophageal speech was the presence of an incompetent distal esophageal sphincter. Poor speakers or those who had not acquired esophageal speech complained of one or more of the following symptoms: heartburn, regurgitation, chest pain, a sensation of food sticking in the throat, and a watery esophageal voice quality. These researchers speculated that hernia and reflux were likely present in this group of laryngectomees prior to surgery and that their attempts to learn esophageal speech aggravated the condition. Thus, they recommend that, when complaints warrant, the possibility of hiatus hernia be investigated prior to the initiation of esophageal speech training. If hiatus hernia is confirmed, they suggest use of an artificial larynx or that an antireflux hernia-plasty be performed.

Numerous authors (Berlin, 1964; Diedrich and Youngstrom, 1966; Greene, 1964; Hoople and Brewer, 1954; Martin, Hoops, and Shanks, 1974; and Svane-Knudsen, 1959) have either surmised or reported evidence to indicate that pure tone levels and speech reception thresholds are related to the acquisition of esophageal speech. Unanimous agreement among these individuals must be considered significant and cannot be overlooked when considering factors that adversely affect esophageal speech skill. Apparently adequate hearing is necessary to monitor output of esophageal voice and speech; also, it is necessary to monitor the loudness level of stoma noise. Consequently, laryngectomees who demonstrate hearing impairment should receive aural rehabilitation to maximize their opportunity to acquire esophageal speech.

Other medical problems such as recurring fistulas, senility, arthritis, cleft or paralysis of the palate, pulmonary disease, colostomy, and neurological disorders have also been mentioned as reasons why laryngectomees cannot learn esophageal speech. Although objective data are not available to support most of these assertions, logic prevents an argumentative reaction.

Psychological Characteristics.   The fact that psychological adjustments to laryngectomy are necessary is not disputed by anyone. However, the list of characteristics required to make such adjustments varies from writer to writer and is usually supported by case studies or responses to interview sessions. Several controlled investigations, wherein psychological test measurements were utilized (Amster et al., 1972; Barton and Hejna, 1952; Beamer, 1954; DiBartolo, 1971; Keith et al., 1974; Webb and Irving, 1964) have not yielded a psychological profile that can differentiate between an alaryngeal group and a normal group or between good or poor esophageal speakers. However, data from them have been interpreted to indicate that specific factors such as younger age, higher educational level, favorable self-concept, good body image, high achievement level, less depression, and lower levels of anxiety are related to good esophageal speech. Shames and associates (1963) and Goldstein and Salmon (1978) apparently are the only investigators to report that esophageal speakers can be differentiated from artificial larynx speakers. Shames and associates stated that esophageal speakers showed greater need to conform and to influence others and less need to work hard at a task. Goldstein and Salmon reported that esophageal speakers scored higher on a measure of motivation than did artificial larynx speakers. This finding from Goldstein and Salmon conflicts with a portion of that reported by Shames and co-workers if motivation can be interpreted as similar to endurance. Thus, despite the numerous psychological characteristics that have in the past been suggested as related to esophageal speech rehabilitation, only a few have been shown to have such a relationship.

It can be concluded from a review of the literature that few factors have been shown conclusively to influence the acquisition or proficiency of esophageal speech. As Martin (1976) stated, "In all likelihood, there are multiple co-existing factors which interact in a complex manner to facilitate or hinder the development of esophageal speech" (p. 32).

When a group of artificial larynx speakers were asked why they thought that they had not acquired esophageal speech, their answers were varied. Some responses were (1) I was undergoing extensive cobalt therapy, postoperatively; (2) I did not want to learn; (3) I had to talk immediately to go back to work; (4) an air intake caused a build-up of air on my stomach, a constant sore throat, and a general irritation in my neck and shoulder areas; (5) I had a fear of irritating an area in my pharynx and esophagus that has already been weakened by cancer; and (6) I do not like the sound of it and the feelings of discomfort I have when I am with esophageal speakers who make it appear so effortful.

These comments are shared only to underscore that reasons for not acquiring esophageal speech are highly individualized and should be considered as such when discussing the topic with each laryngectomee.

QUESTIONS

1. Do you think type and extent of surgery are influential factors in speech development following laryngectomy?
2. What do you think are the absolute minimum anatomical and physiological requirements of the esophageal speech mechanism for speaking with an esophageal voice?
3. Describe the psychological attributes you would like to see in a potential client who comes to you for esophageal voice lessons.

REFERENCES

Amster, W. W., Love, R. J., Menzel, O. J., Sandler, J., Sculthorpe, W. B., and Gross, F. M. (1972). Psychosocial factors and speech after laryngectomy. *J. Commun. Disord., 5,* 1–18.

Barton, J., and Hejna, R. (1963). Factors associated with success or nonsuccess in acquisition of esophageal speech. *J. Speech Hearing Assoc. (Virginia), 4,* 19–20.

Beamer, M. W. (1954). *A qualitative study of the personality adjustment of laryngectomized subjects.* Unpublished master's thesis, Texas State College for Women, Denton.

Berlin, C. I. (1964). Hearing loss, palatal function, and other factors in post-laryngectomy rehabilitation. *J. Chron. Dis., 17,* 677–684.

Bozymski, R. M., and Pharr, S. Y. (1972). Esophageal manometry and speech proficiency in post-laryngectomy patients (abstract). *Gastroenterology, 62,* 726.

Crouch, Z. B. (1974). *The relationship of intraluminal swallowing, resting, and phonation pressures to esophageal phonation "goodness" and maximum duration of phonation.* Unpublished doctoral dissertation, University of Kansas, Lawrence, KS.

Damsté, P. H. (1958). *Oesophageal Speech.* Groningen: Gebr. Hoitsema.

Dey, F. L., and Kirchner, J. A. (1961). The upper esophageal sphincter after laryngectomy. *Laryngoscope, 71,* 99–115.

DiBartolo, R. (1971). Psychological considerations in the attainment of esophageal speech. *J. Surg. Oncol., 3,* 451–466.

Diedrich, W. M., and Youngstrom, K. A. (1966). *Alaryngeal speech.* Springfield, IL: Charles C Thomas.

Duguay, M. J. (1979). How do you perceive the role of the lay teacher in laryngectomee rehabilitation? *Texas J. Audiology Speech Pathol., 4,* 12–13.

Gardner, W. H., and Harris, H. E. (1961). Aids and devices for laryngectomees. *Arch. Otolaryng., 73,* 145–152.

Goldstein, L. P., and Salmon, S. J. (1978). The relationship between adience-abience scale scores and judged communication. *Laryngoscope, 88,* 1855–1860.

Greene, M. (1964). *The voice and its disorders.* (2nd ed.). Philadelphia: J. B. Lippincott.

Heaver, L., White, W., and Goldstein, N. (1955). Clinical experience in restoring oral communication to 274 laryngectomized patients by esophageal voice. *J. Am. Geriat. Soc., 3,* 687–690.

Hodson, C. J., and Oswald, M. V. (1958). *Speech recovery after total laryngectomy.* London: E. & S. Livingstone.

Hoople, G. D., and Brewer, D. W. (1954). Voice production in the laryngectomized patient. *Ann. Otol. Rhinol. Laryngol., 63,* 640–650.

Horn, D. (1962). *Laryngectomee Survey Report.* Eleventh Annual Meeting, International Association of Laryngectomees, Memphis, TN.

Hunt, R. B. (1964). Rehabilitation of the laryngectomee. *Laryngoscope, 74,* 382–395.

Ingelfinger, F. J. (1958). Esophageal motility. *Physiol. Rev. 38,* 533–584.

Keith, R. L., Ewert, J. C., and Flowers, C. R. (1974). Factors influencing the learning of esophageal speech. *Brit. J. Disord. Commun., 9,* 110–116.

Kirchner, J. A., Scatliff, J. H., Dey, F. L., and Shedd, D. P. (1963). The pharynx after laryngectomy. *Laryngoscope, 63,* 18–33.

Kitzing, P., and Toremalm, N. G. (1970). The situation of the laryngectomized patient. *Acta. Otolaryng., 263,* 119–123.

Martin, D. E. (1976). The relationship between esophageal speech proficiency and selected measures of auditory function. In *Proceedings of the Laryngectomee Rehabilitation Seminar: A Supplement.* Rochester, MN: Mayo Clinic.

Martin, D. E., Hoops, H. R., and Shanks, J. C. (1974). The relationship between esophageal speech proficiency and selected measures of auditory function. *J. Speech Hearing Res., 74,* 80–85.

Putney, E. J. (1958). Rehabilitation of the post-laryngectomized patient. *Ann. Otol. Rhinol. Laryngol., 67,* 544–549.

Robe, E. Y., Moore, P., Andrews, A. H., Jr., and Holinger, P. H. (1956). A study of the role of certain factors in the development of speech after laryngectomy: 1. Type of operation, 2. Site of Pseudoglottis, 3. Coordination of speech with respiration. *Laryngoscope, 66,* 173–186 (Part 1), 382–401 (Part 2), and 418–419 (Part 3).

Salmon, S. J. (1965). *Pressure variations in the esophagus, pharyngeal-esophageal constriction and pharynx associated with esophageal speech production.* Unpublished doctoral dissertation, State University of Iowa, Iowa City.

Schwab, W. (1957). X-ray cinematographic investigations in substitute speech after a laryngectomy. *Acta. Oto. Rhino. Laryng. Iber. Amer., 8,* 270–273.

Seeman, M. (1958). Zur pathologie der Osophagusstimme. (Contribution to the pathology of the esophageal voice.) *Folia Phoniat., 10,* 44–50.

Shames, G. H., Font., J., and Matthews, J. (1963). Factors related to speech proficiency of the laryngectomized. *J. Speech Hearing Dis., 28,* 273–287.

Svane-Knudsen, V. (1959). The substitute voice of the laryngectomized patient. *Acta Oto-Laryng., 52,* 85–93.

Vrticka, K., and Svoboda, M. (1961). A clinical and x-ray study of 100 laryngectomized speakers. *Folia Phoniat., 13,* 174–186.

Webb, M. W., and Irving, R. W. (1964). Psychologic and anamnestic patterns characteristic of laryngectomees: relation to speech rehabilitation. *J. Am. Geriat. Soc., 12,* 303–322.

Winans, C. S., Reichbach, E. J., and Waldrop, W. F. (1974). Esophageal determinants of alaryngeal speech. *Arch. Otolaryngol., 99,* 10–14.

Wolfe, R. B., Olson, J. E., and Goldenberg, D. D. (1971). Rehabilitation of the laryngectomee: the role of the distal esophageal sphincter. *Laryngoscope, 81,* 1971–1978.

Chapter 31

Extras in Rehabilitation: Smelling, Swimming, and Compensating for Changes After Laryngectomy

P. Helbert Damsté

Apart from esophageal speech, which is of course a most important aspect of laryngectomy rehabilitation, there are a number of lesser details that are also of interest for the patient and all others concerned with his restoration to a normal life. Many such details have been described by Gardner (1971), and Gardner and Harris (1961). Some possibilities that are not well known and that can make much difference in the lives of many laryngectomees now and in the future are described in this chapter.

SMELLING

The sense of smell is apparently lost after laryngectomy. The sense, however, is usually intact; it is only that the sensory epithelium is high up in the nose between the eyes and cannot be reached by the air that carries odorous vapors. When the airstream through the nose is re-established, the capacity to smell will be restored.

The same pumping action that is taught in the first stages of esophageal speech training is used to restore the sense of smell. By movements with the bottom of the mouth and the base of the tongue it is possible to displace enough air to cause a good ventilation of the nose. For the purpose of smelling, the air is not pumped into the esophagus but, by lowering the velum, into the nasal cavity. Most people can learn to sniff in this way. It is helpful in the first stage of practice to close off the greater part of the external nasal orifices by having the patient loosely apply his thumb and forefinger. A hissing sound tells when air is passing, an audible feedback that the attempted maneuver has been successful. Some patients have become so adept at this maneuver that they can even blow their nose.

There is a difference in our appreciation of odors entering through the nostrils and odors entering from behind when food is being chewed and swallowed. This gustatory sense of smell blends with the taste sensation elicited in the oral cavity. The gustatory smell is present in most patients but is reported to improve when the pumping action is applied during meals. The restoration of smell and taste may seem trivial to some, but it is not. These senses are, with the sense of touch, the primary means of orientation in a world that must be scanned for sources of agreeable, attractive, dangerous, or poisonous things. To be deprived of these signals is maybe not as bad as being blind or deaf, but it is a fundamental loss of exciting messages and feelings. Because it is not difficult to restore the function, this practice should not be omitted in the therapy program.

SWIMMING

As the laryngectomees become more enterprising and clinicians become more and more familiar with the handicap, the limits of what laryngectomees can do gradually widen. The usual advice to stay away from (deep) water and to avoid boating, fishing, and swimming can now be given with the revision that with simple equipment and some practice the laryngectomee can again enter deep water if he used to swim before his operation.

The first demonstration of swimming by laryngectomees on record was at the congress of the European Federation of Clubs for the Laryngectomized at the Lake of Geneva in 1974, thanks to an initiative of Paul Hauwaert, the active president of the Belgian Society of Voice Handicapped. The Belgian swimming instructors trained Dutch colleagues and together they gave a demonstration at a postlaryngectomy seminar on England's south coast in 1978.

In this way a new discovery by patients is propagated. The propagation will be more successful if the idea is supported by the professionals involved in laryngectomee rehabilitation. It is a necessity that these professionals be well informed about the possibility. Lack of interest or a doubtful remark by the surgeon can make an end to a good intention. From the patient, after all, it demands some courage and one more extra

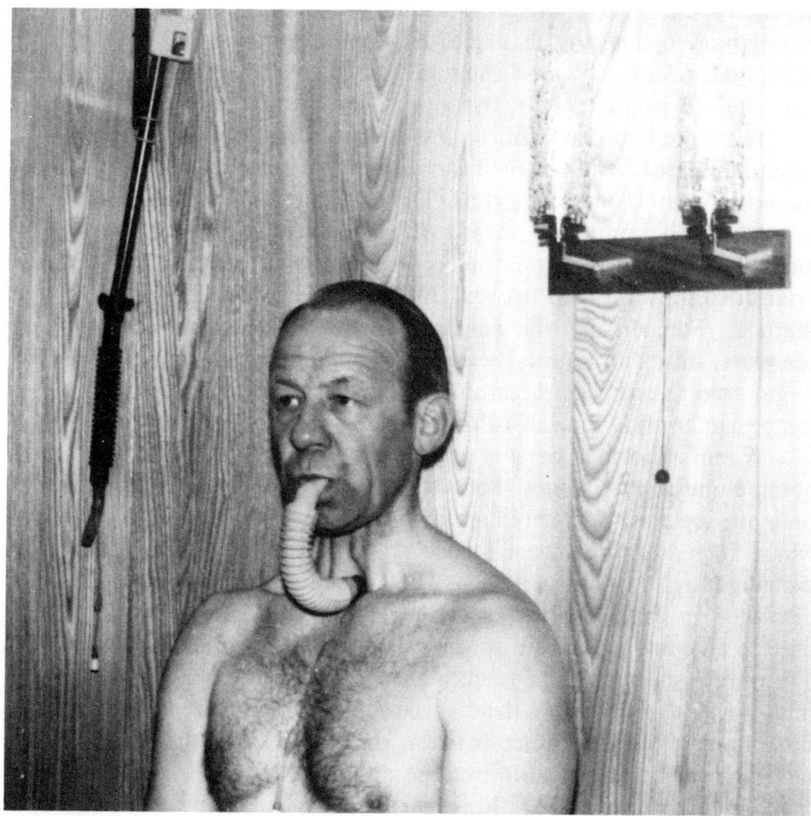

Figure 31–1.   Air tube used by a laryngectomee for swimming.

effort. It is in the interest of his general health and well-being that he be encouraged to follow his intention to receive instructions about swimming, if he wants it.

First come the preparations on dry land: the laryngectomee must get used to breathing through the air tube or snorkel. After a good expectoration to remove secretions from the trachea, a tracheal cannula with an inflatable cuff is inserted into the stoma (Fig. 31–1). The cannula should be of the correct size. The first time a surface anesthetic is needed; after one or two experiences this can be omitted. The cuff is then filled with air by means of a syringe; the filling tube has a self-sealing end and remains hanging outside the stoma on the chest wall. A bulging balloon in the middle of the filling tube allows a regular check of the degree of inflation of the cuff. The cuff should completely close off the space between the cannula and the wall of the trachea. This is checked by inspiratory and expiratory movements while the cannula is closed by a finger; when a hissing noise betrays the passing of air, a more complete filling of the cuff is required or a larger-sized cannula is needed. When the cannula has a watertight fit in the trachea, the snorkel can be connected.

There are two possibilities. One is the snorkel, an air tube tied with a band against the side of the head and sticking out above the surface of the water when the wearer swims. The other possibility is connecting the cannula to the mouth by means of a flexible tube of about 15 centimeters (cm) ending in a mouthpiece that fits in the oral vestibule and has extensions that are held between the teeth. The airway is then through the nose. For persons who have not been breathing through their nose for years, this is an unusual sensation. It requires daily practice at home to get used to effortless breathing through the nose before the laryngectomee can confide himself to the water.

When a normal person uses a snorkel, he does so in order to observe underwater scenes. The snorkeler experiences a deepening of his breathing because a 35 cm long tube is connected to his respiratory tract, which increases the "dead space" (space that is not used for gas exchange) by 175 milliliters (ml). This is the extra volume that has to be displaced in each respiratory cycle. The laryngectomee by contrast is used to an extra small dead space: no nasal, oral, and pharyngeal cavity, and only a short piece of trachea; hence the need to prepare for swimming by getting used to a dead space that automatically leads to deeper breathing. As to the choice between the snorkel and the person's own nasal airway, it is probably not the added volume of dead space that makes the difference but the higher resistance of the air when it is breathed through the nose. The nasal passages have lost the habit of adapting rapidly to changes in air flow, and they have a limited flow capacity anyway.

There is now little risk when the swimmer steps down in the pool. He will prefer to begin in the shallow part of the pool (1.20 meters deep). With the solid floor still under his feet, he checks once more whether the cannula fits water- and airtight in the trachea; when on blowing out against closed nostrils no trace of bubbles is seen coming from the submerged neck, all is ready for the start. It depends on his skill and physical condition whether he stays in the shallow part or ventures into the deeper part.

Some have jumped or dived from the diving board, with one hand holding the tubes so that the impact of the water will not pull them from the stoma. And what if that should happen? With a few strokes the swimmer will reach the rim of the pool. His reserve of air is sufficient to blow the water that might have intruded into the stoma out with an elegant squirt. Several laryngectomees have had this experience when washing the neck or when showering.

Can all laryngectomees who want it participate in swimming? Quite a few patients are troubled by excess secretions from the stoma or by shortness of breath. These conditions need not stand in the way. The moist air in the pool will prevent dried-out secretions from plugging the airways. The deeper breathing movements will help to remove excess mucus. Persons who are short of breath because of emphysema will be wise and habituate themselves very gradually to longer ranges and greater efforts. Only a too-narrow stoma that will not accommodate a cannula with cuff can be a real obstacle. Indeed, it is always sensible for the patient to discuss the intended swimming activity with his surgeon.

The advantages of engaging in swimming are many. Participating in activities that one used to do before the operation reduces the sense of being handicapped. One restriction less is one more gain for rehabilitation. Bathing and swimming can be continued to an advanced age. They can be a contribution to mental and physical health and compensate for the loss of other gratifying functions that are incompatible with the laryngectomized condition. The fishing addict may now consider wearing a cannula with snorkel or mouthpiece as long as he is on board his motorboat, rowboat, or canoe. Even sculling and sailing would come within reach, although preferably in the company of a nonlaryngectomized person who can swim. Even when on vacation at the beach, well-equipped and prepared laryngectomees can swim in the sea.

QUESTIONS

1. Damsté seems to think that laryngectomees can smell again. What is the method he describes for getting air to pass through the nose?
2. The author describes the use of a snorkel-like device for swimming and a second device that permits breathing through the nose. For either, what seems to be the most important factor?

REFERENCES

Gardner, W. H. (1971). *Laryngectomee speech and rehabilitation.* Springfield, IL: Charles C Thomas.

Gardner, W. H., and Harris, H. E. (1961). Aids and devices for laryngectomees. *Arch. Otolaryngol., 73,* 145–152.

Chapter 32

Clinical Considerations in Management of the Laryngectomee

Douglas E. Fox

The initial considerations of knowing and understanding the laryngectomee influence the success of rehabilitation efforts. Educating the laryngectomee concerning all aspects of rehabilitation is important to success. A systematic approach helps the clinician plan the course of comprehensive teaching and management. The purpose of this discussion is to create an awareness of certain clinical considerations and to introduce a tool for data collection.

Knowing the laryngectomee as a patient comes through review and understanding of his medical treatment to date. By careful review of the medical chart the clinician becomes familiar with the contents of consultation, surgical, and laboratory reports; medical history and status; and the nature of correspondence between the patient and medical personnel.

The following chart review (Fig. 32–1) is introduced for possible use in collection of important information. The form is adapted from Baker and Cunningham (1980).

The following are considerations in the process of completing the form. Some knowledge about each section of the form will assist the speech pathologist in developing a comprehensive view of the patient's needs.

AGE

With increasing age there are special factors that influence the vocal rehabilitation process. In the elderly, the abdominal and general muscu-

LARYNGECTOMY ASSESSMENT FORM

Name _________________________ Birthdate _______________ Age _________

Address _____________________________ Phone # _____________________________

Sex _________ Race ___________ Marital Status: S M W D Religion ___________

Family members ____

Nearest kin _______________ Phone # _______________ Relationship _____________

Others living in home ____

Occupation history (including present occupation and address) ________________
____

Importance of speech to occupation ____

Education ____

Ability to read and write ____

Medical Background

Illness and treatment ____

Previous hospitalizations ____

Allergies ____

First indication of laryngeal problem ________________________________

Metastasis sites ____

Therapy

Surgery: Date _______________ Place __________________________________

Surgeon _____________________________ Hospital ______________________

Site of lesion____

Radical neck dissection____

Time in hospital ____

Complications following surgery ______________________________________

Radiation:

   Past area ____

      Amount ____

      Complications ____

   Present area ____

      Amount ____

      Complications ____

Chemotherapy:

   Past agents ____

      Response ____

      Complications ____

   Present agents ____

      Response ____

      Complications ____

Problem/System Review

Neurological/Sensory

  Deficit ____

  Hearing ____

  Speech (pronunciation prior to surgery) _______________________

    Previous speech therapy (when/by whom) ____________________

    Procedures ____

    Success ____

    Artificial devices used __________________________________

    Ability to belch voluntarily ______________________________

Gastrointestinal

  Appetite ____

  Diet ____

  Nausea (when occurs, relief measures) ________________________

  Fluid intake ____

  Difficulty swallowing____________________________________

  Difficulty eating_______________________________________

  Elimination____

Respiratory (chronic obstructive pulmonary disease)

  Problems/treatment _____________________________________

Cardiovascular

  Problems/treatment _____________________________________

Skin

  Problems/treatment _____________________________________

Musculoskeletal

  Problems/treatment _____________________________________

Pain

  Location _________________________ Relief measures _________

Infection

  Location _________________________ Treatment _____________

Hematologic

  Hgb _____________ WBC _____________ Platelets ___________

Sleep/rest patterns ____

Sexuality ____

Health Behaviors

Understanding of disease ____________________________________

Understanding of therapy (medical and speech) ___________________

____

Expectations of therapy (medical and speech) ____________________

____

Counseling before surgery/by whom ___________________________

Counseling after surgery/by whom _______________________________

Attitude before surgery _______________________________________

Attitude after surgery ____

Present attitude toward laryngectomy (depressed, frustrated, eager to develop speech)

____

____

Degree of dependency ____

Other personality traits or problems ___________________________

  (silent, outgoing, talkative) _________________________________

Previous contact with other laryngectomees ____________________

____

Attitude of family and friends ________________________________

Hobbies/life styles before laryngectomy ________________________

____

Alteration of life style due to laryngectomy ___________________

____

Use of tobacco and alcohol (amount, type, onset, duration) ______

____

Other services involved (social, visiting nurse, etc.) ___________

____

Impressions:

Recommendations:

Initial

Interviewer ___________________________

Date ___________________________

Discharge update/revision

Interviewer ___________________________

Date ___________________________

Figure 32–1.   Laryngectomy assessment form.

lar tone frequently decreases, lungs lose elasticity, the thorax loses its distensibility, the mucosa of the vocal tract atrophies, nerve endings are reduced in number, and psychoneurological functions differ.

Gardner (1978) summarized four studies that showed that success in acquisition of esophageal voice was a function of age. Gardner's data showed that for the age group 21 to 40 years there was almost 100 per cent chance of success; for 40 to 60 years, a 75 per cent chance of success; and for 61 years and older, a 50 per cent chance. The age factor in esophageal voice acquisition may now be of lesser importance with the development in recent years of tracheoesophageal puncture (TEP) techniques. These techniques allow for alternate methods of voice restoration in patients who otherwise might have failed to acquire voice.

OCCUPATIONAL HISTORY

Occupational history gives insight into the patient's "stick-to-it-iveness," work interests, and the importance of speech for the occupation. In noisy environments an electrolarynx may provide the best method of communication. Group presentations may require voice amplifiers. Dust, irritants, and fumes in the work environment may increase secretions and require special suction equipment at work. Keith, Ewert, and Flowers (1974) reported that persons who have special needs for oral communication in their vocational life tend to learn esophageal speech more readily than other persons. Fifty per cent of the relatively good speakers in their study were engaged in a type of work in which speech seems essential, and only 28 per cent of poor speakers were so employed.

EDUCATION

Keith and co-workers (1974) also reported that education correlated with speech proficiency but not to a high degree. They found a nonsignificant correlation between intelligence and learning esophageal speech. They suggested that other more critical factors may influence the acquisition of esophageal voice, including time devoted to practice, postoperative anatomical and physiological characteristics, the family's and friends' moral support, and the patient's communication needs.

PSYCHOLOGICAL FACTORS

Psychological factors reported in the literature to be critical include a catastrophic reaction to having the larynx removed, impressions of physical unattractiveness, and constant fear of recurrence of cancer and death. Some authors have suggested the use of anti-depressant drugs; however, one must keep in mind that depression may be a natural consequence of life's events and may be appropriate. Keith and colleagues (1974) reported that the Depression Scale of the Minnesota Multiphasic Personality Inventory (MMPI) was the only test scale correlating with the learning of esophageal speech but that the correlation was low. Perhaps depression is not as great a factor as has been suggested in some of the literature.

ALCOHOLISM

Alcoholism has also been noted to be detrimental to learning new skills such as esophageal speech because of difficulties in retaining information, cooperating and concentrating in therapy, and socializing normally outside of treatment when practicing communication skills.

MEDICAL BACKGROUND

Understanding the medical background is essential in knowing the laryngectomee patient and his previous illnesses, treatments, and hospitalizations. History of the psychoneurological system may reveal that there were subtle prelaryngectomy voice changes that may be a sign of neurological disease. A history of voice fatigue or changing pitch range may give insight into the amount of neck muscle control and tension prior to laryngectomy. Allergies involving the upper respiratory system may cause irritation to the esophagus and increase secretions in the laryngectomee. The laryngectomee's health-seeking behaviors at the first indication of laryngeal problems, and his initial reaction to diagnosis of cancer, give insight into mechanisms of denial versus confrontation of the condition.

SITE OF CANCER

Information on diagnosis and sites of metastasis offers prognostic information. The patient's knowledge of metastasis can influence his motivational state, especially if there are limitations in his physical ability to work at rehabilitation.

Squamous cell malignancies tend to appear in the throat or neck before they metastasize elsewhere. Cancer invading the lymphatic channels may have spread to the lymph glands of the neck and beyond to the chest or lungs. Thorough review and understanding of cancer type, size of lesion, metastasis, and structures removed at surgery are important to the speech-language pathologist's understanding of the laryngectomee.

Generally, supraglottic cancers occur from the laryngeal ventricles to the tip of the epiglottis including the false cords. These tend to be less differentiated, grow toward the base of the tongue, and have positive neck nodes in 50 per cent of patients at the time of diagnosis. The nodes are usually of the superior cervical group. Extension to the aryepiglottic fold, pyriform sinus, or base of the tongue is associated with poorer prognosis.

Glottic cancers extend from the laryngeal ventricles to 1 centimeter (cm) below the margin of the true cords, including the true cords. These are about twice as common as supraglottic cancers. They spread concentrically, slowly, toward and around the anterior commissure, and they metastasize late. Reduced or absence of movement of the cords reduces survival rates.

Subglottic cancers extend from the laryngeal ventricles to 1 cm below the margin of the true cords to the lower border of the cricoid cartilage. These are rarely primary and are usually extensions from glottic primary cancer. Transglottic cancers involve two or more of the above. The results of the treatment will vary with size, location, and tissue type. Small lesions of the true cords are routinely cured in over 90 per cent of the patients. Patients with advanced lesions with palpable nodes have 5 year survival rates of about 35 per cent.

SURGERY

Surgical experiences vary among laryngectomees. Some laryngectomies are done without preoperative consultation by the speech-language pathologist. Unfortunately, it is not uncommon for patients to consult a speech pathologist for the first time 1 month after surgery. The number of surgeries done at a medical center may make a difference in the level of care. A surgeon's individual interest in restoring a good postoperative voice results in varied surgical techniques. Some physicians perform laryngectomies without full knowledge of or interest in requirements for the best possible postsurgical voice.

Site of lesion, cancer type, and treatment prognosis should be familiar to the speech pathologist. Tumor Registry Staging Classification forms, such as that shown in Figure 32–2, are frequently found in the medical record and should be reviewed.

Laryngeal cancer constitutes about 4 per cent of all the cancers diagnosed in the United States each year. About 80 per cent occur after age 40 with a mean age of 59 and a male-to-female ratio of 7 to 1. Second primaries, usually of the airways, occur in about 10 per cent. The pathology is squamous cell carcinoma in 98 per cent of the cases, varying from carcinoma-in-situ to well differentiated to poorly differentiated.

What the laryngectomee is told about speech and survival may influence his attitudes. McNeil, Weichselbaum, and Pauker (1981) interviewed 37 nonlaryngectomized healthy individuals concerning their preferences regarding longevity and voice preservation. In view of the survival rates, 20 per cent of those interviewed chose radiation instead of surgery to save the voice. The investigators suggested that treatment choices should be made on the basis of a patient's attitudes toward quality of life as well as the chance of survival.

TUMOR REGISTRY STAGING CLASSIFICATION
LARYNX

Patient name ____ Date _______________

Medical record number ___________________________________ Age _______ Sex _______

Time of classification: Clinical _______ Surgical _______ Pathological _______

Re-treatment _______ Autopsy _______

Location of Tumor	Site of Origin	Sites Also Involved
Supraglottis		
Ventricular band	_______	_______
Arytenoid	_______	_______
Suprahyoid epiglottis	_______	_______
Infrahyoid epiglottis	_______	_______
Aryepiglottic fold	_______	_______
Glottis		
Vocal cords (including commissures)	_______	_______
Subglottis	_______	_______

Primary Tumor

_______ TX = Tumor cannot be assessed

_______ T0 = No evidence of primary tumor

_______ TIS = Carcinoma in situ

Supraglottis

_______ T1 = Tumor confined to site of origin with normal mobility

_______ T2 = Tumor involving adjacent supraglottic site(s) or glottis without fixation

_______ T3 = Tumor limited to larynx with fixation or extension to involve postcricoid area, medial wall of pyriform sinus, or pre-epiglottic space

_______ T4 = Massive tumor extending beyond the larynx to involve oropharynx or soft tissues of neck or to cause destruction of thyroid cartilage

Glottis

_______ T1 = Tumor confined to vocal cord(s) with normal mobility

_______ T2 = Supraglottic or subglottic extension with normal or impaired cord mobility

_______ T3 = Tumor confined to larynx with cord fixation

     _______ T4 = Massive tumor with thyroid cartilage destruction or extension beyond the confines of the larynx

Subglottis

     _______ T1 = Tumor confined to the subglottic region

     _______ T2 = Tumor extension to vocal cords with normal or impaired cord mobility

     _______ T3 = Tumor confined to larynx with cord fixation

     _______ T4 = Massive tumor with cartilage destruction or extension beyond the confines of the larynx, or both

Nodal Involvement

_______ NX = Nodes cannot be assessed

_______ N0 = No clinically positive node

_______ N1 = Single clinically positive homolateral node 3 cm or less in diameter

_______ N2 = Single clinically positive homolateral node more than 3 cm but not more than 6 cm in diameter or multiple clinically positive homolateral nodes, none more than 6 cm in diameter.

_______ N3 = Massive homolateral node(s), bilateral nodes, or contralateral node(s)

Distant Metastasis

_______ MX = Not assessed

_______ M0 = No known distant metastasis

_______ M1 = Distant metastasis present

  Specify: Pulmonary ______ Osseous ______ Hepatic ______

  Brain ______ Lymph Nodes ______ Bone Marrow ______ Pleura ______

  Skin ______ Eye ______ Other ________________________________

Histopathology

_______ Squamous cell carcinoma

_______ Undifferentiated carcinoma

_______ Adenocarcinoma

_______ Other — Specify

Grade

_______ Grade 1 = Well differentiated

_______ Grade 2 = Moderately to well differentiated

_______ Grade 3-4 = Poorly to very poorly differentiated

Residual Tumor

_______ R0 = No residual tumor

_______ R1 = Microscopic residual tumor

_______ R2 = Macroscopic residual tumor

Patient Performance Status

```
_______  100  =  Normal, no complaints and no evidence of disease
_______   90  =  Able to carry on normal activity; minor signs or symptoms
_______   80  =  Normal activity with effort; some signs or symptoms of disease
_______   70  =  Cares for self; unable to perform normal activity or active work
_______   60  =  Requires occasional assistance; is able to care for most of needs
_______   50  =  Requires considerable assistance and frequent medical care
_______   40  =  Disabled; requires special care and assistance
_______   30  =  Severely disabled; hospitalization indicated; death not imminent
_______   20  =  Very sick; hospitalization and active support are necessary
_______   10  =  Moribund; fatal processes progressing rapidly
_______    0  =  Patient expired
```

Figure 32–2. Laryngeal tumor registry staging classification.

COMPLICATIONS FOLLOWING SURGERY

Postoperative considerations relate to structures removed, as in radical neck procedures, glossectomy, mandibulectomy, and gastric pull-through; nerves involved; and other surgical complications. Damage to cranial nerves (X, the vagus; XII, the hypoglossal; and V, the trigeminal) may result in impairment of oral sensation and tongue movements. Oral-tactile feedback and execution of some air injection techniques for esophageal speech may become impossible.

There are two main complications postsurgically. The first of these is airway obstruction, signs of which are restlessness, tachycardia, tachypnea, and fitful or labored breathing. The second is carotid artery blow-out, which may occur because of infection in the wound that leads to extensive necrosis of the skin, which in turn exposes the carotid artery wall, which may rupture. Saliva may also eat away at the carotid artery.

Fistula formation is another postoperative complication. Small fistulas are not uncommon following laryngectomy. Larger fistulas are usually managed with separate surgical procedures. The physician's willingness to manage fistulas is necessary in tracheoesophageal shunting procedures done as primary procedures. Other postsurgical complications include sloughing of the skin flap, delayed or inadequate suture-line healing, and lower respiratory tract infection.

Radiation is also relevant to the development of esophageal speech. Richardson (1981) studied postlaryngectomy communication and its relationship to total laryngectomy and the use of radiation therapy. For those learning esophageal speech, the quality of speech was not affected by the extent of surgery, except in the case of extensive surgeries involving the esophagus or pharynx. The relationship between radiation and communication was not statistically significant. Nonradiated patients were expected to do the best but did not. Those doing best received radiation only before the operation. Those radiated only after the operation did worst. Richardson also reported that nonclosing fistulas and radical neck procedures were not strong determinants of mastery of esophageal speech.

Gates and Hearne (1982) found that postoperative radiation had a direct effect on learning speech. Pain and dryness were reported, and patients tended to discontinue therapy during radiation and would not return. Gates also concluded that patients with pyriform sinus cancers were less likely to develop esophageal speech than those with glottic and supraglottic primaries. Dysphagia was present at the rate of 30 per cent in glottic and supraglottic cancers.

The speech-language pathologist often is the first professional the laryngectomee may ask about the effects of radiation or chemotherapy treatment. Once the physician has made a recommendation for one or both of these as a treatment choice, the laryngectomee may have additional questions to which the speech pathologist can provide answers. Two excellent sourcebooks are available that discuss complications associated with both treatments (National Cancer Institute, 1981a, 1981b).

Other postsurgical complications relate to abnormalities in the anatomy that may affect esophageal speech. Simpson, Smith, and Gordon (1972) discussed strictures and pouches. They found patients with double constriction or a further narrowing between the esophagus and oral pharynx in addition to the pharyngoesophageal narrowing. Three types are described: permanent organic strictures above the pharyngoesophageal (PE) segment, pseudostrictures, and strictures due to voluntary contraction. Permanent organic strictures above the PE segment were seemingly related to loss of excised mucosa or fibrosis secondary to delayed healing. Pseudostrictures were due to bulging of the posterior pharyngeal wall into the lumen of the hypopharynx. They also found pouches or diverticula (i.e., localized forward bulging of the anterior pharyngeal wall beyond the normal configuration). High pouches were found just at the base of the tongue at the hyoid level and low pouches were located between the hyoid and PE segment. Air or mucus and saliva may be trapped in the pouches, making the quality of voice wet or bubbly.

Nayar, Sharma, and Arora (1984) have reported a study done in the Otolaryngology service of Nehru Hospital, Chandigarh, India. They studied the hypopharyngeal anatomy of 20 postlaryngectomy patients with endoscopy and radiological contrast medium. The pharynx was found to be essentially a featureless tube with mucosal rugosities running alongs its axis. They found no correlation between the endoscopic and radiological appearance of the pseudoepiglottis or between present and postoperative complications or the acquisition of esophageal speech. A low incidence of postoperative dysphagia was also noted. The less textured diet in India may account for the low incidence of dysphagia. The average Indian diet of soft boiled rice curds and grain is easier to masticate and swallow than meat and boiled vegetables, which form the staple Western diet.

The following two cases were investigated by the author with videofluoroscopy when progress with esophageal speech production suggested possible esophageal problems.

Case 1, C. R.

White male patient, age 63, with a cancer type T2-N1-Mo squamous cell carcinoma, underwent a total laryngectomy and right radical neck dissection on July 15, 1981. Two cycles of chemotherapy were given presurgically, including Cis Platinum and bleomycin. Esophageal speech training began in August 1981. Within 2 months C. R. was producing three to five syllables per air charge and could prolong the single air charge further in producing all five vowels (a-e-i-o-u) three times through. By November, 1981, a "wet quality" in the voice appeared, and he indicated concern about swallowing problems. Neither of these concerns was present at the time he began esophageal speech training. C. R. reported difficulty swallowing food and liquid and was able to identify where the foods would get stuck. There was also a visible anterior bulging of neck tissue appearing with air intake for speech and during swallowing. Digitial pressure and the use of neck bands reduced the wetness of the voice quality and improved the duration of esophageal sound. Digital pressure also improved the swallowing. On April 19, 1984, a videofluoroscopic air-insufflation test and a test of sound production without air insufflation were completed.

Figure 32–3 (lateral view) demonstrates his esophageal configuration. There are two points of narrowing above and below a bulging positioned to the right of midline. This finding is visualized much more easily in the movement on ¾ inch videotape recording than is demonstrated in the still figure presented here. On phonation there was vibration at both narrowings, suggesting two vibratory sound sources, more clearly demonstrated on videotape. Figure 32–4 shows the residual liquid barium, at rest, thought to account for some of the "wet" quality of the esophageal voice. Figure 32–5 shows another view of the irregularity of the esophageal tract.

On June 18, 1982, C. R. underwent surgery for reconstruction of the diverticulum and had two fistulas develop postsurgically. Eventually these healed, and C. R. reported significant improvement in swallowing. The esophageal speech improved markedly, with reduction of the wet quality and increased duration on each air charge. Figure 32–6 shows the postsurgical videofluoroscopic results in the anteroposterior view. Note the surgical tie-off of the bulging slightly to the right of center with clearing of the barium. Again the irregular esophageal shape is seen.

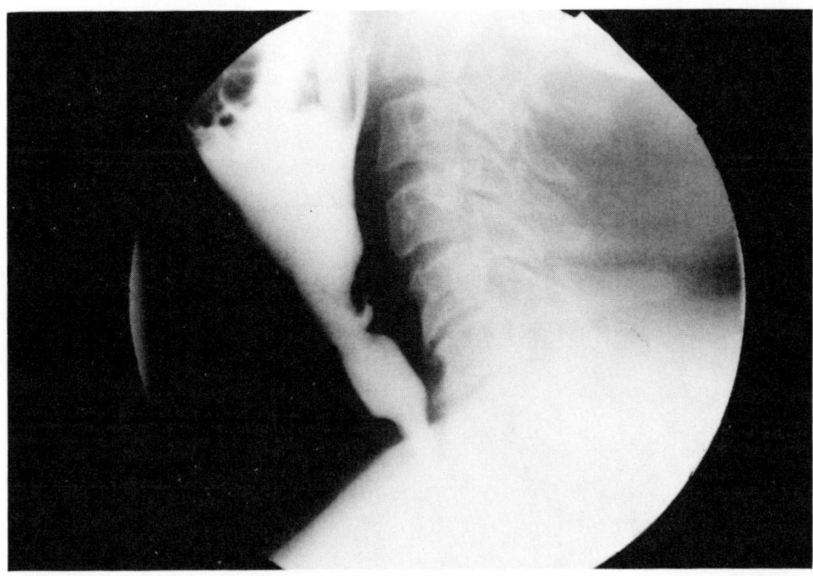

Figure 32–3. Case C. R. Radiograph demonstrates barium outlining esophageal narrowing at two positions, one above and the other below an area of bulging not clearly seen in lateral view. Both narrowings show vibration as potential sound sources when viewed on videotape recording.

Case 2, B. B.

White female patient, age 57, underwent a total laryngectomy in May, 1984. Following surgery she complained of difficulty with all food substances, with liquid, soft foods or chewable foods "sticking" immediately after the swallow. Food was brought back up after each meal. The esophageal voice lacked duration and volume and suggested the possibility of a loose PE segment.

Figure 32–7 shows the videofluoroscopic swallow results, with a portion of a bolus passing through the cricopharyngeal sphincter and the other portion collecting in the pouch. Figure 32–8 demonstrates the residual collection in the pouch after the completed swallow. Swallows of liquid barium, Esophatrast paste, and a cookie coated with Esophatrast paste all resulted in about one half of the substance falling into the anterior pouch. Esophageal sound attempts under videofluoroscopy suggested that the pouching was pulling anteriorly away from the PE segment, resulting in a loose segment. It was also felt that air injection filled the pouch during sound attempts. Both these factors contributed to the poor voice quality. At the time of this writing the patient was undergoing a course of post-surgical radiation. Her physician is also considering possible surgical reconstruction of the pouch in the future.

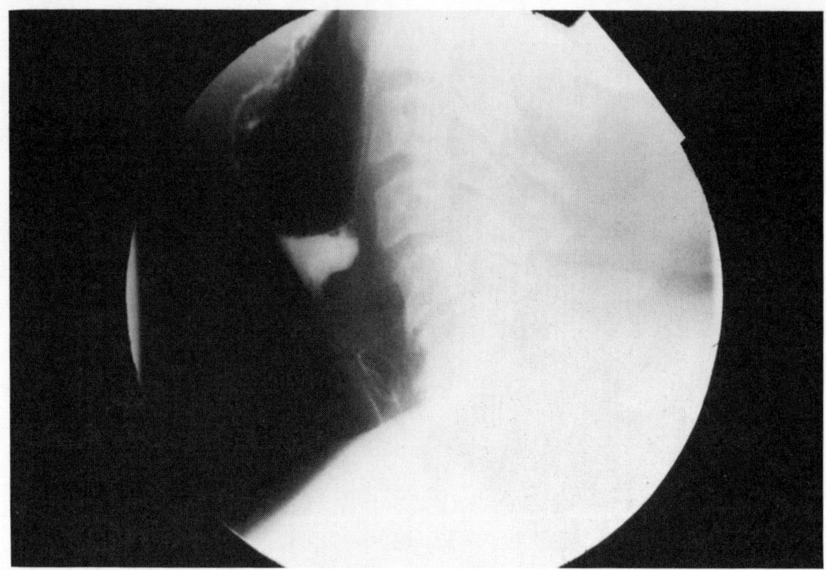

Figure 32–4.   Case C. R. Residual barium, at rest, thought to be contributing to a "wet" esophageal voice quality.

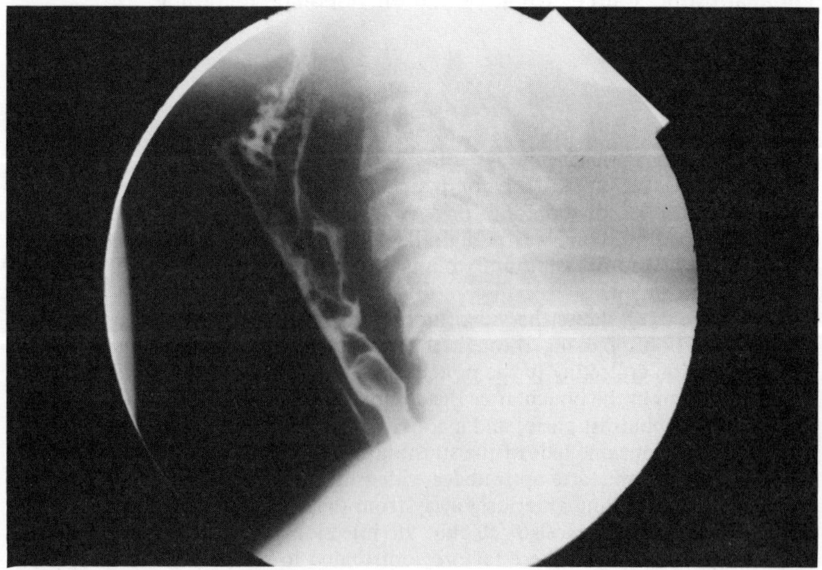

Figure 32–5.   Case C. R. View of irregularity in esophageal tract.

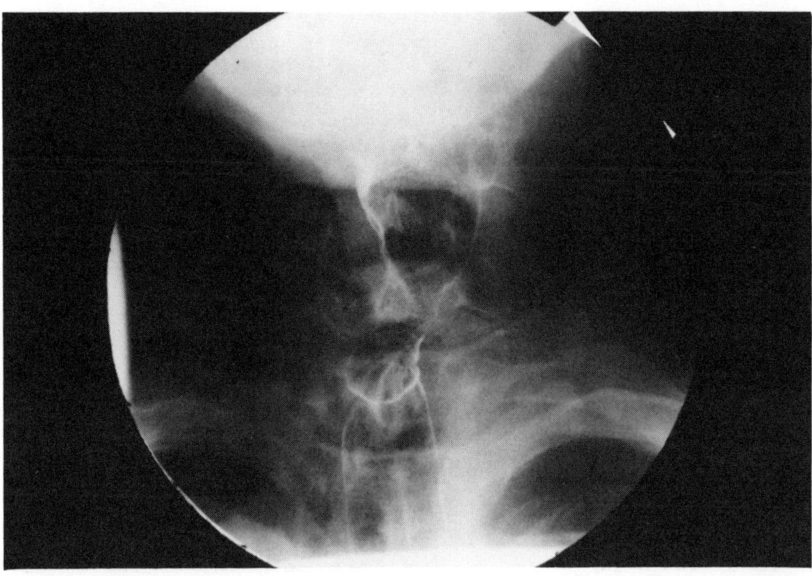

Figure 32–6. Case C. R. Anteroposterior view of postsurgical tie-off of the bulge slightly to the right of the center with no residual barium. Note the irregular shape of the esophagus.

Both case studies represent problems in both swallowing and sound production and could be clearly diagnosed only with videofluoroscopy. The speech-language pathologist should use such techniques to investigate when the esophageal voice is not making reasonable progress and when there is reason to suspect abnormalities in esophageal anatomy.

Vincent, Robbins, Walsh, and Vaughan (1984) suggested the use of barium swallow examinations in tracheoesophageal puncture procedures. A preoperative barium swallow can provide anatomical information that may alert the surgeon to intraoperative complications as well as establish a baseline. Evidence of tight stricture that would prevent the passage of an endoscope could lead to cancellations of the tracheoesophageal puncture until after stricture dilatation. An abnormal cricopharyngeal opening alerts the speech pathologist to potential difficulties in alaryngeal speech and the surgeon to the possible need for a future cricopharyngeal myotomy.

These authors suggest for laryngectomees with postoperative fever a minimum of anteroposterior and lateral neck films as well as chest radiographs. In vocalization problems the radiological examination may reveal a remediable cause, such as abnormal position of the valve tip or abnormal cricopharyngeal opening.

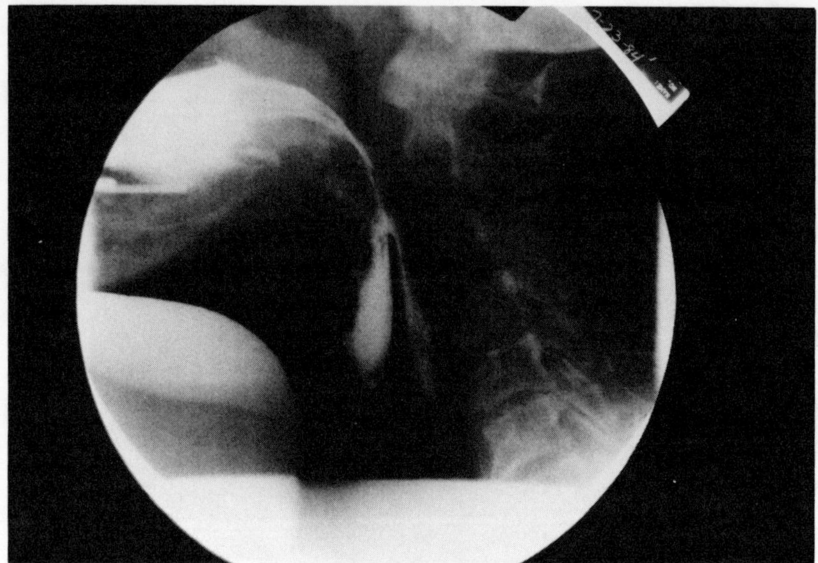

Figure 32–7. Case B. B. Videofluoroscopic swallowing study with a portion of bolus passing into the esophagus and a simultaneous collection in the pouch.

Julian, Noscoe, and Berry (1981) have discussed a xeroradiographic study of the larynx. Xeroradiography is a technique that allows both soft tissue and denser bone to be visualized in the same image. The image is transferred to paper as in a paper photocopier. The technique is also being applied to the laryngectomee to view changes in the esophageal tract at various stages of esophageal voice training. Figure 32–9 shows a postlaryngectomy view with the PE segment at rest. Figure 32–10 demonstrates esophageal voicing at 8 months postoperative. Note the opening of the PE segment and inflation of the air-charged esophagus just below the PE segment. (Both prints are taken from slides obtained in this author's personal communications with Frances MacCurtain, speech therapist at the Royal Ear, Nose, and Throat Hospital in London, England.)

Postsurgically the inability to relax the PE segment and upper esophageal spasm can result in voice failure. There is considerable literature addressing this special problem. Singer and Blom (1981) discussed the use of selective myotomy when investigation found an airtight closure of the PE segment. McGarvey and Weinberg (1984) have discussed the use of the air-insufflation test in the normal human esophagus to document the degree to which normal adults can consistently produce and continuously

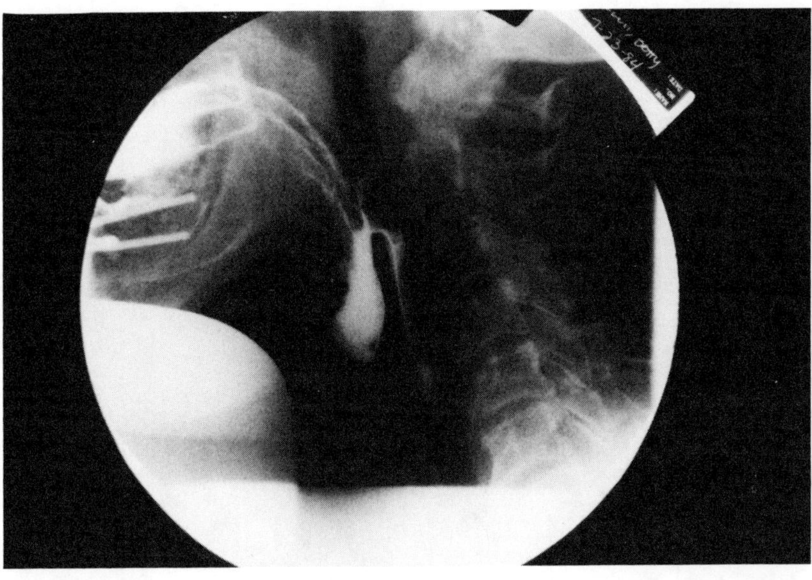

Figure 32–8.   Case B. B. Pouch filled with barium anterior to the PE segment after the swallow is completed.

sustain esophageal voice. Their results were interpreted to support two views; first, that the "normal function of the PE segment represents an influence detrimental to the ultimate acquisition of functionally service-able esophageal or tracheoesophageal speech" (p. 272); second, "laryngectomized patients having airtight closure of the pharyngeoesophageal segment during insufflation testing exhibit a normal esophageal response" (p. 272). They further commented that postsurgically the upper esophagus must function as a valve and suggested the need for further investigation of reflux in laryngectomees who have undergone a surgical myotomy procedure. In some centers surgical myotomies are now being done as primary procedures at the time of laryngectomy. Further investigation of tonicity of the PE segment and its relationship to air-pressure levels at the segment in both esophageal speech and tracheoesophageal speech is needed. The relationship of tonicity of the PE segment and pressure levels at the stoma site may prove beneficial in fitting the correct type of prosthesis in tracheoesophageal shunting techniques.

Postsurgically, the distal cardiac sphincter must be considered because an incompetent sphincter may result in difficulty in retaining air in the esophagus. This sphincter separates the stomach from the esophageal lumens.

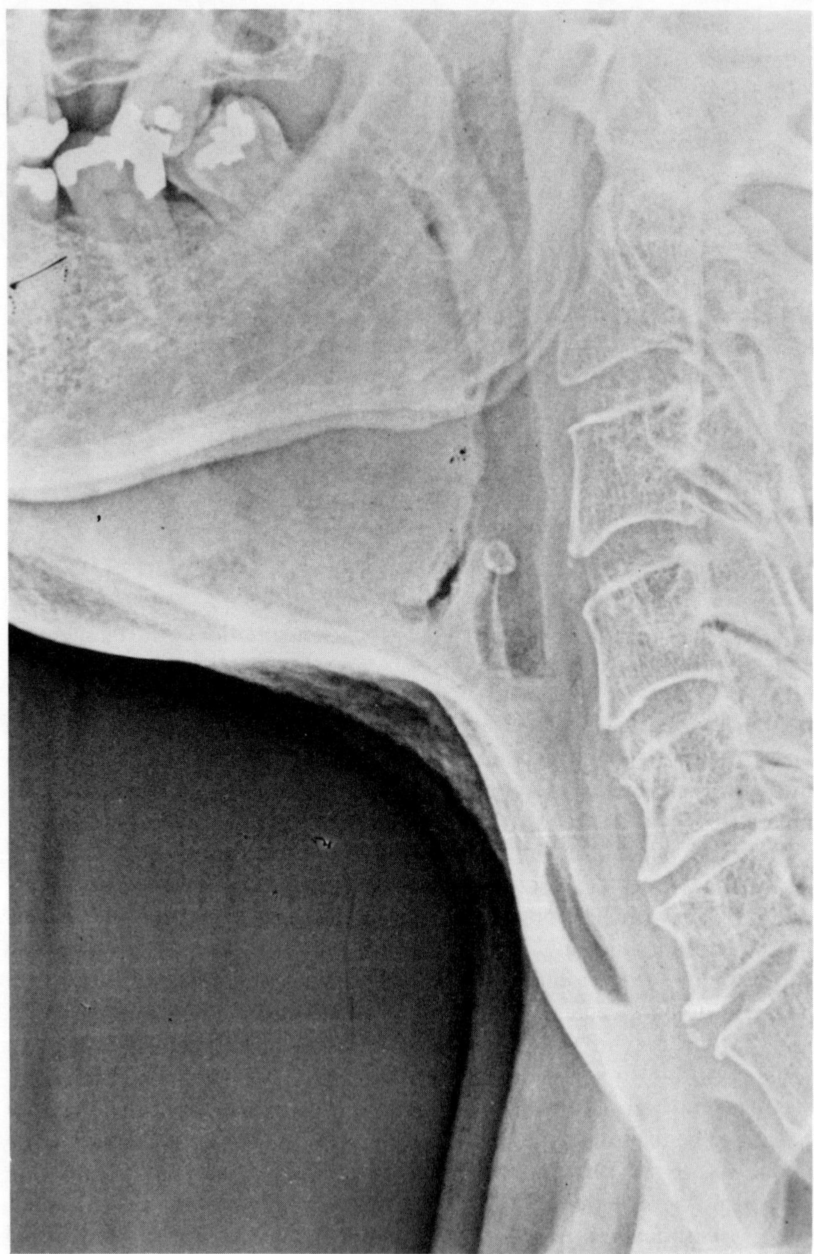

Figure 32–9. Xeroradiography showing PE segment at rest. (Courtesy of Frances MacCurtain.)

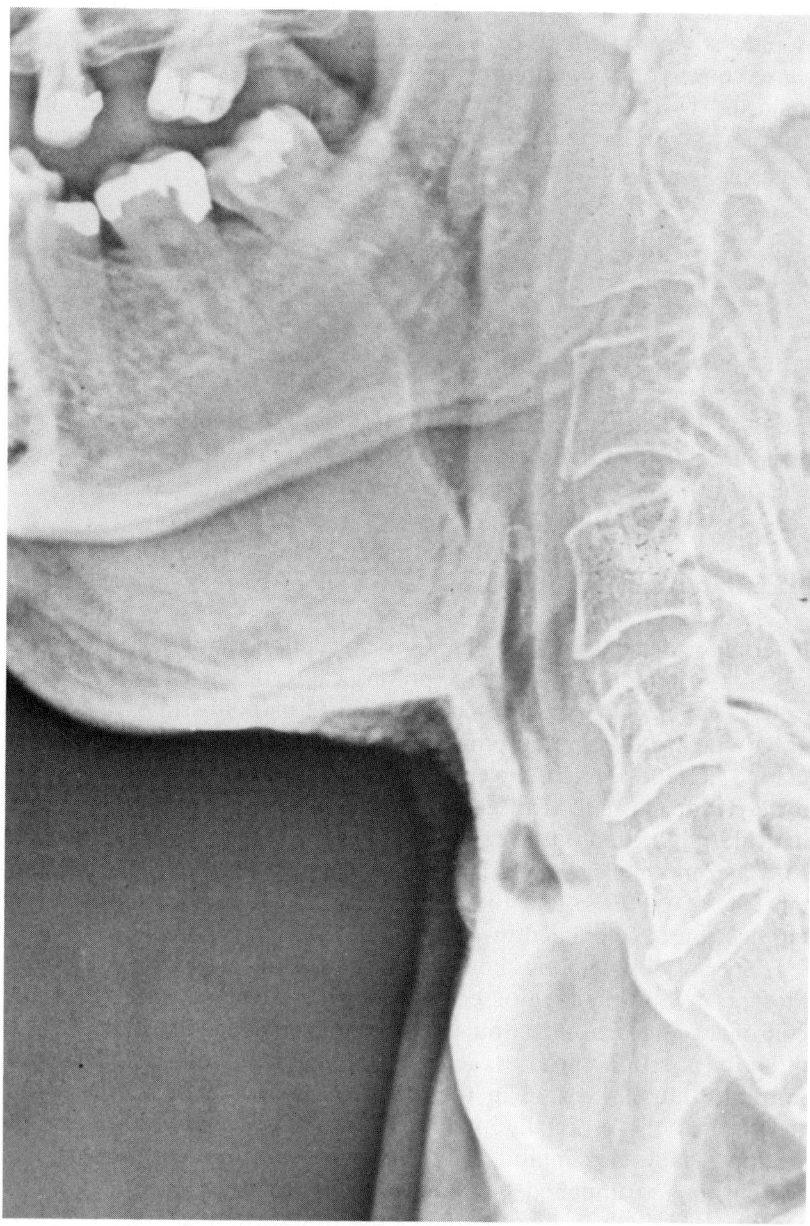

Figure 32–10. Xeroradiography showing esophageal voicing at 8 months postoperative with the air-charged esophagus just below the PE segment. (Courtesy of Francis MacCurtain.)

Problems with achalasia postsurgically may inhibit progress with esophageal speech. In this condition the lower esophagus may not be relaxed owing to incoordination of the muscles in this area and the lower sphincter. Symptoms may include difficulty swallowing, weight loss, pain, and regurgitation. Correction of the problem may be overcome by bougienage to dilate the esophageal tract or surgery.

PROBLEM-SYSTEM REVIEW

Central and peripheral deficits must be considered in planning the treatment course postsurgically. Berlin (1964) concluded that high-frequency hearing losses may impede both acquisition of esophageal speech and use of the artificial larynx. Stoma noise is high frequency and may be difficult to hear with high-frequency losses. It is also difficult to monitor speech with some artificial larynxes because of sound masking.

SPEECH PRIOR TO SURGERY

It is important to share the family's perception of presurgical speech patterns. An audio- or videotape presurgical recording will be beneficial to both the patient and the speech-language pathologist. A formal test battery before surgery can provide information about speech rate, articulation, loudness, pitch, dialect, breathing patterns, posture, voice quality, eye contact, and use of gestures. All these are important to consider in achieving a good postsurgical voice.

Oral mechanism examinations pre- and postoperatively are important. Perry (1983) offers the oral speech mechanism examination for laryngectomees presented in Appendix 32-A.

Special observations should be made of tongue and lips for hypoglossal involvement, glossectomy, and edema as these relate to consonant-linked air injection. Loose dentition may inhibit tongue relaxation for injection purposes. Temporomandibular joint dysfunction may introduce muscle tension in the head and neck. There may be excess tongue activity, especially pulling of the tongue posteriorly. Palatal weakness may also inhibit injection techniques, and artificial larynx speech may be impaired by changes in intraoral air pressure. A high maxillary arch may influence tongue position with injection. In the area of the neck, factors such as neck size or position of the stoma may influence placement of an artificial larynx.

GASTROINTESTINAL SYSTEM

Appetite, diet, nausea, difficulty swallowing, and elimination must be considered both pre- and postoperatively. Complications in these areas may be due to course of chemotherapy or radiotherapy and also to some of the problems mentioned earlier such as hernia, sphincters, and pouches.

RESPIRATORY SYSTEM

Considerations should be given to respiratory tract infections, postnasal drip, allergies, infections, sinusitis, humidification, and breathing patterns. Difficulties with these may influence voice quality, resulting in a "wet" quality in the case of any drainage from the nasal passages into the upper esophagus, where the sound source for esophageal speech is located. Nasal sounds m, n, and ng, already difficult sounds for the laryngectomee because of reduced nasal airflow, may become even more difficult to produce with any nasal obstruction, such as allergies or sinusitis. Chronic respiratory problems such as asthma or bronchitis can result in excess stoma noise and noisy breathing, which is a distraction to the esophageal sound production, making it difficult to hear the speech.

CARDIOVASCULAR SYSTEM

Heart conditions may need monitoring postoperatively. Effort and fatigue levels will influence progress in esophageal speech development.

MUSCULOSKELETAL SYSTEM

Control of the musculoskeletal system is primary in initiation of esophageal voice work. Subtle musculoskeletal adjustments may produce stress and muscle tension—inhibiting esophageal speech.

PAIN

Severe pain is not a common complaint with laryngectomy. The laryngectomee may complain of pain in the back of the neck owing to hyperextension of the neck during surgery.

SLEEP AND REST PATTERNS

Special note of oversleeping should be made because it may be a result of depression, radiation, or chemotherapy. Alterations in sleep patterns may influence time in practice of voice restoration.

HEALTH BEHAVIORS

The laryngectomee's overall health behaviors may have an impact on the ability to learn and contribute to his motivation and readiness to learn esophageal speech. Laborwit (1981) introduced the "Inventory for Assessment of Laryngectomy Rehabilitation," a 72-item inventory of multiple-choice questions developed on the hypothesis that "the more functional information a laryngectomee possesses, the greater will be his capacity to act upon that information optimizing his achievement of rehabilitation goals" (p. 2).

PRE- AND POSTOPERATIVE COUNSELING

Johnson, Casper, and Lesswing (1979) reported that patients and families felt that rehabilitation could have been facilitated if they had been better informed preoperatively. They undertook a study to better understand and identify specific problems encountered by laryngectomized patients. Structured interviews were devised to obtain consistent sources of information from alaryngeal patients in an atmosphere of confidentiality. In their interviews the otolaryngology professionals reported that they adequately informed their patients and that speech pathologists or rehabilitated laryngectomees were often called in preoperatively. The patient and family expressed a desire for exposure to a speech pathologist for a successfully rehabilitated patient. They go on to report that a paradox exists in that professional people have not been successful because patient and family do not retain information in a crisis situation. Too much information is given by the professional in a single session, and the manner of information given may not match the patient's level of understanding. All those interviewed stated that they had been inadequately prepared to deal with their loved ones postoperatively. An inventory such as that of Laborwit may be a useful tool in addressing this concern.

ATTITUDES

Attitudes before and after surgery, depression, frustration, anger, and eagerness to develop the postoperative method of communication will influence progress. The degree of dependence on a spouse and certain personality traits (i.e., silent, outgoing, talkative) influence progress. Attitudes will also be influenced by contacts with other laryngectomees, attitudes of family and friends, hobbies, life styles, and alterations in life style due to the laryngectomy.

OTHER SERVICES

The speech-language pathologist must also be aware of the laryngectomee's need for other community services and assist in making appropriate contacts with agencies for social, nursing, and medical services.

COST OF SERVICES AND PRODUCTS

The speech pathologist also has a special role in understanding third-party reimbursement of services and supplying this information to the laryngectomee. The American Cancer Society has recently published a pamphlet entitled *CANCER—Your Job, Insurance and the Law* (American Cancer Society Publication No. 4585). The pamphlet is for individuals who want to go back to work and feel they are being discriminated against because of their history of cancer. It gives information about Sections 503 and 504 of the Rehabilitation Act of 1983, which lists cancer as a disability.

Speech-language pathologists assume the responsibility of introducing the electrolarynx and stoma coverings. Numerous companies manufacture these products; the speech pathologist should be sensitive to the needs of the laryngectomee to whom the product is dispensed. There is also a responsibility to the third-party payer for selection of the most appropriate product at a reasonable cost. It is important to ask laryngectomees about their evaluation of products to aid in future selection and recommendation for products. The speech-language pathologist also has the responsibility of informing the manufacturer of products that are not appropriate for the laryngectomee either in quality or cost. This author has developed two questionnaires for such data collection. The first, Appendix 32–B, "Questionnaire: Electrolarynx," addresses the artificial aid. Appendix 32–C, "Questionnaire: Stoma Coverings," addresses products for stoma protection.

This chapter by no means addresses all possible clinical considerations in working with laryngectomees. The variables are numerous, and it is the responsibility of the speech-language pathologist to attempt to address any variable affecting the rehabilitation process of the laryngectomee patient. This constant answer-seeking behavior of the speech-language pathologist is the key to successful rehabilitation for the laryngectomee.

QUESTIONS

1. Considering that hearing function may decline with advancing age, try to give a possible explanation of Gardner's 1978 findings of decreasing success rates for speech as a function of age.
2. Which represents a glottal cancer that might have the less favorable prognosis for a patient's developing serviceable postlaryngectomy esophageal voice, a T1-N2 or a T4-N2 lesion?
3. On what variables do Richardson (1981) and Gates (1982) seem to disagree regarding the influence of those variables on speech development?
4. How might a stricture above the PE segment affect speech production?
5. Why do you think Fox speculates that palatal weakness might interfere with speech development for some laryngectomees? You might consider air charge as a factor.
6. Fox lists seven aspects that should be considered that involve the respiratory system. List them and then for each try to indicate some characteristics of speaking that might manifest problems with these aspects.

APPENDIX 32–A. ORAL PERIPHERAL EXAM FOR LARYNGECTOMEES

Evaluation of Laryngectomee's Oral Physical Mechanism
Preoperative and Postoperative Assessment

Use: Torch   Date preoperative assessment ___________

      Stopwatch   Date postoperative assessment __________

      Spatula   Examiner ______________________________

Name ____

Age ____

Hospital No. _________________________________

Occupation __________________________________

1. Lip movements

    (i) Lips at rest

        Note any facial weakness   preoperative   postoperative
          Right
          Left
          Normal

    (ii) Lip rounding and spreading

        Ask patient to say oo-ee five times as fast as possible.
        Time second attempt.   preoperative   postoperative
          T =

    (iii) Lip seal

        Ask patient to hold air in his cheeks for as long as possible.
                      preoperative   postoperative
          T =

2. Tongue movements

    (i) Tongue appearance   preoperative   postoperative
        (a) at rest
        (b) on protrusion

    (ii) Tongue deviation

        Ask patient to protrude tongue. Note any deviation.
                      preoperative   postoperative
          Right
          Left
          Normal

    (iii) Protrusion or retraction

        Ask patient to protrude or retract tongue five times.

        Time second attempt.   preoperative   postoperative
          T =

    (iv) Elevation and depression

Ask patient to put his tongue up toward his nose and down toward his chin five times, as quickly as possible.

Time second attempt.   preoperative   postoperative
   T =

  (v)   Lateral movements

Ask patient to move his tongue from side to side as fast as possible.

Time second attempt.   preoperative   postoperative
   T =

  (vi)   Tongue strength

Ask patient to push against spatula using

(a) Tip of tongue
(b) Lateral movements   preoperative   postoperative
     Right
     Left
Note any weakness or lack of resistance

3. Dentures

Present   preoperative   postoperative
  Yes
  No
  If yes: well fitting
        poorly fitting
  Comments

4. Palate

  (i)   Ask patient if fluids ever come down his nose.
               preoperative   postoperative
     Yes
     No

  (ii)   Ask patient to phonate on /a/ and note palatal elevation: is it uniform or is there palatal weakness?
               preoperative   postoperative

  (iii)   Ask the patient to suck water through a straw and note performance.
               preoperative   postoperative

5. Mandibular and maxillary arches

  (i)   Ask the patient to open and close mouth as wide as possible. Note movements.
               preoperative   postoperative

6. Neck status

  (i)   Normal: Fibrosis:
       Edema: Cicatrix:
              preoperative   postoperative

  (ii)   Range of movements:

     Elevation or depression
     Lateral—circular R and L
     Ear to shoulder R and L
     Bilateral shoulder elevation
     Arm elevation—right, left, bilateral

7. Articulation or rate of speech

8. Voice quality preoperatively
    Normal   Husky   Hoarse   Harsh

9. Accent preoperatively

10. Breathing   preoperative   postoperative

APPENDIX 32–B. ELECTROLARYNX QUESTIONNAIRE

Speech Pathology Services North Memorial Center, Robbinsdale, Minnesota 55422

The purpose of this questionnaire is to collect data about patient evaluation of electrolarynx usage or other communication aid following laryngectomy. Your assistance is appreciated.

Patient Name ____ Age ____________

Address ____ Sex ______M ______F

City ____________________ State ____________________ Zip ______________

Name of Electrolarynx ____

Company Name ____

How long have you used your current electrolarynx? ______________________________

What other electrolarynx have you used? ______________________________

How long did you use it? ____

Why did you choose your current electrolarynx? ______________________________

____

Do you use esophageal speech? Comment ______________________________

____

Please rate the following aspects of your current electrolarynx by circling the appropriate number.

		Poor	*Fair*	*Good*	*Excellent*
1.	Your overall ability to use it comfortably	1	2	3	4
	Comments _______________________________				
2.	Quality (tone)	1	2	3	4
	Comments _______________________________				
3.	Ability to physicially handle the aid (hold it)	1	2	3	4
	Comments _______________________________				
4.	Rating of how quiet (no extra noise)	1	2	3	4
	Comments _______________________________				
5.	Ability to change pitches	1	2	3	4
	Comments _______________________________				
6.	Ability to change loudness	1	2	3	4
	Comments _______________________________				
7.	Ease of placement against the surface of the skin	1	2	3	4
	Comments _______________________________				
8.	Weight	1	2	3	4
	Comments _______________________________				
9.	Size	1	2	3	4
	Comments _______________________________				
10.	Ease of carrying around with you	1	2	3	4
	Comments _______________________________				

		Poor	Fair	Good	Excellent
11.	Cost of the aid	1	2	3	4
	Comments ___________________				
12.	Life of the battery	1	2	3	4
	Comments ___________________				
13.	Ease of changing batteries	1	2	3	4
	Comments ___________________				
14.	Cost of battery	1	2	3	4
	Comments ___________________				
15.	Ease of purchasing batteries	1	2	3	4
	Comments ___________________				
16.	Durability (needed repairs)	1	2	3	4
	Comments ___________________				
17.	Availability of repairs	1	2	3	4
	Comments ___________________				
18.	How do others rate your speech with the aid?	1	2	3	4
	Comments ___________________				

Would you recommend this electrolarynx for others?   Yes __________ No __________

Do you have any suggestions for modification of the aid? ____________________

____

Thank you.

APPENDIX 32–C. STOMA COVERINGS QUESTIONNAIRE

Speech Pathology Services, North Memorial Medical Center, Robbinsdale, Minnesota 55422

The purpose of this questionnaire is to collect data about patient evaluation of stoma coverings. Your assistance is appreciated.

Patient Name ____ Age ____________

Address ____ Sex ______M ______F

City __________________ State _______________ Zip _______________

Name of Stoma Covering ____

Company Name ____

How long have you worn this covering? ____

Please rate the following aspects of the stoma covering by circling the appropriate number.

		Poor	Fair	Good	Excellent
1.	Overall comfortableness	1	2	3	4
	Comments ______________				
2.	Ease of breathing	1	2	3	4
	Comments ______________				
3.	Thickness	1	2	3	4
	Comments ______________				
4.	Ability to use with other clothing	1	2	3	4
	Comments ______________				
5.	Size	1	2	3	4
	Comments ______________				
6.	Shape	1	2	3	4
	Comments ______________				
7.	Durability	1	2	3	4
	Comments ______________				
8.	Cleaning	1	2	3	4
	Comments ______________				
9.	Color	1	2	3	4
	Comments ______________				
10.	Ease of removal and replacement	1	2	3	4
	Comments ______________				
11.	Availability (how easy to replace)	1	2	3	4
	Comments ______________				
12.	Cost	1	2	3	4
	Comments ______________				

Do you recommend this covering for other laryngectomees? Yes _______ No _______

Comments ____

What are the major advantages of the covering? ____

What are the major disadvantages of the covering? ____

Do you have any recommendations for modification of stoma coverings? _________

REFERENCES

Baker, B., and Cunningham, C. (1980). Vocal rehabilitation of the patient with a laryngectomy. *Oncology Nursing Forum, 7*(4), 23–36.

Berlin, C. (1984). Hearing loss, palatal function, and other factors in post-laryngectomy rehabilitation. *J. Chronic Dis., 17,* 677–684.

Gardner, W. (1978). *Laryngectomee speech and rehabilitation.* Springfield, IL: Charles C Thomas.

Gates, G. A., Hearne, E. M., III. (1982). Predicting esophageal speech. *Ann. Otol. Rhinol. Laryngol., 91,* 454–457.

Johnson, J., Casper, J., and Lesswing, J. (1979). Toward the total rehabilitation of the alaryngeal patient. *Laryngoscope, 89,* 1813–1819.

Julian, W., Noscoe, N., and Berry, R. (1981). Xeroradiographic tomography of the larynx. *Clin. Radiol., 32,* 577–583.

Keith, R., Ewert, J., and Flowers, C. (1974). Factors influencing the learning of esophageal speech. *Brit. J. Comm. Dis., 9,* 110–116.

Laborwit, J. (1981). Inventory for the Assessment of Laryngectomy Rehabilitation. Tigard, OR: CC Publications.

McGarvey, S., and Weinberg, B. (1984). Esophageal insufflation test in nonlaryngectomized adults. *J. Speech Hearing Dis., 49,* 272–277.

McNeil, B., Weichselbaum, R., and Pauker, S. (1981). Speech and survival tradeoffs between quality and quantity of life in laryngeal cancer. *New Engl. J. Med., 305,* 982–987.

Nayar, R., Sharma, V., and Arora, M. (1984). A study of the pharynx after laryngectomy. *J. Laryngol. Otol., 98,* 807–810.

Perry, A. (1983). Assessment: What, why, how, and when to measure social, physical, communication and psychological improvement. In Y. Edels (Ed.), *Laryngectomy: Diagnosis to rehabilitation.* London: Croom Helm.

Richardson, J. (1981). Surgical and radiological effects upon the development of speech after total laryngectomy. *Ann. Otolaryngol., 90,* 294–297.

Simpson, I., Smith, J., and Gordon, M. (1972). Laryngectomy: The influence of muscle reconstruction on the mechanism of esophageal voice production. *J. Laryngol. Otol., 86,* 961–990.

Singer, M., and Blom, E. (1981). Selective myotomy for voice restoration after total laryngectomy. *Arch. Otolaryngol., 107,* 670–673.

U.S. Department of Health and Human Services, Public Health Service, National Institute of Health. (1981a). *Chemotherapy and you: A guide to self-help during treatment* (Publication No. 81–1136). Bethesda, MD: National Cancer Institute.

U.S. Department of Health and Human Services, Public Health Service, National Institute of Health. (1981b). *Radiation therapy and you: A guide to self-help during treatment* (Publication No. 81–1117). Bethesda, MD: National Cancer Institute.

Vincent, M., Robbins, A., Walsh, M., and Vaughan, C. (1984). Evaluation of Blom-Singer voice prosthesis. *Amer. J. Radiol., 143,* 745–750.

Chapter **33**

Airway Maintenance and First Aid for Laryngectomees

Douglas E. Fox

Medical emergencies for the laryngectomee are similar to those in the general population. The permanency of a tracheostoma necessitates special considerations in maintaining an adequate airway and especially so for cardiopulmonary resuscitation (CPR) in the event of a cardiac arrest. The following discussion will first address the maintenance of an airway and then address CPR for the laryngectomee. It is critical that the speech-language pathologist and others working with this population have the knowledge to manage a medical emergency of this kind.

HISTORY OF THE TRACHEOTOMY

The first tracheotomy was reportedly performed 124 years before the birth of Christ by a physician in Rome (Portex, 1976). Three hundred years later a physician, Antyllus, performed a transverse incision between the third and forth tracheal rings. Physicians performing these early airway procedures in the laryngeal population feared the tracheal rings would not heal. Until the sixteenth century, tracheotomy was performed reluctantly. However, with more successful experience it gradually gained acceptance as a safe procedure and the design of the first cannula to keep the airway open then followed. Originally, the cannula was short and straight and had two wings to prevent it from slipping into the trachea, and it was secured around the neck by tapes. Later a physician, Casserius, suggested a curved cannula. By the nineteenth century, 28 successful operations had been recorded usually for trauma, foreign bodies, or inflammation leading to acute obstruction of the upper respiratory tract. Further development of the tracheotomy tube is attributed to Bourdellat in 1852, Durham and Guy's Hospital in 1869, and Parker's tubing of children in 1880. Methods of extracting blood and mucus from the trachea, such as the use of quills and feathers, were introduced. Greater recognition of the signs of respiratory distress improved the technique and designs of tracheotomy tubes, and ventilators have made the procedure commonplace in modern medicine.

Theodore Billroth performed the first successful laryngectomy for cancer in 1873. The postoperative deficits left in early procedures taxed the medical management of the wounds at that time in medicine. The wounds in early laryngectomies were frequently left open in the hope that the pharynx would close spontaneously and the tracheostomy would remain open. In laryngectomy procedures, the permanent airway is diverted to the neck with the tracheal stump being brought anteriorly and sutured to the skin, creating a permanent stoma; however, it was not until 1892 that this principle was introduced by Solis-Cohen. The early design of the cannula was also applied to the laryngectomee. It is common practice today to use the tracheal cannula immediately postoperatively, although newer surgical techniques may eliminate the need for the cannula in some laryngectomees. Special problems created by the new airway have been reported elsewhere in the literature and will not be repeated in this discussion.

ANATOMY AND PHYSIOLOGY OF THE TRACHEA

The trachea is tubular and approximately 4 to 5 inches in length. It extends from the larynx where it joins at the level of the sixth cervical vertebra (C6) and bifurcates, about the level of the fifth cervical vertebra (C6), into the right and left bronchi to the lungs. There are 15 to 20 C-shaped rings of cartilage separated by the fibrous muscular tissue that forms its supporting framework. A fibroelastic membrane extends across the open portion of the trachea where the cartilages are incomplete on the dorsal end. There are four layers to the tracheal structure, including mucosa, submucosa, cartilage, and adventitia. The submucosa is loose connective tissue containing glands that secrete mucus. In laryngectomees, these glands become somewhat hypersecretive until the airway adjusts to its new exposure via the neck, which lacks the filtering system provided by the nose and mouth prior to laryngectomy.

MAINTAINING THE AIRWAY

Most laryngectomees adjust well to the shortened airway, but the air is no longer filtered, warmed, or moistened by the lining of the nose and throat. Reflux coughing may occur, encrustation may cause restriction in breathing, and secretions may increase, as the trachea and lungs usually secrete a great deal of mucus. For several days postoperatively excessive serum and tissue fluid are secreted under the skin in the operative site. These are all concerns in maintaining an airway.

There are a number of factors reported to contribute to an inadequate stoma, including a small trachea. Actually, the stomal size may need to be only the diameter of one nostril for survival purposes alone. Other factors include enlarged thyroid, relative deficit of anterior cervical skin, irradiation, excessive tracheal resection with tension, poor approximation of the mucocutaneous junction, type of stoma reconstruction, postoperative infection and fistula, and the presence of a foreign body such as the tracheal cannula, which may form excessive granulation tissue and consequently contribute to stenosis.

A report on tracheal stomal stenosis after laryngectomy by Griffith and Luce (1982), involving 89 patients, showed 22 per cent incidence of tracheal stenosis overall. Other associated events included postoperative radiation (36 per cent), preoperative radiotherapy (19 per cent), combined pre- and postoperative radiotherapy (17 per cent), and retention of the tracheal cannula for longer than one week (25 per cent). The technique of stomal construction was an important determinant of stomal stenosis: the highest incidence of stenosis (29 per cent) occurred in procedures with a simple circle of straight transection of the trachea; stenosis occurred in 15 per cent with a beveled technique; and the lowest incidence of stenosis (8 per cent) occurred in a primary plastic or flap construction technique. Other important factors include handling of the tracheal mucosa, poor approximation of mucocutaneous tissues impinging on the stoma, excessive tension at the suture line, devascularization of the trachea, enlarged thyroid lobes, and incomplete removal of strap muscles. Once tracheal stenosis occurs, management becomes a problem. Management may require dilatation by introducing progressively larger laryngectomy cannulas or tracheostomy buttons. Operative resection may be required in some instances. Some individuals may permanently require cannulation or a stoma button.

The surgical management for maintenance of an airway is crucial. In some instances, a second surgical procedure to reconstruct the stoma site may be indicated. Proper instruction for weaning the patient from a cannula is important because misunderstanding by the laryngectomee on occasion results in a tendency for stenosis. Tubes can usually be weaned in about 6 weeks if the stoma is of sufficient size. The tube may be left out one hour at a time and the time gradually increased as long as there is no shrinkage of the stoma. Resistance to reinsertion of the tube means that the stoma is closing. Irritation and bleeding of the tracheal mucosa may occur if forceful insertion is required; in such instances reinsertion for 24 to 48 hours may be necessary before again starting the weaning process.

THE TRACHEOSTOMA TUBE

The main purpose of the tracheostoma tube is to keep the airway open. Probably the most popular tube has been the silver Jackson tube (Fig. 33-1). The silver tube is designed without a fixed or bonded cuff and is used for long-term tracheostomy. The tube components include the obturator, which is designed to insert the outer cannula to prevent damage to the tracheal wall. The inner cannula is inserted into the outer cannula once the obturator has been removed. The inner cannula is withdrawn for cleaning to prevent secretions from obstructing the tube, whereas the outer cannula maintains patency of the airway. The outer cannula is secured in place by a fabric tape around the patient's neck. A

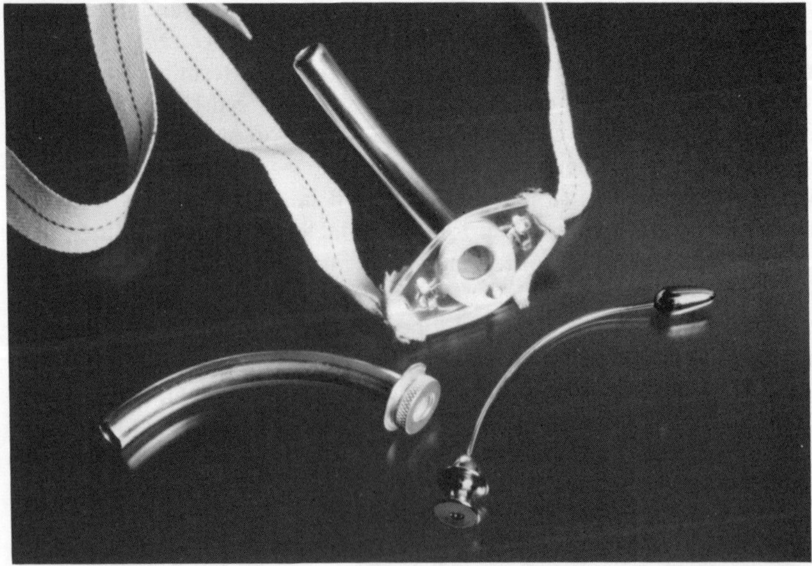

Figure 33-1. Outer cannula with strap (top), inner cannula (lower left), and obturator (lower right).

cuffed tracheostoma tube is not necessary with laryngectomy because of the separation of the airway from the esophagus, thus eliminating the concern for aspiration during eating. In laryngeal patients, the inflated cuff seals the area between the trachea and the lower portion of the outer cannula. This permits positive-pressure ventilation, prevents aspiration, and positions the tube centrally in the trachea.

Examples of some other tracheostomy tubes are also shown to give greater understanding of the tube designs not only for maintaining an airway but also for communication purposes.

1. The Shiley low-pressure cuff (Fig. 33–2) is used with the nonlaryngectomee. This is a plastic tube and is shown with the cuff for comparison with the silver tube used with the laryngectomee. Cuffed tubes are not necessary with the laryngectomee because the airway is out the neck and any substance given orally could not spill into the airway, as it would for the nonlaryngectomee. The cuffed tube is designed to protect the airway from secretions or food during swallowing in the nonlaryngectomee.

2. The Lara Med plastic cannula (Fig. 33–3) and the Teflon cannula (Fig. 33–4) are lighter in weight than the silver cannulas and are reported to be more flexible and fit more comfortably and easily.

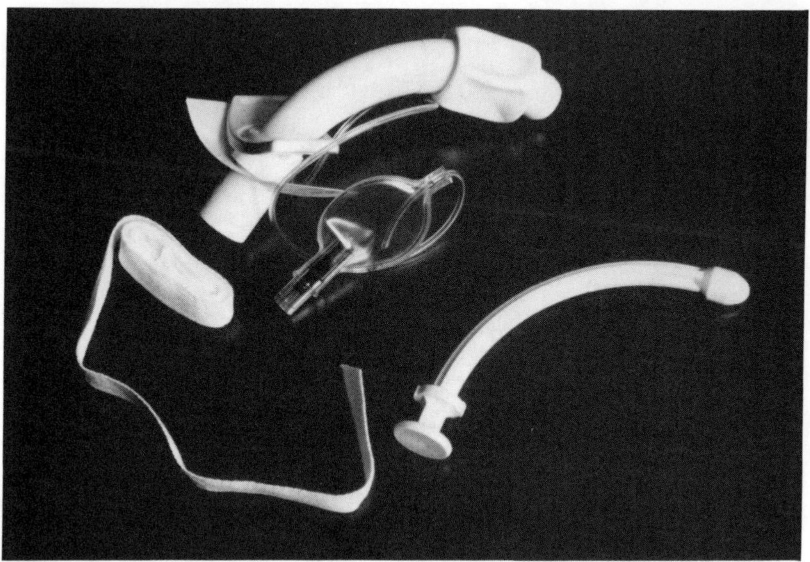

Figure 33–2. The Shiley low-pressure cuffed tracheostoma tube. Inner cannula in place with cuff inflater attachment, obturator, and strap.

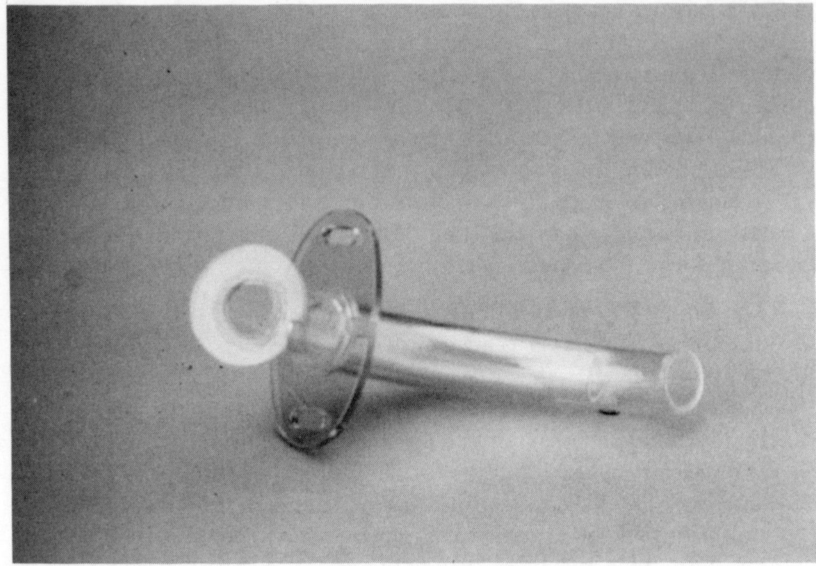

Figure 33–3. The Lara Med plastic cannula.

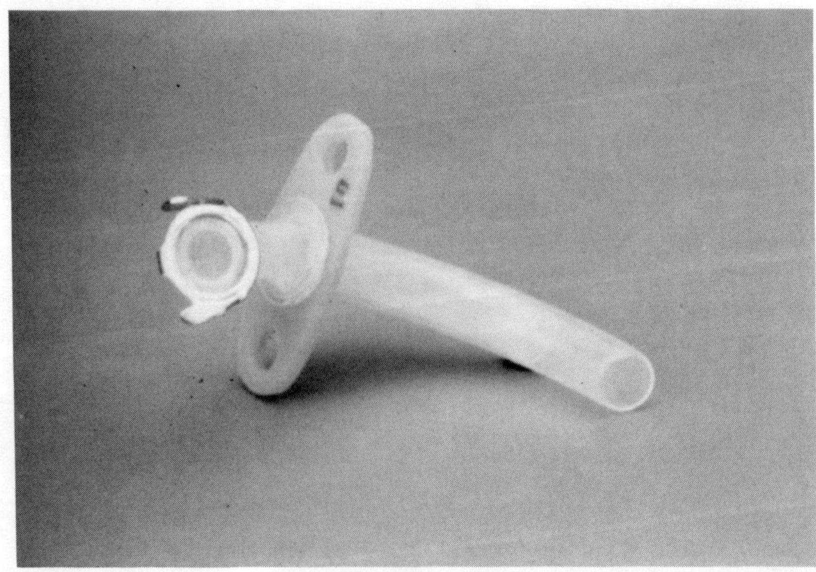

Figure 33–4. The Lara Med Teflon cannula.

The Teflon cannula is generally thin walled and can be worn longer than the conventional plastic tube because it retains its dimensions and interchangeability for years. These tubes are also used with the laryngectomee. (These cannulas are available from Lara Med, Ltd., Post Box 1588, Kelowna, B.C., V1Y 7V8.)

3. The fenestrated tracheostomy tube (Fig. 33-5) is used for laryngeal speakers and is shown for comparison with tubes used with the laryngectomee. The air port on the superior portion of the curve in the tube is to shunt air past the vocal cords for sound production.

4. The Communitrach (Figs. 33-6 and 33-7), also for laryngeal speakers, is another example of a speaking tracheostomy tube designed for individuals requiring ventilator assistance. The inner cannula connects to the ventilator for life-support breathing. A separate air source feeds the outer cannula with air for speaking, which is directed between the inner and outer cannula upward through several air ports past the vocal folds. The purpose of the design is to minimize blockage by secretions. A second person is required to clamp an air feeder hose to shunt the air between the inner and outer cannula for voicing. The phonation is acoustically perceived as a room whisper. (The Communitrach is available from Implant Technologies, Inc., 7800 Metro Parkway, Suite 217, Minneapolis, MN 55420.)

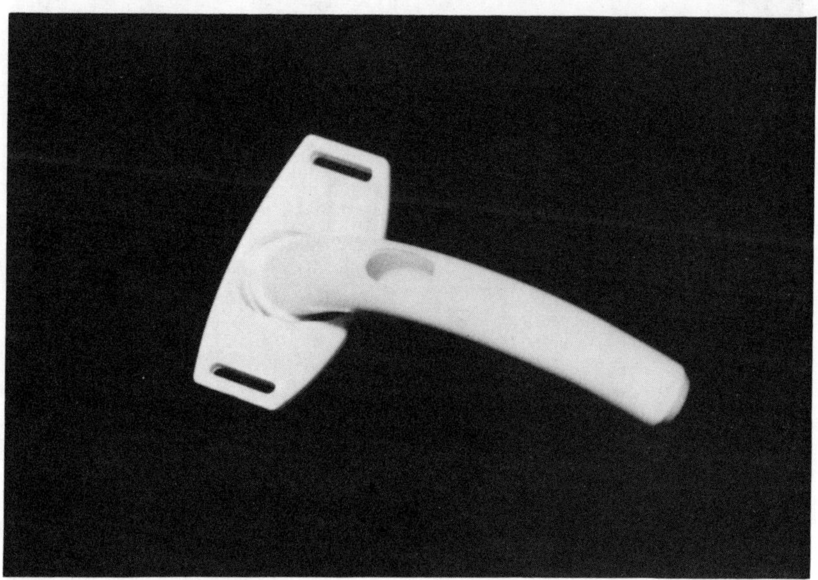

Figure 33-5. The fenestrated tracheostomy tube.

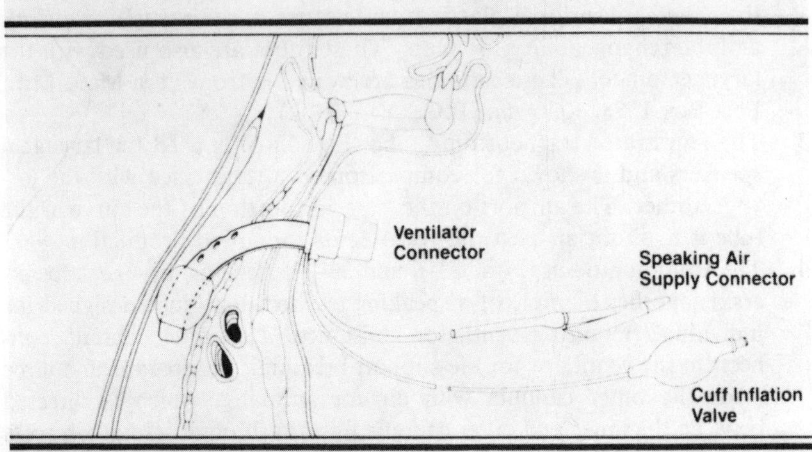

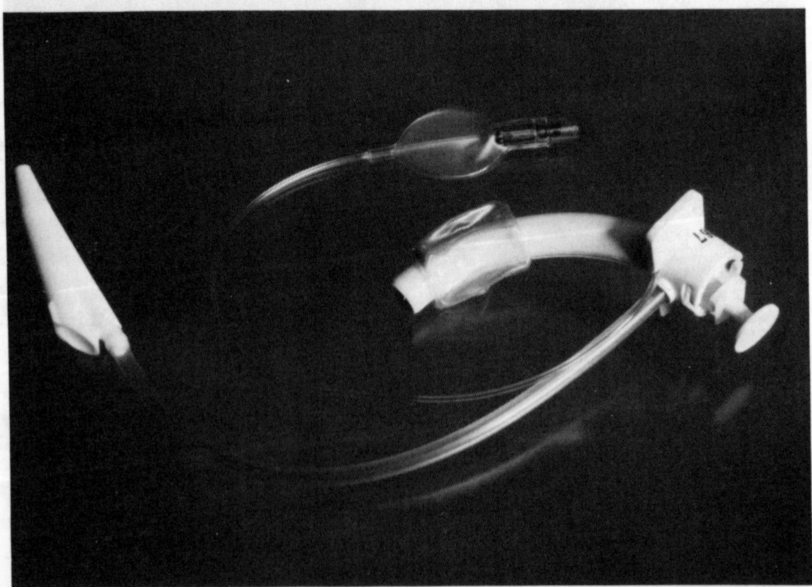

Figure 33–6. The Communitrach.

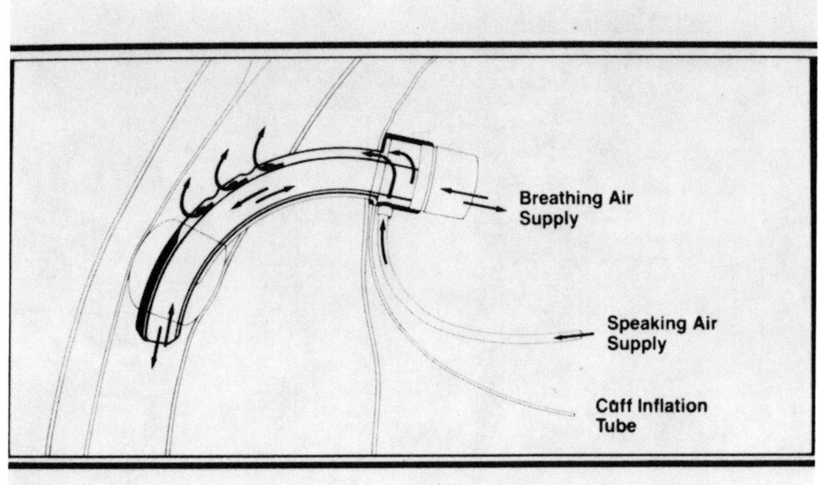

Figure 33–7. The Communitrach, showing direction of air flow for breathing and speaking.

STOMA BUTTONS

Stoma buttons resemble a short tracheostomy tube and serve a similar function of preventing stoma stenosis. They are usually not used immediately after surgery because (1) they fit tightly and the stoma site is too tender, and (2) they are difficult to keep in place until the rim that develops in postoperative healing is formed, this rim contributing to adherence of the button. Stoma buttons are worn to keep the stoma size from shrinking. In some individuals they may need to be worn permanently; however, once the stoma has healed most laryngectomees do not require a stoma button. Stoma buttons are generally worn all day; occasionally only a few hours of insertion at a time are required to maintain the stoma size. Some stoma buttons may soften and slip if worn in a heated shower and so must be worn with caution. In addition to maintaining an airway, stoma buttons have proven useful in assisting the seal in tracheoesophageal puncture techniques. In tracheoesophageal punctures, the stoma may be irregular in shape or slightly large; the stoma button may help create a stoma site that gives a good air seal when digital pressure is used to shunt the air posteriorly. Use of sesame oil, olive oils, salad oils, or K-Y Jelly might be required for insertion.

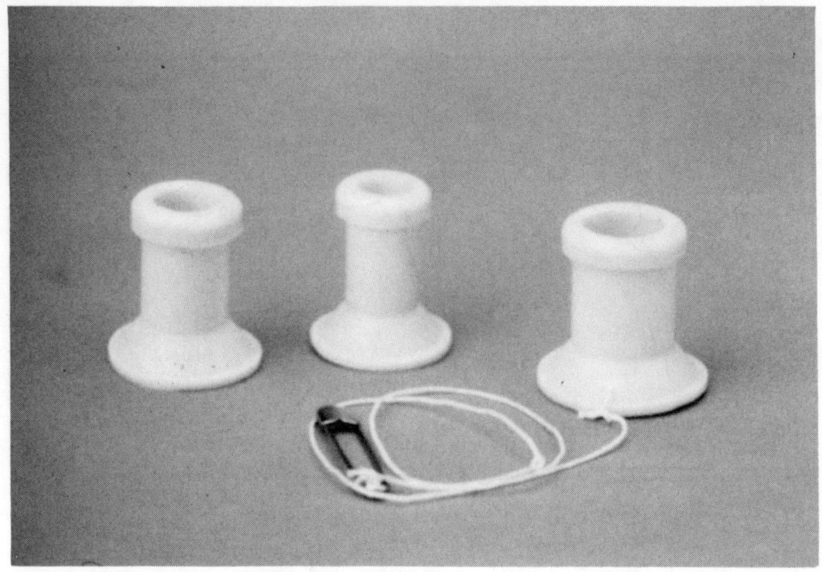

Figure 33–8. Lara Med "Stoma Open."

Stoma buttons have become popular items among a number of companies manufacturing products for the laryngectomee. Lara Med sells a stoma button in three sizes, called "Stoma Open" (Fig. 33–8). Charles F. Thackery (175-X New Boston St., Woburn, MA 01801) sells stoma studs (Fig. 33–9) with radiopaque substance for easier observation under radiography in the event they are aspirated. The stoma stud is made from medical grade silicone so that there will be no allergic reaction when worn. A hole has been made on the outer flange to allow a cotton thread to be attached and pinned to clothing so the stud will not be lost if expelled through coughing. The studs are available in 8 mm, 10 mm, 12 mm, and 14 mm sizes. The Bivona Tracheostoma Vent (Fig. 33–10) is all silicone. It is available in six sizes (outside dimensions 12 mm, 13.5 mm, 15 mm, 17 mm, 20 mm, 24 mm) and four lengths (18 mm, 27 mm, 36 mm, 55 mm) (Bivona, Inc., 5700 West 23rd Avenue, Gary, IN 46406). The illustrations are not meant to be an exhaustive listing of all the commercially available stoma buttons.

The speech-language pathologist should be familiar with insertion and cleaning techniques for both tracheostomy tubes and stoma buttons. There is a good description of insertion and cleaning techniques in Keith, Shane, Coates, and Devine (1984).

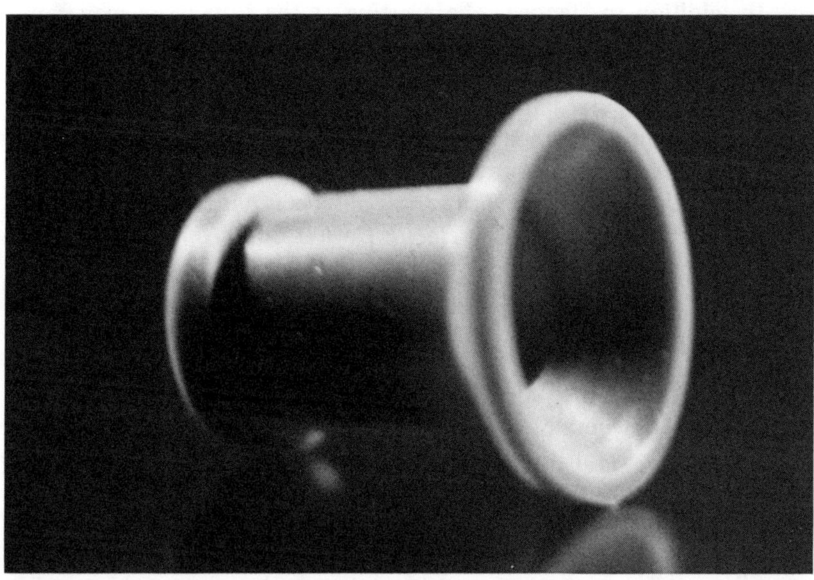

Figure 33–9. The Charles F. Thackery Stoma Stud.

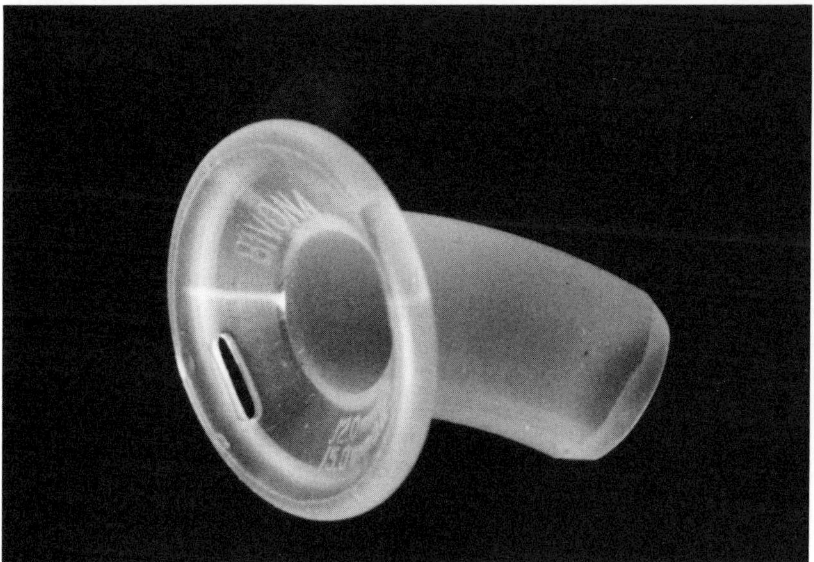

Figure 33–10. The Bivona Tracheostoma Vent.

In addition to stenosis, the crusting at the stoma site may cause airway restriction. A number of suggestions have been offered to prevent crusting. These include application of petroleum jelly (Vaseline) around the stoma site; regular bathing; forceful coughing and deep breathing to remove secretions from the lungs; and adequate humidification. The role of stoma coverings for airway protection and humidification should be familiar to those working with laryngectomees. Further discussion of humidification can be found in *Health Devices Sourcebook* (May, 1983).

OBSTRUCTION TO AIR FLOW

Signs of obstruction to air flow include stridor, retraction, indrawing, and wheezing. Generally, to reduce any air-flow obstruction the laryngectomee will rely on the cough first. Secretions are usually managed unless there is a history of chronic infections. In such instances, cleaning the airway every 5 to 10 minutes may be necessary. The speech-language pathologist should be familiar with such techniques for the laryngectomee. Some laryngectomees are known to travel with portable suction equipment or a portable oxygen tank.

The American Cancer Society has available bedside signs, posters, and information sheets that alert individuals encountering the laryngectomees to the fact that they are neck breathers: poster No. 4528.02 (Fig. 33–11), bedside sign No. 4528 (Fig. 33–12), and information guideline sheet No. 4528.01 (Fig. 33–13).

CARDIOPULMONARY RESUSCITATION (CPR)

Over 650,000 persons die from heart attacks each year, with 350,000 of these deaths occurring outside the hospital, usually within 2 hours after onset of the attack. Over 40 per cent can be successfully resuscitated if CPR is begun promptly; however, without a bystander this percentage drops to 21 per cent. There are over 30,000 laryngectomees in the United States. The laryngectomee is included in this population, and the fact that his respiration is separated from the nose and mouth could be an important lifesaving feature during emergencies should heart activity and breathing cease. In many emergencies, the laryngectomee may have a better change of survival than the mouth breather because expelled stomach contents cannot spill over into the airway. Professionals working with laryngectomees, other laryngectomees, spouses, and family members should become knowledgeable about CPR procedures for the neck breather in the event of a medical emergency.

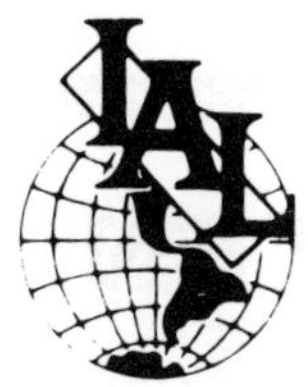

NECK BREATHERS
NEED YOUR SPECIAL HELP

HERE IS WHAT TO DO

1. Keep neck opening clear, clean—wipe away any discharge.

2. Do not plug up neck opening.

3. Do not allow any liquids to enter neck opening.

4. Patient may not be able to speak face-to-face or on intercom, but may be able to indicate yes or no by head shake, eye blink, or hand squeeze.

5. Watch facial expression for evidence of discomfort.

6. Pulmonary resuscitation must be administered through neck opening (not mouth).

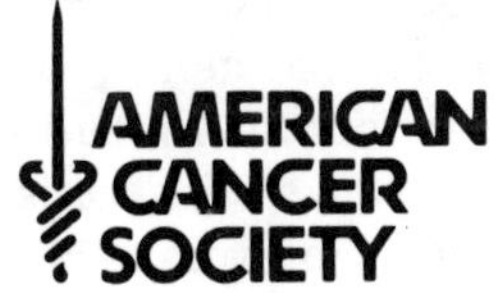

Figure 33–11.   American Cancer Society poster No. 4528.02.

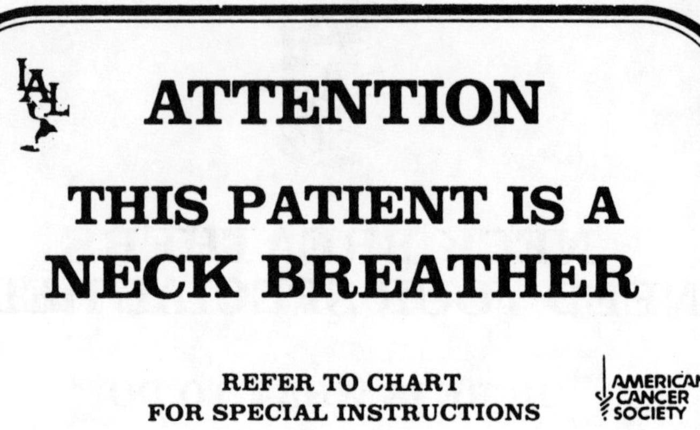

Figure 33–12.   American Cancer Society bedside sign No. 4528.

The person finding a laryngectomee with possible cardiac arrest may not immediately know that he is a neck breather unless he or she has known the individual. A Medic Alert bracelet or neckpiece or pocket identification will identify the victim as a neck breather (Fig. 33–14). A metal or plastic tube or stoma button may or may not be in place. Removal of these is not necessary to start CPR and it wastes valuable time (Fig. 33–15).

All constrictive clothing down to the sternum should be loosened and encrustation and mucus from the stoma site quickly cleaned to establish an airway (Fig. 33–16). The head should be tilted back with some support under the shoulders with an article of clothing to allow access to the stoma for mouth-to-stoma breathing (Fig. 33–17).

The resuscitator may feel that mouth-to-stoma contact is not sanitary. Actually, it is more sanitary than mouth-to-mouth contact because the air coming directly from the stoma site is cleaner than that coming through the mouth. Contents of vomit cannot be discharged to the mouth as is possible in mouth-to-mouth resuscitation (Fig. 33–18).

Airway, breathing, and circulation are monitored in the same manner as in CPR for the nonlaryngectomee. Once the airway is established and lack of breathing or insufficient breathing is noted, then mouth-to-neck breathing should be started immediately. There is no need to cover the nose or mouth as in standard CPR. If the resuscitator were to

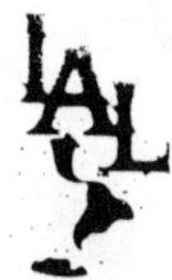

NECK BREATHER GUIDELINES
FOR MEDICAL PERSONNEL

1. Keep neck opening clear. clean—wipe away
   any discharge.

2. Do not plug up neck opening.

3. Do not allow any liquids to enter neck opening.

4. Patient may not be able to speak face-to-face or
   on intercom. but may be able to indicate yes or
   no by head shake. eye blink. or hand squeeze.

5. Watch facial expression for evidence of
   discomfort.

6. Pulmonary resuscitation must be administered
   through neck opening (not mouth).

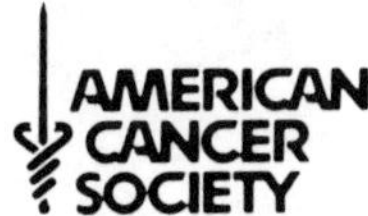

(Permission is granted to reproduce as needed)

Figure 33–13. American Cancer Society information guideline sheet No.
4528.01.

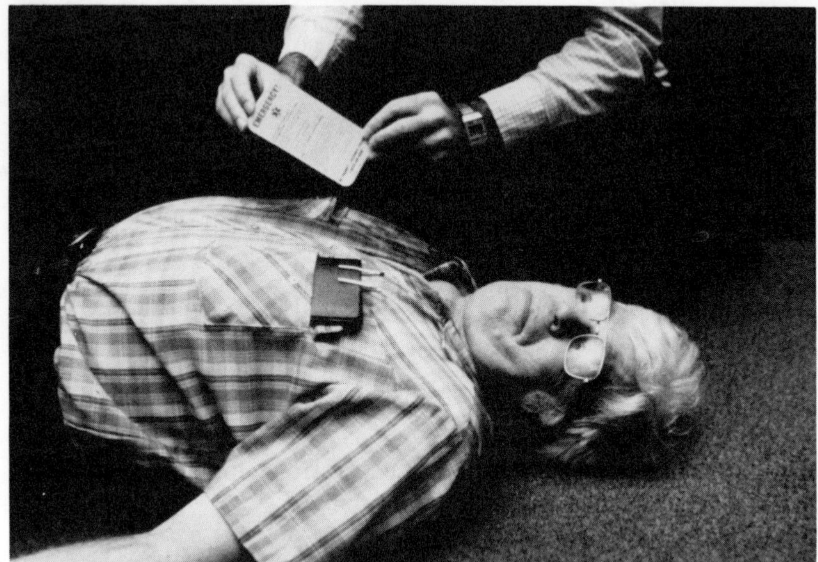

Figure 33–14. Emergency identification.

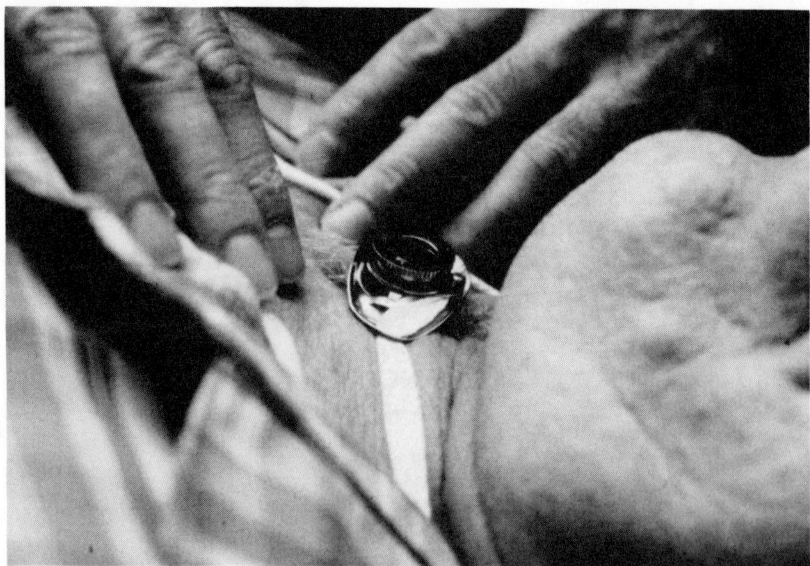

Figure 33–15. Tracheostoma tube in place.

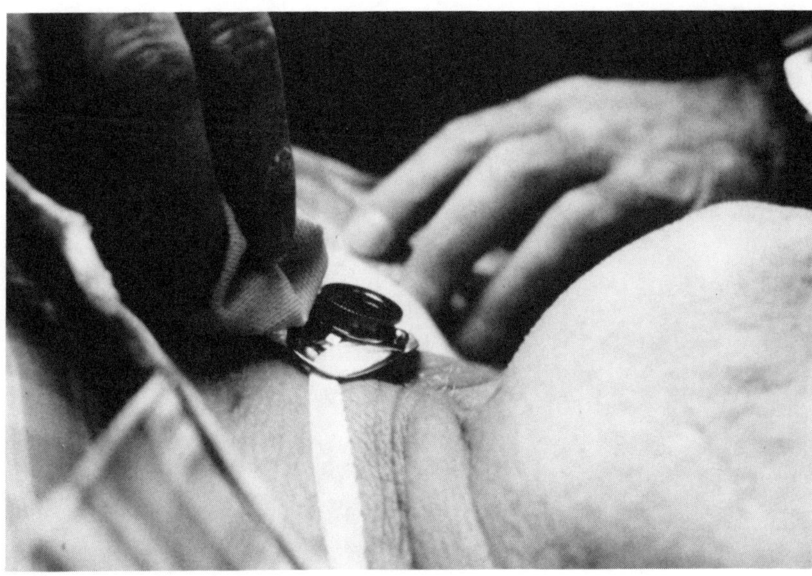

Figure 33–16. Cleaning the stoma to establish airway.

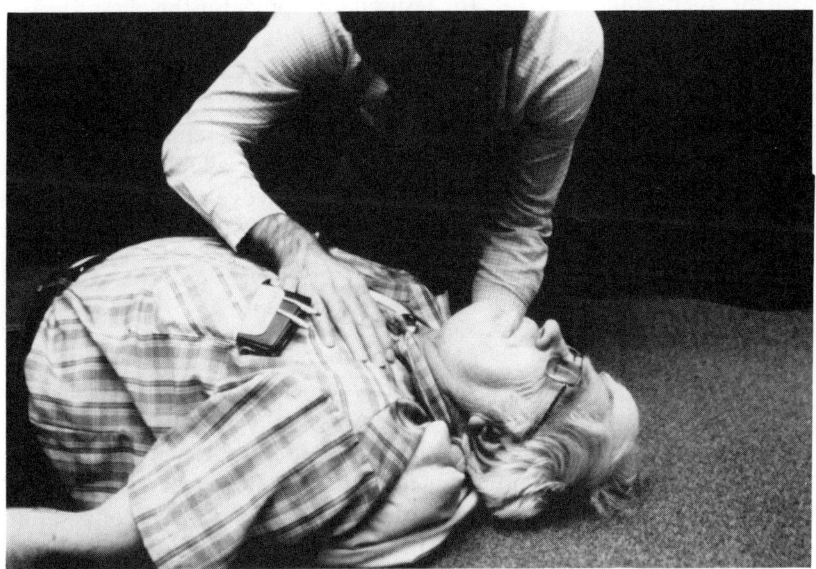

Figure 33–17. The head tilted back to allow access to the stoma.

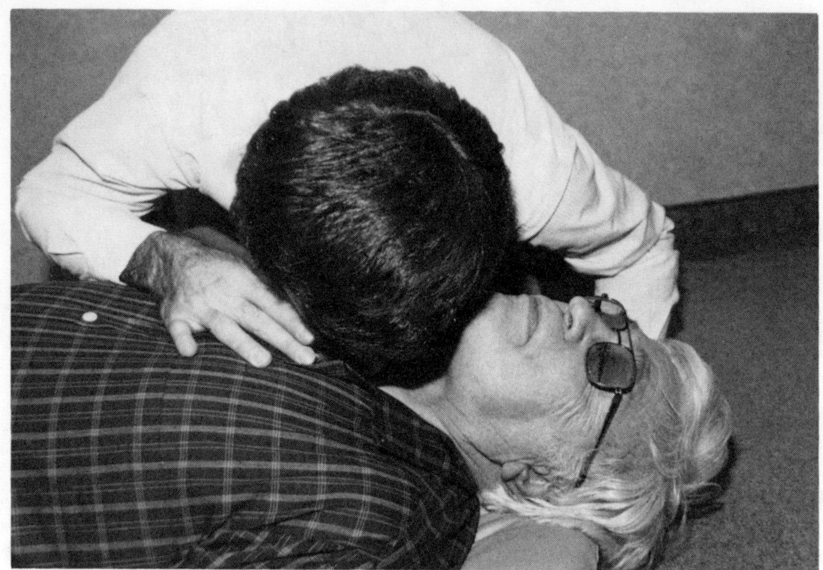

Figure 33–18. Mouth-to-stoma breathing.

breathe into the nose or mouth, he or she would only fill the stomach with air. As in standard CPR, the resuscitator looks for the chest to rise, indicating that the lungs are being filled with air. The techniques for establishing circulation are the same as in standard CPR. For one-person CPR, the rate of compressions to breathing is 15 to 2, and for two-person CPR, it is 5 to 1. Once spontaneous breathing returns, a portable oxygen supply may be applied to the stoma site if available (Fig. 33–19), but only if the rescuer has experience and knowledge of this equipment and settings for air-flow rates.

Partial Neck Breathers

If a victim is encountered with a stoma tube in place, the tube does not necessarily mean that he is a laryngectomee and a total neck breather. There are other individuals with a tracheostomy tube in place to establish an airway; however, they may breathe only partially through the neck.

This should be noted immediately if the airway is clear and the chest does not rise when air is blown into the stoma and air is felt coming out the nose and mouth (Fig. 33–20). In this instance, the mouth and nose are sealed with one hand, with the head tilted backward to help seal the tongue against the palate (Fig. 33–21). Mouth-to-stoma breathing is then started; the chest should rise and the necessary steps in CPR can follow.

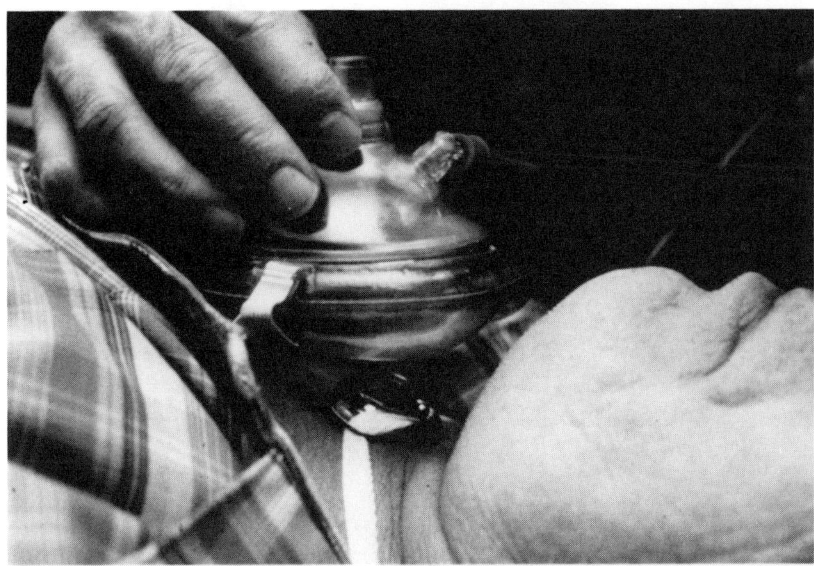

Figure 33–19. Oxygen supply to stoma.

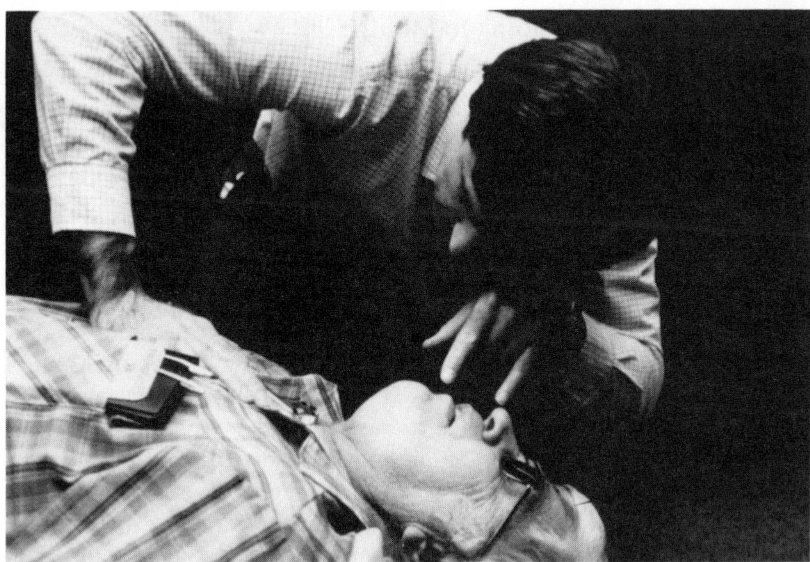

Figure 33–20. Checking for air through nose or mouth to determine whether patient is neck breather if the chest fails to rise.

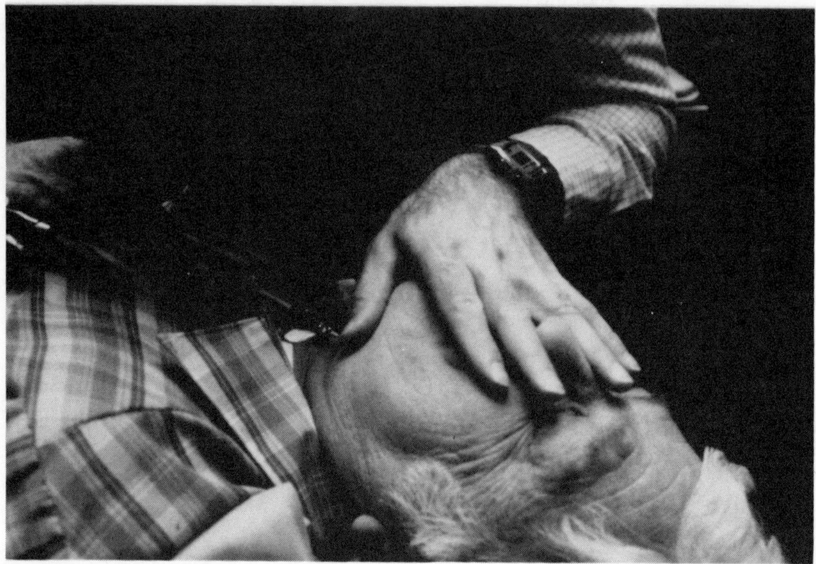

Figure 33–21.   Seal off mouth and nose with head tilted back to get a palate seal for partial neck breathers.

Stoma-to-Stoma and Stoma-to-Mouth CPR

Because of the amount of time laryngectomees spend together there may be the need for stoma-to-stoma resuscitation. The laryngectomee may also encounter a laryngeal victim and can become the rescuer.

The International Association of Laryngectomees (I.A.L.) published an article in the I.A.L. Newsletter (American Cancer Society, 1982) addressing the question "Can Laryngectomees Really Do Artificial Respiration?" The article stated, "The laryngectomees are as proficient in using CPR with the exception of artificial respiration" (p. 1). It was suggested that "if the laryngectomee is alone and needs to resuscitate, then the American Red Cross older chest pressure, Silvester Method of Resuscitation, be used" (p. 1). This method has not been used in CPR since the early 1970s, when it was replaced by the more effective mouth-to-mouth procedure. The author also stated that "resuscitation requires exceptional lung power, a resource that laryngectomees usually are short on. If you combine that with an age factor and the difficulty of achieving a tight seal between the stoma and the victim's mouth, you could end up with two emergencies instead of one. . . . The most effective way of administering CPR is with two people, one doing chest compressions and the other mouth-to-mouth resuscitation. A laryngectomee can easily do the compressions'' (p. 3).

In the Silvester method the airway is established in the usual manner. The rescuer kneels at the top of the victim's head, grasps the victim's wrists, and brings them over the lower chest. Then the rescuer rocks forward until the arms are approximately vertical and allows the weight of the upper part of the body to exert steady, even pressure downward (Fig. 33–22). This action should cause air flow out of the victim's lungs. The pressure is released by rocking back and pulling the victim's arms outward and upward over the victim's head and backward as far as possible. This should allow air to flow in (Fig. 33–23). This cycle is repeated about 12 times per minute, with the victim's mouth being checked occasionally for obstruction.

In response to the I.A.L. article, a number of laryngectomees throughout the United States of America initiated CPR training in stoma-to-stoma and stoma-to-mouth procedures to demonstrate that the laryngectomee can become proficient in CPR. Finchem (1982) has expressed the opinion that the individual with a stoma should be able to perform CPR stoma-to-mouth. In their CPR training for laryngectomees they found two concerns. The first of these was the time factor, in that the time spent with the laryngectomee student on airway manage-

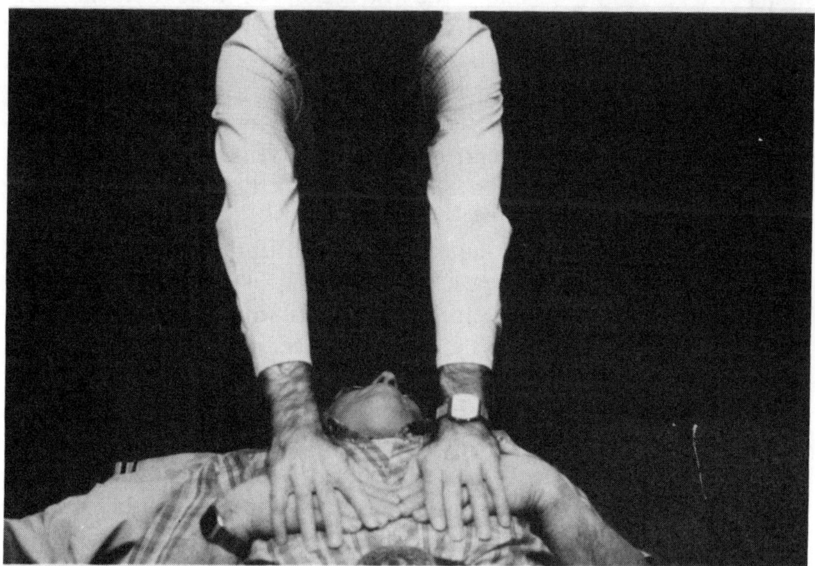

Figure 33–22. Silvester method causing air to flow out of the lungs.

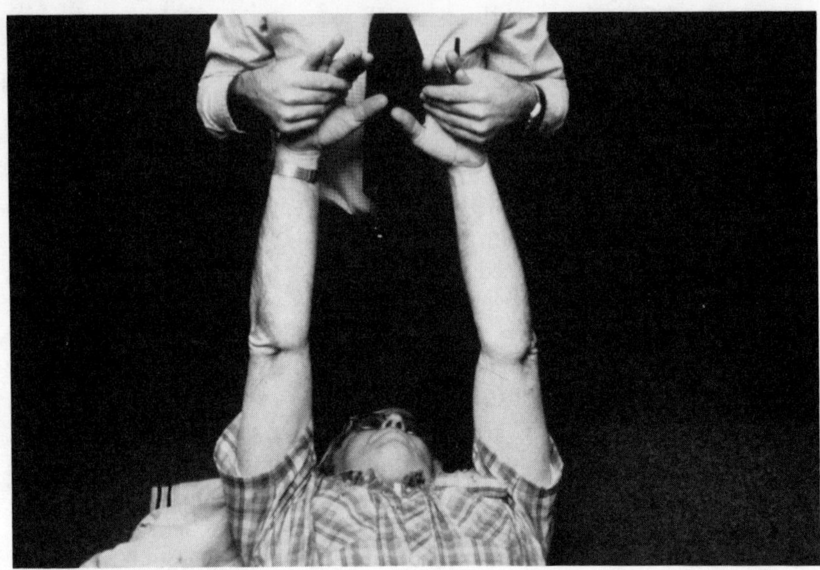

Figure 33–23. Silvester method allowing air to flow into the lungs.

ment and ventilation may have to be doubled depending on the type of stoma or its location. Secondly, the instruction has to be more individualized. Adjunctive equipment to create a better stoma-to-mouth or stoma-to-stoma seal may be useful. Pocket masks, baby bottle nipples, and foam rubber padding are a few of the items being tried. The paper also stated that ". . . in their training work, the majority of laryngectomees displayed no unconquerable difficulty in ventilation with Resuscitation Annie, no need for exceptional lung control, nor was there a problem with age" (p. 4).

Most medical settings require CPR certification of all personnel working with patients. The speech-language pathologist need only apply this knowledge to the laryngectomee. For those working in settings without these requirements, it is advisable to become CPR trained in an authorized program usually sponsored by a local Red Cross.

Laryngectomees are taking the initiative and are working with medical and paramedical personnel to develop training techniques and assistive devices to help the neck breather conduct CPR. Individuals living or working with laryngectomees would be thankful for the assistance of the laryngectomee should they themselves need it in a medical emergency. Speech-language pathologists should make attempts to become as comfortable with CPR for the laryngectomee as for any other individual.

QUESTIONS

1. Why do some laryngectomees wear a stoma button?
2. Contrast stoma buttons and laryngectomee tubes.
3. How might a nonlaryngectomee give CPR to a laryngectomee?
4. What are some signs that indicate a patient's stoma may be too small?
5. Why do laryngectomees not require a cuffed tracheostomy tube?

REFERENCES

American Cancer Society (1971). *First aid for neck breathers,* Pamphlet.
American Cancer Society (1982). *IAL News, 27,* 1.
American Cancer Society (1984). *IAL News, 30,* 1.
American Cancer Society, *First aid for laryngectomees,* Supplemental Pamphlet.
American Red Cross (1980). *CPR module, respiratory and circulatory emergencies.*
Finchem, M. (1982). *Modification of CPR for the laryngectomee.* Unpublished paper.
Griffith, G., and Luce, E. (1982). Tracheal stomal stenosis after laryngectomy. *Plas. Recon. Surg., 70,* 694–698.
Health devices sourcebook (1983–1984). Heat and moisture exchanges (pp. 155–167). Plymouth Meeting, PA: ECRI.
Keith, R., Shane, H., Coates, H., and Devine, K. (1984). *Looking forward . . . A guidebook for the laryngectomee.* New York: Thieme-Stratton.
Keith, R., and Shanks, J. (1983). Laryngectomee rehabilitation: Past and present. *Speech and language: Advances in basic research and practice,* Vol. 9, Orlando, FL: Academic Press.
Long, J., and Newfield, P. (1976). *Tracheostomy care handbook.* Wilmington, MA: Portex.
Montgomery, W., and Herrin, T. (1981). *Cardiopulmonary resuscitation, student manual for basic life support.* Dallas: American Heart Association.
Portex, Inc. (1976). *Tracheostomy care handbook, a concise guide for the care of a patient with a tracheostomy.* Wilmington, MA: Author.

Chapter **34**

The Psychosocial Concomitants of Laryngectomy

Stuart I. Gilmore

A person is disabled when unable to perform functions that are desired personally or required by the environment (Stolov, 1981). The specific problems that result constitute the person's total disability. Disability problems may arise from the person's disease, the person's psychology, social functioning or vocational functioning, or from the interaction of these four parameters. Disability removal (i.e., rehabilitation) is achieved through attacks on the disease, enhancement of the person's psychology, and direct modification of the interface between patient and environment.

King, Fowlks, and Pierson (1968) suggested that none of the many tumors affecting humans is of greater importance to the rehabilitation worker than laryngeal cancer. They attributed this importance to at least three factors associated with laryngeal cancer: (1) an increasing incidence, suggesting a growing number of patients requiring help; (2) a good prognosis for life, with more than half of the laryngectomized population living for a good number of years; and (3) the unique nature of the disability, including the loss of voice, with its many psychological, social, and economic implications.

This chapter presents a review of literature concerning the psychosocial concomitants of laryngectomy. It is organized in reference to four important functional domains: physical, social, occupational, and psychological. This organization presents a framework within which the unique array of disability problems experienced by laryngectomized individuals can be appreciated as a basis for both clinical management and further research.

PHYSICAL CONCOMITANTS

Speech

Physical problems, involving impaired or lost functions, constitute the major source for the entire array of disability problems. Many authorities consider speech loss the most traumatizing handicap associated with being laryngectomized and speech acquisition the major adjustment problem (Gates, Ryan, Cooper, et al., 1982a; Gates, Ryan, and Lauder, 1982c; Gilmore, 1961; Jesberg, 1956; King, Marshall, and Gunderson, 1971; Laguaite, 1957; Levin, 1967; Natvig, 1983a; Ryan, Gates, Cantu, and Hearne, 1982).

Speech Privation, the Major Problem.   The loss of the voice is probably the primary physical problem associated with removal of the larynx (King et al., 1968) because of its effect on so many social, occupational, and psychological functions. Hunt's (1964) review of responses from 85 consecutive private patients indicated that their concern for their loss of voice was even greater than their concern for the diagnosis of cancer.

Davis (1981) suggested that not only is loss of voice the single most debilitating handicap associated with laryngectomy but that it comes at a time when individuals need to communicate their anxieties about the diagnosis of cancer. Blanchard (1982) found that the most common problem listed by 115 subjects drawn from laryngectomee clubs throughout the United States was loss of oral communication and subsequent difficulty with learning esophageal speech.

Speech Acquisition.   The literature indicates that many laryngectomized individuals do not acquire esophageal speech and that a significant proportion do not acquire any form of usable oral communication. Putney (1958) surveyed 440 patients and found that 37.7 per cent (166) failed to develop useful voice. Based on a questionnaire survey of 209 patients in 145 Veterans Administration hospitals, Johnson (1960) determined that 57 per cent used esophageal speech, 21 per cent used artificial larynxes, and 22 per cent used only written or whispered modes of communication. Fourteen per cent of Johnson's esophageal speakers reported using conversational speech in 1 month, but the average length of time required to learn this mode of communication was 3 months. Johnson's esophageal speakers reported an average of six syllables per air intake. Slightly over half of these individuals reported having some difficulty with telephone conversation.

A study involving the largest sample (Horn, 1962) indicated that of the 3,366 laryngectomized persons surveyed 64 per cent spoke entirely with esophageal speech, 50 per cent with esophageal and artificial laryngeal speech, and 10 per cent with artificial larynxes only. Twelve per cent of the subjects did not speak at all, and the remainder fit into miscellaneous classes. Gardner (1966) established that of 240 laryngectomized women from 36 of the United States and Canada, 77 per cent were intelligible in face-to-face conversation and 66 per cent in telephone conversation. Murry (1974) stated that in general, after laryngectomy, 15 per cent of the patients will use esophageal speech with excellent intelligibility, 55 per cent will develop an average level of communication, and 30 per cent will require a mechanical aid or will remain aphonic.

Studies conducted in the last decade have reported successful esophageal speech in from 26 to 68 per cent of their subjects, the average being 50 per cent. Goldberg (1975) found that of his 62 subjects, 56.4 per cent were esophageal speakers, 1.5 per cent used artificial larynxes, and 33.9 per cent were restricted to written communication. The remaining 8.2 per cent had partial laryngectomies and reportedly had no speech impairment.

Wallen and Webb (1975) surveyed 2,000 subjects from various laryngectomee organizations and Veterans Administration hospitals, selecting 100 each from male and female subjects for their preliminary report. Based on this sample, 67 per cent of the male subjects and 71 per cent of the female subjects reported using esophageal speech, and 13 per cent of both sexes reported being unable to learn esophageal speech.

Kommers and Sullivan (1979) analyzed questionnaire responses by 45 wives of laryngectomized men. They found that 38 per cent of the men used esophageal speech as their primary communication mode, 11 per cent used artificial larynxes, and 51 per cent wrote, whispered, or used pharyngeal or buccal speech. Forty per cent of the wives considered their husbands to be readily intelligible 3 months postoperatively. Only 53 per cent reported currently understanding their husbands well, and 22.2 per cent reported that their husbands were not yet understandable in person-to-person situations. Sixty-four per cent of the wives reported less phone use by their husbands since surgery. The wives also indicated the following problems while their husbands were attempting to learn esophageal speech: 22.2 per cent of their husbands lacked the desire to learn esophageal speech; 51 per cent were unable to relax; 20 per cent lacked physical strength; and 2.2 per cent did not try to learn it. Approximately 16 per cent of the men were introduced to artificial larynxes 2 to 6 months postsurgically, 6.7 per cent were introduced to it 1 to 2 years postsurgically, and 35.6 per cent were never presented with this option.

Volin (1980) reported that 40 per cent of 72 patients laryngectomized at the New York City Veterans Administration Medical Center developed neither esophageal nor artificial laryngeal speech. Davis (1981) concluded that at least one third of laryngectomized patients do not acquire esophageal speech, and considerably more do not acquire superior speech skills. Additionally, some also do not use artificial larynxes competently. Blanchard (1982) surveyed 115 subjects up to 12 months postsurgically, finding that 50 per cent used esophageal speech as their predominant communication mode, 22 per cent preferred esophageal speech augmented by an artificial larynx, 19 per cent used artificial larynxes only, one person depended on written communication, and eight subjects (less than 10 per cent) had either failed to develop a viable communication mode or were still in the process of acquiring it.

Gates, Ryan, Cooper, and associates (1982a) concluded from a review of the literature that from 43 to 98 per cent of laryngectomized patients acquire esophageal speech, the average being 64 to 69 per cent. Consistent with this trend, they found that 62 per cent of their 40 retrospectively studied subjects acquired esophageal speech. In contrast to this, however, only 26 per cent of their 47 prospectively studied subjects used esophageal speech in daily communication when observed 6 months after completing cancer therapy, and three of these subjects chose to use an electrolarynx when they were tired or in need of increased rate or loudness. Thirty-four per cent of the prospective group used electrolarynxes exclusively, 34 per cent depended on writing, and 6 per cent depended on signing. Only 74 per cent (34) of these 47 prospective patients attempted to learn esophageal speech.

The substantial and unexpected difference between the proportion of retrospective versus prospective subjects who acquired esophageal speech stands out as an important finding of the Gates, Ryan, Cooper, and colleagues (1982a) study. This difference is particularly remarkable considering that the prospective subjects were known to have received quality rehabilitation services. In explaining the basis for this difference, Gates, Ryan, Cooper, and co-workers proposed that the use of radiotherapy and conservative surgery for early lesions has reduced the number of "ideal" candidates for learning esophageal speech. They noted that today's laryngectomized patients are more likely to be older and to have advanced tumors that are treated with multiple, intensive therapies. Consequently, this population is more likely to experience complicated sequelae and functional difficulties (Gates and Hearne, 1982), increased treatment morbidity, and a poorer prognosis than did their 1960 counterparts (Gates et al., 1982c). "Thus, fewer patients are able to learn esophageal speech" (Gates and Hearne, 1982), and ". . . the real potential for success in acquiring esophageal speech and achieving rehabilitation goals is much less than was reported in the past" (Gates et al., 1982c). Indeed, less than half of the prospective subjects interviewed by Gates and associates (1982c) before treatment had received total laryngectomies, thus restricting the prospective sample to the ostensibly more severely impaired patients.

Richardson (1983) reported that of his 60 Los Angeles area subjects, evaluated 6 to 42 months postsurgically, 55 per cent used esophageal speech, 28 per cent used artificial larynxes, and 17 per cent wrote, gestured, or mouthed.

Natvig (1983c) personally interviewed and evaluated the speech of 189 subjects, almost the total population of Norwegian laryngectomees. He found that 63 per cent had socially acceptable esophageal speech and 27.5 per cent were unable to produce any esophageal speech. Five of Natvig's subjects were tracheoesophageal shunt speakers, 17 per cent (32) used electrolarynxes satisfactorily, and 8.5 per cent remained speechless. Cross-sectional data indicated that speech continued to improve for 36 months. Fifty-two per cent of the artificial larynx users had obtained their instruments more than five months postsurgically, usually when it was obvious that they would not acquire esophageal speech. Only 39 per cent (74) claimed no serious difficulties with speech acquisition.

In a later article, Natvig (1984) indicated that 46 per cent of his 189 subjects felt that speech was still their greatest problem. Sixty-seven per cent reported that people, even their spouses, mistook them for being deaf and talked loudly or shouted at them. Moreover, people sometimes stopped talking to them, addressing their spouses instead. Interruptions while speaking were also common, and 15 per cent of Natvig's subjects reported feeling hurt by them. Natvig commented that interruptions by spouses were frequent during his interviews, often with no apparent relation to the subject's speech capabilities.

Temporary speech deterioration had been experienced by 82 per cent of Natvig's subjects, reflecting nervousness (24 per cent), poor voice in the morning (24 per cent), infection and cold weather (9 per cent), and combined factors (35 per cent). No deteriorating factors were reported in the speech of only 18 per cent of the subjects. Deterioration of speech intelligibility with the passage of time was observed in some subjects by Diedrich and Youngstrom (1966), and by Amster and associates (1972).

The recent literature on speech loss and acquisition has begun to address the successes and failures associated with surgical voice restoration procedures. In general, the numbers of cases reported have been small, and success rates have often been higher when reported by specialists who developed the procedures than when reported by those replicating them. Shunt procedures have often been complicated by stenosis, deteriorating deglutition associated with better voice production, aspiration, flap necrosis in irradiated subjects, fistulization, esophagotracheal reflux, and concern for local recurrence rates (Singer, 1983; Singer, Blom, and Hamaker, 1983). Similar problems have plagued approaches to conservative surgery (partial laryngectomy), in addition to restrictions in candidate selection inherent in tumor stage and location and success rates based on small series and short postsurgical follow-up durations, especially with newer procedures. With regard to reed-fistula speech, a number of speech and biomedical liabilities precluding its consideration as a routine approach to speech restoration have been described (Shedd, Schaaf, and Weinberg, 1976; Weinberg, Shedd, and Horii, 1978).

In the past five years the literature focused on tracheoesophageal puncture (TEP) procedures, which utilize silicone prostheses to stent the puncture, prevent aspiration of esophageal contents into the trachea, and enable the use of pulmonary air (rather than small quantities of air trapped in the esophagus) for speech production. Early reports suggested that problems associated with TEP often reflected inappropriate candidate selection (e.g., patients having insufficient motor control to insert or care for the prosthesis or to occlude the stoma or patients having cricopharyngeal spasms and needing myotomies). Additional problems associated with TEP included the necessity for using the thumb to occlude the stoma, difficulties related to excessive prosthesis airway resistance or prosthesis retention or both, occasional prosthesis aspiration, questionable angulation of the fistula tract, spontaneous fistula closure, tracheal mucositis, and esophageal tearing (Blom, Singer, and Hamaker, 1985; Shapiro and Vadakkencherry, 1982; Singer and Blom, 1980; Singer, Blom, and Hamaker, 1981; Weinberg and Moon, 1984; Wetmore, Grueger, and Wesson, 1981).

Primary among the advantages of the TEP procedure are its simplicity, its effectiveness with patients having difficulty developing esophageal speech, the relative ease and rapidity of learning to use TEP speech, its cost-effectiveness, and its relative absence of complications (Singer and Blom, 1980; Singer et al., 1981). The major advantage of the TEP appears to be its success rate in voice restoration, which Robbins, Fisher, Blom, and Singer (1984a) determined to be as high as 93 per cent in their literature review. The largest series reported (Singer et al., 1983) established that successful voice acquisition occurred in 113 of 129 patients (88 per cent) managed with TEP.

Hamaker, Singer, Blom, and Daniels (1985) reported recently on speech acquisition and related problems in a series of 48 patients with whom TEP was used as a primary restoration procedure at the time of laryngectomy. Satisfactory speech resulted in 69 per cent of their patients, increasing to 75 per cent following revision surgery. Among the 15 patients an assortment of problems were noted: four were able to use the prosthesis but did not, two allowed the puncture to close after 13 months of nonuse except in the physician's office, one had a psychiatric problem resulting in the removal of the prosthesis because of nonuse, one did not want to place "a dirty thumb" on his stoma, one maintained but seldom used the prosthesis, three failed due to CNS dysfunction, four were impaired by residual cancer and its associated treatment, two developed fistulae unrelated to the puncture, one learned and preferred esophageal speech, one triggered coughing spasms on touching the stoma, and two required secondary myotomies to obtain success.

The literature also indicates that along with its high success rate, the acoustical, aerodynamic, and intelligibility characteristics of TEP speech often equal or exceed those of superior standard esophageal speech and that TEP speakers show greater similarities in these parameters to laryngeal than to esophageal speakers (Weinberg, Horii, Blom, and Singer, 1982; Robbins, 1984; Robbins, Fisher, Blom, and Singer, 1984b).

In summary, the numbers of laryngectomized individuals acquiring esophageal speech vary considerably, the general figure being somewhere between 60 and 70 per cent. Moreover, a significant portion may be aphonic, lacking the ability or desire to use an artificial larynx. Additionally, relatively few esophageal speakers (perhaps 15 per cent) achieve the intelligibility and fluency necessary to be judged excellent, and about an equal proportion are not readily intelligible. The extent to which this variability is accounted for by physical factors or psychological factors is a puzzle that pervades the literature. Recent writings suggest that surgical voice restoration procedures may eliminate this puzzle to a significant extent.

Aside from the literature on speech acquisition and privation, the literature on speech deals with the responses of the laryngectomized person to that loss; the physical and psychological factors influencing speech development, especially esophageal speech; the procedures for teaching speech to the laryngectomized; and the importance of speech in patient rehabilitation. Several temporally oriented themes occur in articles on patient responses: shock and mortification upon hearing that the voice must be sacrificed; fear, frustration, and emotional reactions accompanying the sudden and complete postsurgical loss of spoken communication; and the difficulties, frustrations, and embarrassment associated with speechlessness, the acquisition of a new communication mode, or both. These topics and the relationship of speech to rehabilitation are considered in the following sections. Additional chapters deal with the factors influencing speech development and with teaching procedures.

Responses to Speech Loss. McNeil, Weichselbaum, and Pauker (1981) provided a significant insight into how people feel about the potential loss of their laryngeal voices and the substitution of esophageal speech. They interviewed 50 normally speaking male volunteers, including 25 middle- and upper-management executives and 25 firefighters, having an average age of 40, to determine who would prefer radiation alone, or radiation possibly followed by salvage surgery, to immediate removal of the larynx. Prior to answering questions, each subject listened to tapes of one excellent and one typical esophageal speaker. Utility curves were then constructed, summarizing the subjects' attitudes toward survival for various periods. In essence, the subjects specified how many years of survival they would be willing to give up or trade off to retain their normal speech.

McNeil and co-workers (1981) found that the amount of time that the subjects were willing to trade in order to retain laryngeal speech varied with survival time and that a subject might not be willing to give up any time if survival were sufficiently short. For most durations explored, the utility of survival with esophageal speech was lower than that of survival with laryngeal speech, and for the remaining survival durations the values were equal. Overall, the average reduction was 14 per cent. Although most subjects were willing to accept some decrease in long-term survival to maintain speech, virtually none would accept a decrease below 5 years. With regard to treatment choice, practically no subjects would decline surgery for the average results of radiation therapy, a 3 year survival of 30 per cent. For 3 year, 40 per cent survivals, the percentages changed appreciably, with 19 per cent choosing radiation and 24 per cent radiation followed by salvage surgery, if necessary. McNeil and colleagues concluded that "patients' attitudes toward morbidity are important, and survival is not their only consideration" (p. 87). Although the subjects in this study were not actually experiencing the stress of having laryngeal cancer, their responses indicated that, within the restrictions discussed, maintenance of laryngeal voice can be as important as life itself.

Bisi and Conley (1965) acknowledged voice to be one of the most important and central facets of a person's identity and maintained that its loss deprives the individual of an organ that has served a number of important functions since early childhood: communication with others, expression of emotions, mastery of innumerable situations in the external world, defense, gratification, and carrying out sublimation. Laryngeal loss, they stated, signifies both a mutilation and a deprivation of very important functions necessary to adaptation. They indicated further that some patients will not be reconciled to substituting esophageal voice.

McDonald (1949) held that deprivation of speech disrupts the patient's pattern of living, and Laguaite (1962) expressed concern for its interpersonal and vocational implications. Levy and Abramson (1983) maintained that speechlessness is a psychological devastation for both the patient and the family. Kommers, Sullivan, and Yonkers (1977) determined from a survey of 45 wives that their fear that their husbands would never speak again was an important element of their experience.

Gardner (1961) and Lerman (1966) discussed the emotional trauma and shock experienced by a laryngectomized individual when he realizes he cannot talk. The loss of ability to communicate with others was described by King and associates (1971) as having a "unique nightmare quality" and as causing feelings of isolation; and the loss of the larynx as creating body image problems that contribute considerably to depression. The result, they contend, is a constellation of uncertainties about the future, including (1) effects on economic, social, and family life; (2) job loss, inability to find work, or accepting employment with less income, prestige, and ego satisfaction; (3) becoming dependent on others; and (4) evoking disgust, fear, or pity in others.

Substantial effects on emotional health, social interaction, and self-image accompanying voice loss were acknowledged by Gates and co-workers (1982a). Similarly, Heaver, White, and Goldstein (1955) commented on the anxiety pervading patients who can no longer talk. A number of authors discussed the emotional implications of speechlessness: frustration and emotional reactions (Laguaite, 1962); severe mental depression and even suicide (Goldberg, 1975); emotional disturbance (Davis, 1981); anxiety and depression (Gilchrist, 1973); and loss of prestige, introversion, and withdrawal (Gardner, 1971).

Morrison (1941) reported that when leaving the hospital and returning to their families, many patients face numerous problems of social contacts and work resumption, and

> realize fully the meaning of the total loss of the power of intelligible speech. They find themselves cut off from friends and relatives and from business or professional associates by the barrier of total aphonia. Many develop profound depression and worries about financial security and obligations, which may make them unhappy indeed.

J. Greene (1947) suggested that loss of the larynx may affect the whole personality and that people depend on voice for vocation. For example, salesman and teachers may suffer greater than average ego deflation. He contended that the resulting fear and anxiety may even interfere with the acquisition of a substitute voice. This contention was supported by Greene and Faulkner (1940), who studied 13 laryngectomized subjects. They found that spasms of the esophagus could be increased and that the pharyngoesophageal lumen could be narrowed by suggestions arousing grief, anxiety, anger, fear, and apprehension and that the spasms relaxed and the lumen widened with suggestions arousing happiness, elation, contentment, security, and enthusiasm. Additionally, Blake (1974) found that subjects who had discontinued speech therapy before 4 months demonstrated statistically significantly higher depression and hysteria.

The most important factor influencing the prognosis for acquiring esophageal speech is the postoperative emotional make-up of the individual, according to Pitkin (1953). Bisi and Conley (1965) went so far as to classify patients in three psychological groups relative to speech acquisition: esophageal speakers who have the emotional status adequate for the demands of adaptation; artificial laryngeal speakers who may prove adequate or inadequate; and laryngectomees who fail to acquire speech. Some research support linking psychological status and speech acquisition was contributed by Natvig (1983c), who determined that low stress vulnerability enhanced speech acquisition, and that subjects judged as having "mastered the laryngectomy event" more frequently acquired speech. Natvig also found that socially acceptable esophageal speech was of great importance for postoperative mastery of the laryngectomy event (Natvig, 1983c).

Many authors have stated that psychological factors play important roles in the failure to acquire speech (Beukelman, Cummings, Dobie, and Weymuller, 1980; Bisi and Conley, 1965; Davis, 1981; Diedrich and Youngstrom, 1966; Fontaine and Mitchell, 1960; Gardner, 1961, 1971; Gates et al., 1982a, 1982b, 1982c; Goldberg, 1975; J. Greene, 1947; Heaver and Arnold, 1962; Laguaite, 1962; Nahum and Golden, 1963; Pitkin, 1953; Putney, 1958; and Stoll, 1958, to name a few). Significantly, several of the psychological factors cited, notably depression and motivation, frequently reflect reactions to the speech loss, suggesting a vicious circle that may maintain speechlessness.

Among the writers contributing to an understanding of the embarrassment and frustration associated with laryngectomy are Bisi and Conley (1965), who described laryngeal loss as a "mutilation," and McNeil and associates (1981), who concluded from their study of 50 normal male subjects that attitudes toward esophageal speech morbidity, and not just survival, are important in rehabilitation planning. After acknowledging the altered respiratory, phonatory, and articulatory systems following laryngectomy, and the low pitch and volume of the esophageal voice, King and co-workers (1971) indicated that these are often sources of self-consciousness, especially in the female speaker. They also suggested that articulation may be affected by tongue innervation problems associated with radical neck dissection, poorly fitting dentures, and hearing loss, all of which may intensify withdrawal and lead to dropping out of speech therapy.

The complications of esophageal speech may be socially embarrassing (King, et al., 1971). McDonald (1949) described feelings of shame or guilt associated with laryngectomy. Stoll (1958) stated that many patients fear rejection by society. Gardner (1961) wrote that loss of prestige and ego status, frustration, and embarrassment are associated with esophageal speech and that the speaker may become discouraged and depressed and withdraw from communication when first attempts are unsatisfactory. Psychological elements were reported by Stoll (1958) to be strong deterrents in women, who disliked being the center of attention, had oversensitive esthetic sensibilities, and felt their new voices made them conspicuous. King and co-workers (1968) found that 50.8 per cent of their laryngectomized subjects, regardless of communication mode (esophageal speech, artificial larynx, writing, or a combination), never used it outside their home.

Gardner (1966) determined from the 240 female respondents he studied that their first esophageal sounds evoked emotional responses varying from hope and happiness in the optimists to embarrassment, frustration, and pity in the pessimists. The pessimists anticipated a hopeless, sad, and doubtful future because of their "frog croaking, hoarse, male voices" (p. 34). A number of writers have discussed the "masculinization" associated with the reduced fundamental frequency of the female voice, and the embarrassment that may result (Gilmore, 1961; King et al., 1971; Laguaite, 1962; Snidecor and Curry, 1960; Weinberg and Bennett, 1971).

Forty-four per cent of Gardner's (1966) 240 laryngectomized women claimed that their husbands were indifferent toward, disliked, or ridiculed early speech attempts. Moreover, the women reported that their husbands did not encourage them or show sympathy or understanding. Many women indicated that people walked away from them, did not listen, became impatient, and often inappropriately filled in what they were attempting to say. The most common complaint was that esophageal speech was not easily understood.

Wallen and Webb (1975) determined that between 23 and 40 per cent of their male and female subjects did not enjoy using the telephone, indicated concern for how their voices sounded, and disliked talking in front of groups. The responses of 45 wives studied by Kommers and Sullivan (1979) established that 23 per cent reported negative first reactions to their husbands' esophageal speech, and 62 per cent to their artificial device speech. Forty per cent reported decreased communication with their husbands, and 68 per cent reported their husbands to be upset (e.g., refusing to repeat or becoming angry, nervous, frustrated, and irritated) when not understood. Ninety-three per cent denied current embarrassment about their husbands' speech. Gardner (1971) found that many laryngectomized patients had a strong desire to succeed in speech in order to regain prestige among friends and business associates as well as to make a living for their families.

Inability to express anger was a frequent complaint of the 50 subjects studied by Brouwer, Snow, and Van Dam (1979). Seventy per cent indicated that they were unable to express emotions; the ability to do so was found to correlate significantly with the patient's own assessment of his speech. Brouwer and colleagues also reported a study by Bauer of 50 European subjects, which determined that early speakers (less than 2 weeks since laryngectomy) were more dissatisfied with their speech than those slower to learn speech. Bauer concluded that their dissatisfaction might reflect the patients' excessively high early expectation and consequent disappointment with further progress.

M. C. L. Greene (1967) commented on the aversion patients have to voice produced with an artificial larynx. Davis (1981) cautioned that a negative bias of health personnel toward artificial larynxes can be easily transmitted to the patient, often to the patient's emotional, social, and financial detriment. Natvig (1983c) contended that any communication mode after laryngectomy is artificial and that a primary and essential step is all rehabilitation with laryngectomized patients is assisting them to accept their forthcoming mode. In more recent years, several writers have expressed the positive values and acceptability of artificial larynx devices as either interim or permanent speech modes. They have indicated that professionals dealing with postlaryngectomy rehabilitation must accept and use them and train patients to use them proficiently (Davis, 1981; Gates, Ryan, and Lauder, 1982c; Lauder, 1970; Minear and Lucente, 1975; Natvig, 1983c; Salmon and Goldstein, 1978).

A review of the literature dealing with patient responses to the loss of speech suggests that these responses are best characterized as traumatic. Not only are the simultaneous loss of spontaneous oral communication and of a major "individualizing" characteristic frightening but the alternatives—esophageal speech or use of an artificial larynx—may be viewed with ambivalence or disdain, both by the laryngectomee and society.

Rehabilitation and Speech.   It might be assumed that a laryngectomized speaker's evaluation or misevaluation of society's attitude toward his speech would be a significant correlate of his feelings of embarrassment and rejection. McDonald (1949) contended that these evaluations are often responsible for reduced motivation to learn more precise speech. He suggested that there may be a vicious cycle of expected rejection resulting in reduced motivation and practice, which results in poor esophageal speech and consequently in rejection. McDonald maintained that motivation, which is indicated by the patient's attitude toward communication, is the chief factor in the intelligibility of speech.

Numerous writers have stressed the importance of motivation to rehabilitation. Among those indicating its salience for speech acquisition were Gardner (1961), M. C. L. Greene (1967), Amster and associates (1972), Goldberg (1975), Stoll (1958), Warner (1971), and others. Stallings (1981) alleged that patients who are not highly motivated are not likely to cooperate to the extent necessary for long-term success. Perhaps Davis (1981) proposed the most cogent argument when she wrote, "It is a common finding that a motivated patient will overcome many obstacles" (p. 348).

Dabul and Lovestedt (1974) studied 14 "poor" and 5 "good" speakers; they were generally unsuccessful in isolating social and motivational differences between the groups. They did, however, find a trend toward good speakers answering more positively. On the other hand, Goldberg's (1975) research findings supported McDonald's equating of motivation with attitude and consequently with speech success. Goldberg determined that his more intelligible speakers had more optimistic outlooks ($r = 0.28$, $p < 0.05$). He established that the presence of speech was one of four factors in his factor analysis study that related to rehabilitation, accounting for 10.8 per cent of the variance in habilitation status.

The importance of speech restoration to rehabilitation is a theme that several authors have addressed. King and colleagues (1971) stated that the fullest rehabilitation requires dealing with physical, psychological, social, vocational, and communication problems. Gray and Konrad (1976) proposed that developing optimal communication abilities as rapidly as possible would reduce to a minimum the social, psychological, and economic problems caused by the loss of laryngeal speech. Morrison (1941) maintained that the way to solve the worst of the problems of the laryngectomized population, and to cure their psychic depression, was to "get them learning to talk again, assure them they'll be able to resume their work and earning power, and return to normal contact with friends and family" (p. 1102). Davis (1981) advocated use of an artificial larynx immediately postoperatively to facilitate communication and return to work and consequently to reduce tensions, frustrations, and anxieties. Davis suggested, moreover, that artificial devices may even enhance esophageal speech rehabilitation. Both Heaver and Arnold (1962) and Ogura and Gerson (1976) contended that relearning a form of communication significantly lessens depression. Heaver and Arnold added that "the essence of rehabilitation of the laryngectomized patient is in the restoration of verbal facility as soon after operation as the surgeon will permit" (p. 16). Natvig (1983c) concurred that speech rehabilitation should be started as early as possible postoperatively, and Stoll (1958) went so far as to propose that "the rehabilitation program is entirely dependent upon speech acquisition" (p. 552).

Research validation for the relationship between speech and general rehabilitation was provided by Goldberg (1975). His study of the vocational and social adjustment of 62 persons with laryngeal cancer determined that the presence of speech had significant correlation with ultimate vocational plans ($r = .32$), immediate vocational plans ($r = .40$), employment status ($r = .36$), frequency of activities ($r = .42$), and organizational participation (r = .35). Persons who were employed tended to possess speech, either esophageal or by means of artificial larynx (x^2 = 7.27, p < .01). Persons having speech participated in more social activities and in more community organizations.

Amidst all the support for speech training, the reader should heed the caution of Gardner (1961) that program quality is critical and that tragedies can be traced to improper patient orientation and to improper teaching. One further caution regarding rehabilitation should also be acknowledged: For some patients there may be positive gains associated with not developing speech. Drummond (1967) discussed several patients who had acquired esophageal speech but did not use it because of the sympathy they gained. Laguaite (1962) and Bisi and Conley (1965) also contended that being without voice has "secondary gains," enabling some individuals to have their dependence needs met and to escape responsibility.

Other Physiological Alterations

As suggested by Hunt (1964), many factors other than speech are important in the laryngectomee's well being. Aside from the loss of normal phonatory function, there are a number of physiological changes associated with laryngeal excision and other medical treatment for cancer. These may include loss of nonspeech emotive and attention-attracting functions; changes in sensation, biological functions, and nonspeech expression; and associated physical limitations. Moreover, laryngeal cancer generally occurs in an older population having a mean age of approximately 55, a significant history of smoking and alcohol consumption, and consequently a probability of associated health problems and disabilities. Recently, Gates and co-workers (1982c) suggested that total laryngectomy is now reserved for patients having advanced tumor, for which radical neck dissection and adjunctive radiotherapy are often recommended, and sometimes chemotherapy. They stated that such patients are likely to have poor prognoses for cancer control, more treatment morbidity, and a less favorable outlook for recovery. Indeed, physical factors can have great significance for the speech and for social, occupational, and psychological status of the laryngectomized individual. As suggested by Jesberg (1965), adjustment to the changed anatomical and physiological state is a problem and is accomplished gradually.

Nonspeech Communicative Functions. Brouwer, Snow, and Van Dam (1979) reported that 74 per cent of their 50 subjects complained of unsatisfactory ability to express emotions, especially inability to express anger. Parvulescu (1970), among others, discussed the trauma due to the inability to shout, laugh, sing, or attract attention or help through yelling or shouting.

Sensory Impairment. Several writers have stated that smell is reduced or lost following laryngectomy, with a consequent reduction in taste sensation (Gates et al., 1982c; Keith and Shanks, 1983; Laguaite, 1962). A number of researchers have confirmed the reduction of smell and taste. Horn (1962) found that 41 per cent of his 3,366 subjects reported taste to be less accurate, and 79 per cent reported reduction in smell. Gilchrist (1973) reported decreased olfactory acuity in "the vast majority" of his 50 patients. Wallen and Webb (1975) found 50 per cent of their 100 male subjects and 48 per cent of their 100 female subjects reported reduced taste sensation and 79 per cent of the male subjects and 72 per cent of the female subjects felt smell was much reduced. Brouwer and associates (1979) established that of the 50 subjects they surveyed, 22 per cent had no olfactory diminishment, 78 per cent could no longer smell or could perceive only strong odors, and 36 per cent had severe loss of taste. Using a three-drop forced choice technique, Kashima and Kalinowski (1979) studied 123 laryngeal cancer patients. They determined that only 2 of the 41 patients exhibited normal detection thresholds pretreatment and that patients with more advanced (T3 and T4) lesions had greater impairment. Seventy patients showing no evidence of disease postsurgically had subnormal mean scores, but the trend in cases of no tumor recurrence was gradual taste recovery. Following laryngectomy, and most often during and after radiation therapy, the absence or profound disturbance of taste was a common complaint. Neither total nor partial laryngectomy, however, had overriding or permanent influence on taste function. Kashima and Kalinowski (1979) reported that a decline in taste performance postsurgically may be a harbinger of tumor recrudescence or the development of a second cancer.

The sense of hearing, which is important both for speech acquisition and for social interaction, has also been found to be reduced in the laryngectomized population. Laguaite (1962) suggested that poor hearing and visual impairment were both related to age. King and colleagues (1971) stated that high-frequency hearing loss may affect discrimination of consonants and their re-establishment in new speech patterns. Responses from the 100 male and 100 female returns selected randomly from Wallen and Webb's (1975) 2,000 questionnaires indicated that 11 per cent of the male subjects and 6 per cent of the female subjects had presurgical hearing problems and 21 per cent of the males and 10 per cent of the females had postsurgical problems. Erskine (1979) described a composite audiogram for her laryngectomized patients indicating that many had presbycusis compounded by acoustic trauma and a sloping loss of 20 to 25 decibels (dB) at 250 and 500 hertz (Hz) down to 55 or 60 dB at 8,000 Hz. Another aspect of the problem, according to Erskine, was the 20 to 25 dB average loss demonstrated in the composite audiogram of the spouses. The literature indicates that reduced auditory acuity on the part of both the laryngectomized individual and the spouse may be a significant variable in speech, occupational, social, and psychological rehabilitation (Berlin, 1964; Diedrich and Youngstrom, 1966; Erskine, 1979; M. C. L. Greene, 1967; Martin, Hoops, and Shanks, 1974).

Biological Function Impairment. A number of writers have discussed altered biological functions associated with laryngectomy, including respiration and associated functions, deglutition and digestion, and physical functions. Gilmore (1961) and Laguaite (1962) noted that respiration is carried on through the tracheal stoma and not the nose or the mouth. Parvulescu (1970) discussed the psychological trauma associated with not being able to breathe "like all other humans." McDonald (1949), Laguaite (1962), and Keith and Shanks (1983, citing Jackson and Jackson, 1937) commented on the associated loss of laryngeal protection against respiratory hazards. Several writers discussed problems associated with having a stoma. Hunt (1964) acknowledged problems with tracheal crusting and coughing. Keith and Shanks (1983), again citing Jackson and Jackson (1937), indicated increased coughing due to its activation by neck stimulation and reduced tussive function due to loss of strong oral air expulsion. Gilchrist (1973) observed that 38 per cent of his 50 patients complained of stomal and tracheal crusting and 30 per cent of being troubled by coughing. He concluded, and clinical experience supports, that cough, sputum, and crusting constitute a considerable problem in many patients. Brouwer and co-workers (1979) confirmed problems with coughing and mucus expulsion, especially at night and in a smoky atmosphere, in 42 per cent of their 50 patients. They also determined that two of their patients could not care for their own stomas and that 16 per cent continued to wear tracheostomy tubes. Blanchard (1982) reported that the second most common problem, indicated by 12 per cent of the 115 subjects he surveyed from throughout the United States, was excessive mucus and an associated problem of stoma hygiene.

Natvig (1984) found the stomal opening and breathing to be the greatest current problem for 25 per cent of his 189 subjects. Fifty-nine per cent were more bothered by stomal problems in winter than in summer. Many were bothered by the need for stomal care and felt disgust and shame in reference to the stomal opening. A tendency was noted for these problems to decrease significantly after the second postoperative year. Twenty-three per cent of Natvig's subjects felt that the stomal opening was too small, and some felt that they got insufficient air while exercising, even with apparently sufficient stomal opening. Spouses viewed stomal cleaning as a nuisance, as noisy, and as time consuming. Practical stomal care was inadequately managed in 26 per cent and hygienic and esthetic precautions inadequate in 13 per cent of the interviewees.

Deglutition, Digestion, and Related Problems. Problems associated with deglutition and the digestive tract are often reported. Sako, Cardinale, Marchetta, and Shedd (1974) noted that hypopharyngeal edema and secretions may hamper speech, and Levin (1940) acknowledged salivation as a problem for users of intraoral speech aids. Warner (1971) mentioned irregularly shaped hypopharynxes often being found in poor speakers, and Damsté (1975) discussed diverticula in the anterior pharyngoesophageal wall that may retain fluid and result in a moist, husky voice quality. M. C. L. Greene (1967) commented on reduced plasticity of muscular structures, scar formation and fibrosis of the pharyngoesophageal segment, fistula, loss of sensation in the throat, and, following block neck dissection, of less-satisfactory muscular mechanisms having flattened and tight contours. Singer and associates (1981) and Blom and co-workers (1985) reported reflex pharyngoesophageal spasm that can impede air flow and voice production.

Putney (1958) noted that advanced disease may require sacrifice of the hypoglossal nerve bilaterally, or removal of part of the tongue, which might result in difficulty with establishing speech or with swallowing. Hunt (1964), King and colleagues (1971), and M. C. L. Greene (1967) mentioned damage to the peripheral nerve supply with sectioning of the hypoglossal nerve during neck dissection, and consequent restrictions in tongue function. Three per cent of the male respondents and 10 per cent of the female respondents among the 200 in Wallen and Webb's (1975) study reported that their surgery included excision of part of the tongue.

Keith and Shanks (1983), citing Jackson and Jackson (1937), reported problems with deglutition, reduced size of an acceptable bolus, and simultaneous speaking and eating. Gates and colleagues (1982b) also acknowledged swallowing difficulties among the laryngectomized. Brouwer and co-workers (1979) found that of their 50 patients, 36 per cent had temporary difficulty swallowing food, 62 per cent reported no change in eating and drinking habits, and 3 had persistent problems. Blanchard (1982) reported that 70 per cent of his 115 subjects experienced chronic dysphagia. Twenty per cent of Natvig's (1983c) 189 Norwegian subjects reported avoiding certain foods because of swallowing difficulties.

Griglione (1981) reported gastrointestinal disorders, and Levin (1940) reported complaints of gastric air bubbles and burping, especially in the beginning of esophageal speech therapy. Diedrich and Youngstrom (1966) reported an increase of gastrointestinal symptoms in 71 per cent of their questionnaire respondents. Gilchrist (1973) acknowledged that flatulence associated with esophageal speech can result in distension, burping, and stomach rumbling. Wolfe, Olson, and Goldenberg (1971) noted difficulty in achieving esophageal speech as well as problems with chest pain, heartburn, and regurgitation, associated with an incompetent distal esophageal sphincter and hiatal hernia. Only 6 of Natvig's (1983c) 189 subjects regarded eating and digestion problems as their greatest, although several were bothered by stomach rumbling and distension that were troublesome enough in some to decrease social activities. Dry mouth, dental problems, edema, and discomfort associated with radiation of the oral area and neck have also been reported.

Physical Limitations. Among the physical limitations associated with laryngectomy are shoulder drop (Hunt, 1964; Gates et al., 1982b) and shoulder pain (Hunt, 1964), which are usually related to radical neck dissection. Laguaite (1962) indicated that physical problems are perhaps more extensive following neck dissection and irradiation. Snidecor (1975) acknowledged decrements in physical capacity that might limit strenuous physical work and continuation of an occupation. Keith and Shanks (1983), citing Jackson and Jackson (1937), mention limitations in thoracic fixation for lifting or exerting effort. Brouwer and associates (1979) determined that 76 per cent of their 50 patients tired more easily and became breathless more quickly postsurgically. Coyne, Stram, Payton, Klein, and Gressler (1968), however, reported that cardiovascular and respiratory function, as well as abdominal muscle efficiency, is not impaired postsurgically and that tasks involving lifting can be performed safely. Gilchrist (1973), after studying 50 British subjects, concluded that physical capacity will not bar laryngectomized patients from pursuing everyday activities, although radical neck dissection may limit physical capacity on the operated side. Keith and Shanks (1983) stated that the physiological consequences for activities of daily living are compensable to a great extent.

Keith and Shanks (1983) commented on postsurgical restrictions on playing wind instruments, to which clinical experience would add whistling, blowing up a balloon, or orally inflating objects. Although frequently assumed to be significant elements in postlaryngectomy adjustment, the presence of significant physical restrictions is disputed both by research findings and patient performance.

Age and Illness. On the average, the individual suffering laryngeal cancer is likely to be in his mid-fifties, and the population to be considered is an aging one. Timiras (1978) proposed that aging results in morphological, functional, and biochemical involution, always regressive and often silent, affecting most organs and resulting in a gradual decline in performance. He stated, moreover, that "it is frequently under stress that failing capacities are revealed'' (p. 607) and that with aging there is a failure of homeostasis and adaptive competence. Surely these are significant concerns for the older laryngectomized population, which is faced with many stressful situations.

Of Horn's (1962) 3,366 respondents, 27 per cent reported fair health, 7 per cent poor, and 23 per cent worse than before surgery. Wallen and Webb (1975) established that of their 100 male and 100 female respondents, 21 per cent of the male respondents and 34 per cent of the female respondents considered their present health to be less good than preoperatively. Laguaite (1962) indicated that the following age-associated problems may be present: poor health; degenerative conditions such as arthritis, cardiovascular disease, and cerebrovascular disease; poor sight and hearing; and dental problems. King and colleagues (1971) also noted frequent edentulousness and poorly fitting dentures. Kommers and Sullivan (1979) noted that 51 per cent of the 45 wives in their survey reported that their husbands had current medical problems other than those associated with the laryngectomy.

Griglione (1981) cited several authors to support her contention that confused mental status is a problem. Sako and associates (1974) suggested that senility may hamper speech acquisition. Davis (1981) indicated that ill health, senility, and alcoholism are factors influencing the ability to concentrate and cooperate and hence affect speech rehabilitation.

Minear and Lucente (1975) believed that the laryngectomized demonstrate greater alcohol abuse than other groups, and King and colleagues (1971) noted that alcoholic problems may intensify following laryngectomy. Barton (1965) determined that 8 of his series of 50 patients developed or increased previous tendencies toward alcoholism. Webb and Irving (1964) established that over half of their 77 patients had "addictive" tendencies to smoking, drinking, and excessive speaking. They proposed that these presented a psychoanalytic orality factor in the genesis of laryngeal cancer. Approximately 30 per cent of the wives in Kommers and Sullivan's (1979) study reported that their husbands drank moderately, and approximately 13 per cent reported excessive drinking. Wallen and Webb (1975) found that 14 per cent of the male subjects and 7 per cent of the female subjects in their sample of 100 from each sex drank ½ pint or more of alcohol daily. The conclusion by King and co-workers (1968) that ". . . the rehabilitation of a significant proportion of laryngectomees will be complicated by serious problems with alcohol'' (p. 195) best summarizes the significance of the literature.

Lowry (1975) determined that 60 per cent of his 100 head and neck cancer patients had drinking problems but that cancer confined to the vocal cord had no association with heavy drinking. Lowry cautioned that it is important to recognize drinking problems in case management, since apart from treating the alcoholism the entire oral cavity and hypopharynx are at risk of cancer. Moreover, he stated that it is hard to find an alcoholic who does not smoke.

Smoking has been established as the major causal factor in laryngeal cancer. King and colleagues (1968) determined from their literature review that from 92.5 to 99.5 per cent of the laryngectomized population smoked in comparison to the 74.3 to 89 per cent of the general population. Both they and Sako and associates (1974) observed that many laryngectomees show chronic pulmonary change and problems (e.g., emphysema) resulting from prolonged, heavy smoking. Both articles indicated that these may impede speech acquisition.

One additional health problem remains to be discussed, that of recurrence. As indicated earlier, recurrence rates in laryngeal cancer are among the lowest of all cancers (40 per cent, according to Gates et al., 1982b). Nonetheless, the dread of recurrence has been acknowledged by many authors (Fontaine and Mitchell, 1960; Gilmore, 1961; King and colleagues, 1971; Laguaite, 1962; Minear and Lucente, 1975; Meyers, Aarons, Suzuki, and Pilcher, 1980; Morrison, 1941; Natvig, 1983b; Wallen and Webb, 1975; and others).

In summary, a wide variety of physical problems other than the loss of speech may compound the rehabilitation problems of the laryngectomized individual. Included are impaired nonspeech communication, sensation, biological function, swallowing, and digestion; also included are physical limitations, age, and illness. Problems with alcohol consumption are relatively frequent. Drummond (1967) and Keith, Ewert, and Flowers (1974) suggested that physical factors may be more influential than psychological factors in esophageal voice failure. As Salmon (1979) suggests, although objective data are not available to support most assertions regarding the effect of physical concomitants on speech acquisition, "logic prevents an argumentative reaction" (p. 507). Certainly many of the physical problems, reported or speculated, would complicate the rehabilitation process.

SOCIAL CONCOMITANTS

Athelstan (1981), writing on the psychosocial aspects of physical disability, stated that it usually causes profound changes in social relationships, including effects on the family and dissolution of predisability friendships. Furthermore, Athelstan stated, "One of the most predictable effects of a visible disability is a change in the social status of the individual. Disabled persons in our society assume a special kind of minority status and occupy a socially devalued role . . . often assumed by others to be less attractive, less desirable, and less capable in ways which are totally unrelated to their disability" (p. 14). Athelstan suggested that loss of social status may also result from the indirect effects of disability, such as its economic consequences, including depletion of family assets to pay medical costs and reductions in earning capacity.

Clearly, having undergone a laryngectomy results in changes in the individual's relation to society and its units, notably the family and the community. Occupation, both vocational and avocational, may also change. It is also clear that laryngectomized individuals may have both depleted incomes and monetary resources as well as readily discernible disability and consequent reduction in social status. Visible signs may include the tracheostoma, scars, residuals of radical neck dissection, use of an artificial larynx or perhaps of a hand to cover the stoma for tracheoesophageal puncture (TEP) speech or for digital pressure to a flaccid pharyngoesophageal segment, and possibly grimaces or visible air trapping. Audible signs may include the acoustical and temporal differences of esophageal, TEP, or electronically or mechanically aided speech, which result from changes in the vibratory source, resonating tract, and air supply. Audible "stigmata," such as klunks and clicks associated with trapping air for speech, background noise due to forceful air escape through the stoma, and poor technique in using an artificial larynx, may also mask content and attract undesired attention (Gilmore, 1974). As indicated by Diedrich and Youngstrom (1966), the laryngectomized individual's differences "become patent when he is asked to speak, cough, breathe, eat, smell, bathe, lift, cry or laugh" (p. 66).

The social concomitants of laryngectomy are of significance for rehabilitation workers. With regard to speech rehabilitation, reduction in social interaction reduces important opportunities for practicing, perfecting, and generalizing the skills being taught in the speech clinic. Perhaps more importantly, reduction in social roles and contacts diminishes the need to talk and consequently the motivation to expend the effort, time, and financial resources required to reinstate speech. Additionally, according to Athelstan (1981), many of the psychological effects of a disability are the results of the social implications of that disability.

Relationships with Spouse and Family

Importance for Rehabilitation.   Several writers have acknowledged the importance of the spouse and the family in postlaryngectomy rehabilitation. J. Greene (1949) stated that the individual's relationship with his family as well as with his physicians, nurses, and friends can impede or hasten rehabilitation. The wife's and family's attitudes toward the husband's handicap and his efforts to talk are important determinants of speech acquisition (Gardner, 1961). The same applies to female laryngectomees, according to Gardner (1966), who moreover determined that more married women than single women adjusted successfully.

Diedrich and Youngstrom (1966) suggested that the family environment, along with personality, motivation, and aspiration levels, may be more important than physical variables in explaining why one third of laryngectomized individuals do not learn esophageal speech. The spouse's importance for speech adequacy, often as an influence to persevere, was reaffirmed by Gilchrist (1973) and by Goldberg (1975), who found that married persons tended to acquire speech more quickly than unmarried persons.

Kommers and Sullivan (1979) concluded from their study of wives' responses that the home environment may be a critical motivating factor for successful rehabilitation. On the basis of their study of ten esophageal speakers, Gibbs and Achterberg-Lewis (1979) described the spousal relationship for highly successful speakers as frank, both partners expressing opposing views openly, and as based on fulfillment of reciprocal rather than similar needs.

Effects on Marital and Family Status.   The literature dealing with laryngectomy-family status reflects a bleaker clinical expectation than is supported by the research. Webb and Irving (1964) found no difference in marital status between their laryngectomized sample and the general United States population: 77 per cent married or widowed, and 23 per cent single, divorced, or separated. Although King and colleagues (1968) commented that the psychological blow of a laryngectomy is tremendous for both the patient and the family, they concluded from their survey of 138 veteran patients that in spite of the stress imposed on the family, marriages tend to remain stable compared with national trends: 61.5 per cent married; 18.5 per cent divorced, most divorces having occurred before the laryngectomy; 11.5 per cent single; 18 per cent widowed.

Amster and associates (1972) found no significant differences in marital status across a 3 year period between their 20 laryngectomized veterans, 8 veterans who had no history of malignancy and 10 who had surgery for malignancies that had no speech or language concomitants. A majority of Gilchrist's (1973) patients reportedly felt little change and no adverse effect on marital stability following surgery. No change in marital status was found by Johnson, Casper, and Lesswing (1979) in their 25 subjects.

Warner (1971) acknowledged the possibility of social problems resulting within the family following laryngectomy. Snidecor (1975) stated, "At best, the normal dynamics of family interaction are altered" (p. 641), with special problems occurring for female patients. Minear and Lucente (1979) also cautioned that patients and families have been dealt tremendous psychological blows resulting in many types of reactions. The contention that wives and families experience stress and adjustment problems was also supported by Gates and colleagues (1982c), who called for continuing support for the spouse and family, the nature of which must change throughout the rehabilitation process to reflect the problems specific to the time.

Gardner (1966) found that his 129 female laryngectomized respondents reported three different answers regarding the effect of surgery on their marriages: 35 per cent reported no change, 47 per cent reported closer relationships with their husbands, and 18 per cent reported that tensions and misunderstandings were aggravated.

Kommers and colleagues (1977) and Kommers and Sullivan (1979) provided research support as well as clarification of the extent and causes of problems faced by wives. They determined from questionnaires returned by 45 wives that 20 per cent experienced a definite negative influence on their marriage postoperatively. The wives reporting negative marital influences were generally younger than the mean age of the total group. All but one affected wife also reported mitigating factors, including family catastrophes, heavy previous drinking, postretirement problems, and other debilitating medical or mental problems. Seventy-five per cent of the older wives and 47 per cent of the younger reported no marital changes, however, indicating that problems are by no means universal.

Postoperative alterations in family life were established in 27 per cent of the 50 male subjects studied in Holland by Brouwer and coworkers (1979), 1 subject of whom experienced a subsequent divorce. Natvig (1984) determined that 7 of his 189 Norwegian subjects divorced postoperatively, and 3 of them felt that the laryngectomy was the cause. Fifteen per cent of Natvig's couples reported increased problems and difficulties, and 15 per cent reported the opposite. Natvig concluded that the more devoted the couple were before surgery, the more they were after, and the converse.

The literature regarding marital and familial status following laryngectomy indicates that family dissolution is not typical, but that specific problems and stress are likely to occur. The remainder of this section on relationships with spouse and family categorizes and reviews the clinical and research literature regarding those problems. The categories, which should be considered as interdependent rather than discrete, include (1) speech-related problems, involving poor intelligibility, embarrassment, and rejection of the new speech mode; (2) sexual problems; (3) problems associated which changes in life style, involving social contacts, finances, occupation, family roles, and health; (4) an array of problems associated with attitudes and behaviors of both the laryngectomized individual and the spouse; and (5) problems arising from inadequate preparation and counseling.

As suggested by Natvig (1984) following his study of 189 laryngectomized subjects and their spouses, the distribution of these family problems varies as a function of time elapsed since surgery, speech capability, employment status, and the patient's mastery of the laryngectomy event. In addition, the research by Kommers and co-workers (1977) and Kommers and Sullivan (1979) indicated that they may be more frequent and more keenly felt in younger families.

Speech-Related Problems. Heaver and associates (1955) established from their questionnaire responses by 224 subjects that it was not unusual for patients to feel that their families and friends were uncomfortable in their presence owing to their having no satisfactory means for oral communication. Fontaine and Mitchell (1960) provided case studies illustrating family difficulties with understanding speech. More than half of 18 spouses of the 50 patients studied by Brouwer and colleagues (1979) found contact with the laryngectomized partner very difficult soon after surgery, and 3 still had unsatisfactory contact with husbands because they did not speak well. Forty-five per cent of the 45 wives in one study reported decreased overall communication following surgery (Kommers and co-workers, 1977).

Sixty-three per cent of the 45 wives studied by Kommers and coworkers (1977) and Kommers and Sullivan (1979) reported negative first reactions to the artificial larynx, and 23 per cent negative reactions to their husbands' esophageal sound. Although 40 per cent considered their husbands to be readily intelligible 3 months postoperatively, only 53 per cent reported currently understanding them in face-to-face situations. Many revealed concern that their husbands might never speak again.

Gates and colleagues (1982c) indicated that adjustment to the new communicative life style was one of the significant adjustment problems faced by the spouse. Thirty-one per cent of the wives studied by Kommers and Sullivan (1979) reported that adjustment to their husbands' voice loss was more difficult than anticipated.

Sexual Problems. A survey of 237 laryngectomized women indicated that 23 per cent believed that surgery made them less feminine; 35 per cent felt that the scars and the stoma made them less attractive to others; and approximately 16 per cent thought they would not be able to express affection as zealously as before (Gardner, 1966). Single women were more likely to feel unwanted and unattractive according to Snidecor's responses from 155 subjects (1970).

One of the postoperative adjustment problems potentially facing the spouse is alteration of sexual life (Gates et al., 1982c). Kommers and Sullivan (1979) determined that some of their 45 wives considered a change in sex life to be a negative result of the surgery, and 20 per cent reported that it had ''robbed their husbands of some of their manhood''

(p. 414). Twenty-one per cent of Snidecor's (1970) 155 respondents admitted difficulty in sexual relations, and 27 per cent made no comment. No sexual contact was among the problems reported by 10 of the 18 wives of 50 patients followed by Brouwer and associates (1979). Natvig (1984) determined that of the 76 couples interviewed regarding sexual questions, 60 per cent claimed no postoperative alterations; 6 spouses blamed the "unesthetic stoma" for cessation of sexual activity; and 14 impotent subjects blamed irradiation and cytostatic treatments, indicating they had been uninformed of this possible side effect. Johnson and colleagues (1979) indicated only that the majority of their 25 subjects reported no changes in sexual activity.

Meyers and co-workers (1980) determined from their 48 subjects, all members of the Colorado Lost Chord Club, and 25 per cent of whom were women, that 33 per cent experienced changes in their sex lives postoperatively, 40 per cent wished "things could be different," and only 1 subject reported discussion by the physician of possible sexual effects of the laryngectomy. The authors concluded from their data that a significant sexual readjustment takes place in a substantial number of patients and that patients may not communicate these sexual concerns to the surgeon, who may feel uneasy about such counseling. They stated that successful rehabilitation requires such counseling, and that the loss of self-esteem that normally follows disfiguring surgery can often be significantly lessened by a loving spouse or caring friend.

According to Darvill (1983), couples having a satisfactory sexual relationship preoperatively can be reassured that minor inconveniences can be overcome with ingenuity and good humor. He indicated that the most frequent sources of difficulty are a needless fear of suffocation, egressive air from the stoma, and occasional breath odor.

Changes in Life Style. Only four authors were found who related changes in social contacts to changes in marital and family relations. Kommers and Sullivan (1979) acknowledged a concern voiced by a number of their responding wives regarding their husbands' refusal after surgery to go places with them socially. Brouwer and colleagues (1979) determined that 7 of their 50 subjects were not keen to return home following surgery owing to fear of loneliness and communication difficulties. Gates and associates (1982c) considered reduction in social contacts one of the postsurgical adjustment problems facing the spouse. Natvig (1984) found that 79 of his 131 married Norwegian couples claimed no significant change in social life, although alteration in choice of social ties had occurred. Of the 52 couples demonstrating increased isolation, 24 related it to old age or diseases unrelated to cancer; 28 said that speech, stomal, or psychic difficulties were the cause. This pattern was similar to that of the 24 single patients showing increased social isolation.

Clinical experience suggests that financial burdens might influence family interaction. For example, the following could exacerbate spouse and family problems: medical expenses, loss of salary during recuperation, reduced income that might accompany employment change or retirement hastened by the laryngectomy, or deprivation of income due to loss of employment. Horn (1962) established that of his 3,366 subjects, 66 per cent had experienced a drop in income, which 60 per cent attributed to their laryngectomy and 40 per cent to their illness in general. Nineteen per cent had to borrow money to cover medical expenses; the group averaged five months' loss of work because of their illness; and 17 per cent needed the spouse's salary to get through.

Strained finances resulting from large medical bills were a source of irritation to the husbands of a number of Gardner's subjects (1966). Males at all salary levels reported income decline, females only a slight decrease, in Wallen and Webb's (1975) 100 male and 100 female sample. Wallen and Webb concluded that income changes are an element of the trauma associated with laryngectomy.

Kommers and Sullivan (1979) noted that the concerns indicated by their 45 wives included uncertainty of their families' future. Eleven per cent of the wives went to work as a direct result of the laryngectomy, and 10 per cent needed to borrow money to pay medical expenses. Twenty-four per cent expressed negative feelings about having to work away from home. Gates and Hearne (1982) determined that 26 per cent of their subjects reported income loss averaging $1,035, illness costs averaging $8,062, and rehabilitation costs estimated at $413. Six per cent of their retrospective patients had to take lesser-paying jobs postoperatively, and one was unable to find any employment. One fourth of their prospective patients were disabled by their illness and unable to work.

Occupational changes, both vocational and avocational, are mentioned in the literature as requiring adjustments by both the laryngectomized individual and the family. These are discussed in a later section. No doubt they are significant contributors to Parvulescu's (1970) observation that problems in maintaining the desired image as a parent, spouse, and provider are a constant threat.

Additional changes in life style reflect health complaints related to restrictions imposed both by the laryngectomy and by aging. These have been described earlier. Their significance is probably best summarized by Natvig's (1984) finding that 23 per cent of his 189 interviewees reported that old age or other diseases and psychic difficulties were their greatest current problems. Additionally, Kommers and Sullivan (1979) determined that approximately half of their 45 wives reported that their own health had deteriorated as a consequence of the increased stress related to their husbands' laryngectomies. Many reported increased nervousness, depression, and higher blood pressure, and 47 per cent reported lowered spirits. Fewer wives of younger men remained optimistic after surgery (Kommers et al., 1977).

Attitudes and Behaviors. The literature has discussed an array of familial problems centering around attitudes and behaviors emanating from the laryngectomy, both on the part of the laryngectomized individual (generally the husband) and the spouse (generally the wife). Fontaine and Mitchell (1960) reported case histories indicating increased patient withdrawal, inaccessibility, and dependency on the spouse as well as family reactions involving protectiveness, frustration, and resentment. Heaver, White, and Goldstein (1955) established from their survey of 225 patients that it was not unusual for patients to feel that their families and friends were uncomfortable in their presence because of their lack of satisfactory means of oral communication. Gardner (1966) found that 65 per cent of his female subjects reported depressing experiences at home, and 40 per cent reported that they received little inspiration from relatives in regaining their speech.

Fifty-eight per cent of Kommers and Sullivan's (1979) 45 wives reported their husbands as being more nervous and irritable postoperatively, and 51 per cent admitted being somewhat more so themselves. Approximately 7 per cent felt the laryngectomy was a form of punishment to themselves or their husbands, and an equal number were unsure. In 69 per cent the greatest fear was cancer spread and death. Other concerns were the husband's possible inability to cope with surgical consequences or the possibility that he might never speak again. Forty-five per cent of the younger and 15 per cent of the older wives were optimistic preoperatively, and 30 per cent of the younger and 50 per cent of the older were optimistic postoperatively, reflecting the heightened concern of the older wives for surgical survival and of the younger for managing family, vocational, and economic adjustments. Thirty-eight per cent of the wives had negative reactions to the first sight of their husband's stoma; only 22 per cent had been unprepared for this by the surgeon. Thirteen per cent reported that their husbands did not care for their stomas independently.

Brouwer and colleagues (1979) reported that the great majority of their 41 married subjects felt that their spouses were supportive and understanding, but 15 per cent were dissatisfied with their support. Ten (25 per cent) of the wives reported family problems due to their husband's changed behavior after surgery (greater irritability, no sexual contact, and so on) and to the more arduous duties of the wife and family.

The authors concluded that there were more problems in the family and the marriage than the patient himself admitted.

Half of Natvig's (1983b) 189 patients and their spouses experienced greater disagreement after discharge. Thirty-three of the 131 spouses felt they were more depressed than their mates. Some wives recalled the time with depressed, frustrated, emotionally unstable partners as a horrifying period when misconceptions and edginess made them tiptoe for months. They also experienced anxiety aroused by silent, snoreless sleep and feelings of disgust for the noisy cough, expulsion of crusts, and possibly contagious mucus secretions. Many reported having no one with whom to share their plight. Sixty per cent felt many of these problems could have been relieved by satisfactory preoperative counseling and postoperative training. Natvig (1984) observed that one quarter of the spouses studied indicated that laryngectomy makes great demands on the spouse. Thawley, Fuller, and Setzen (1983) added to this picture the fact that a number of patients simply cannot learn esophageal speech, which leads to greater frustration on the part of the patient and the family.

Preparation and Counseling. The studies by Kommers and co-workers (1977) and Kommers and Sullivan (1979) provide considerable insight into problems associated with preparation and counseling. Seventy-eight per cent of the 45 wives were present when the husband learned the diagnosis of cancer, and 87 per cent experienced joint counseling sessions to discuss the surgical procedure. Eighty-seven per cent reported that the physician was their primary information source regarding surgery and its consequences, 62 per cent considering themselves fairly well prepared. Only 31 per cent, however, were counseled alone. Eighteen per cent reported that presurgically their husbands met with a speech pathologist; 29 per cent reported meetings with a laryngectomized visitor.

Some of Kommers and Sullivan's (1979) wives felt that emotionality prevented comprehension of the consequences or that they understood but did not accept. Ninety-eight per cent understood that voice would be lost, but 29 per cent did not know their husbands would no longer breathe through the nose. Over 10 per cent were actually unprepared for the outcomes of surgery. Eighty per cent never met a laryngectomee preoperatively, and only 60 per cent met one in the hospital either before or after surgery. Forty per cent of the wives suggested specific preoperative improvements: asking more questions, visits by another wife, and a film on the "final results."

Kommers and Sullivan (1979) concluded that many wives lacked basic understanding of the consequences of a laryngectomy. They indicated a need for early team counseling in order to prevent isolation and despair. They also advocated continued follow-up and counseling postoperatively, especially among younger wives, with information repeated and with input from a variety of disciplines: physicians, nurses, social workers, speech pathologists, and rehabilitation counselors. Kommers and co-workers (1977) stated that "the mental outlook of both the laryngectomized patient and his family must be considered to maximize rehabilitation success" (p. 1965).

Brouwer and associates (1979) determined that 18 spouses of their 45 subjects felt the advice they had been given was not as good as it might have been. Thirty-nine per cent felt insufficiently informed preoperatively of the consequences of the operation, and 3 spouses had no prior information at all. Natvig (1983b) determined that 21 of 131 spouses did not visit the hospital. Seventy per cent of the 98 known to have visited claimed the counseling provided was unsatisfactory, that their needs were not met, and that they felt unprepared and upset. Natvig (1984) concluded that the spouse should also be involved when the patient is advised.

Laguaite's admonishment (1962) summarized well the implications of the reports on preparation and counseling. She stated that the family's understanding of the operation and its results is just as important as the patient's and that pre- and postoperative counseling is just as important to them. Gilmore (1961) added that social restoration, like speech restoration, should begin before the operation.

Relationships With Friends and Community

Withdrawal. A major reaction toward friends and community following the occurrence of a disability is withdrawal. Cogswell (1967, reported in Athelstan, 1981) described the following changes in social adjustment in a group of men having spinal cord injury: dissolution of predisability friendships and marked reductions in social contacts, frequency of entering community settings, and the number of roles played. The clinical and research literature indicates that withdrawal is a significant component of postlaryngectomy psychosocial adjustments as well.

The perception that family and friends were uncomfortable in their presence was not an unusual response from 224 laryngectomized individuals responding to a questionnaire by Heaver and co-workers (1955). Stoll (1958) suggested that negative attitudes toward esophageal speech resulting from its poor intelligibility could eventuate in fears, embarrassment, and insecurity regarding public recognition of the disability. Patient reactions may induce self-imposed isolation, because it is less painful than the fears associated with social contact, according to Bisi and Conley (1965). The result is avoidance of esophageal speech in order to avoid being noticed by others or exposed to anticipated rejection.

Gardner (1966) demonstrated a relationship between speech proficiency and avoidance or withdrawal. He determined that 83 per cent of the 237 laryngectomized women he studied who retained good preoperative social relationships regained speech, compared with only 30 per cent of those without a good social network. Speech was regained by 76 per cent of those who sought to avoid their friends but by 90 per cent of those who refused to avoid them. Blake (1974) also determined that poor speakers tended to be more socially withdrawn and less self-confident.

Darvill (1983) discussed factors resulting in withdrawal, stating "patients report that this operation has a profound effect upon their sense of social acceptability, not only in public places but even among their closest family and friends. They are aware that the unusual quality of esophageal or electronic pseudo-voice tends to attract attention, as does their characteristic and strange-sounding cough. For these reasons, alas, too high a proportion of patients prefer to stay at home" (1983, p. 200). Reductions in social contacts result from failure to attend dinner parties because of difficulties with simultaneous eating and speaking and from loss of friends who are hard of hearing or who enjoy strenuous sports, especially swimming (Snidecor, 1975).

One laryngectomized individual, writing about her own social experiences during the 2 years since surgery seems to have epitomized the problems precipitating withdrawal. Her comments suggested that sensitivity, embarrassment, and defensiveness were significant elements in her interactions with the community. She wrote of her battle to maintain a sense of humor and to accept herself as well as the inquisitive, unknowing, and often intended-to-help behaviors of others.

The research literature exploring withdrawal has relied on summations of responses to questionnaires regarding activities and attitudes. Horn (1962) studied postoperative changes in his 3,366 respondents in both interests and participation in church, civic, political, community service, and other activities. He determined that, depending on the specific activity, only between 8 and 16 per cent of his subjects were participants, the greatest portion being church related. With regard to interests and participation, respectively, 43 per cent and 30 per cent had no change, 29 per cent and 26 per cent indicated decreases, and 6 per cent and 50 per cent indicated increases. These findings indicated both a sizable reduction of activity and a significant increase in passive involvement postlaryngectomy. Moreover, 25 per cent reported a decreased circle of friends, whereas 54 per cent remained the same and 15 per cent enlarged their circle of friends. The decrease conformed with Cogswell's (1967) finding following spinal cord injuries and supports reductions in friendships postdisability among the laryngectomized. The enlargement probably reflected the effect of laryngectomee support groups and reinforces the statement by Fontaine and Mitchell (1960) that they provide a setting that would enlarge social contacts.

King and colleagues (1968) determined that over half of their 138 veteran subjects never went out of their houses socially, and only 33 per cent did so occasionally. They concluded that a large number of their patients reacted by "withdrawing from life" and that the vast majority were withdrawn from society. Those who wrote were more withdrawn than artificial larynx users, and those using artificial devices were more withdrawn than esophageal speakers. Withdrawal was also greater in older persons. The authors concluded that following laryngectomy, withdrawal and avoidance of social contacts may intensify to the point at which many patients remain virtually isolated, with no outside personal contacts, interests, or hobbies. Minear and Lucente (1975) supported this conclusion in their description of the laryngectomized population as one in which "half never get out of their homes socially, and over half have no hobbies and remain socially withdrawn" (p. 201).

Johnson and co-workers (1979) determined that two thirds of their 25 subjects felt that their social lives had remained the same or improved but that one third experienced decreased social activity owing to embarrassment and easy fatigability. Gates and colleagues (1982a) found social activities reduced in 59 per cent of their subjects, whereas 41 per cent noted no change in numbers of friends or social contact.

Only 22 per cent of the wives interviewed by Goldberg (1975) reported that their husbands visited others by themselves; 9 per cent said they seldom did and 27 per cent reported they never did. Twenty per cent of the husbands belonged to New Voice Clubs and 20 per cent of the husbands and wives regularly attended club meetings. Goldberg's findings led him to conclude that laryngectomized persons having greater optimism, realism, and motivation to survive were more likely to resume social and other activities. Persons who maintained or acquired esophageal or electrolaryngeal speech also participated in more community organizations postoperatively.

Acceptance, Rejection, and Stigma. Problems of rejection and social stigma are encountered by laryngectomized individuals at home, with friends, and in numerous community circumstances. Patient concerns and complaints indicate that rejection is not infrequent. Although the literature in this area is sparse, it has considerable significance.

Jesberg (1956) confirmed the importance of this psychosocial dimension when he specified one of the problems of rehabilitation as being public acceptance of rehabilitated laryngectomees back into society. Drummond (1967) acknowledged the problem when she stated that tolerance is an absolute necessity after hospital discharge, when voice-lessness, depression, distressing coughing, and neck breathing occur in a previously normal person.

Research support is meager, but it indicates that families, friends, and the public in general may relegate laryngectomized individuals to inferior status, often covertly, too frequently overtly. Even professionals may reflect inadequate knowledge and experience with laryngectomized persons, as determined by Killarney and Lass (1979) and consequently may harbor attitudes that hamper acceptance and impede rehabilitation.

Gardner (1966) ascertained that 46 per cent of his married female laryngectomized subjects felt that their husbands avoided them, showed excessive pity, or babied them excessively. Reports, such as one of a husband who feared his wife would jeopardize his professional standing, reflected not only the stigma "imposed" by the society but also that "imposed" by the husband.

Gilmore (1974) explored the social and vocational acceptability of esophageal and laryngeal speakers to captive business and professional men. The 480 subjects either saw silent films, heard audiotapes, or saw and heard sound films of two superior esophageal speakers who held prestige positions requiring public contact and two matched laryngeal speakers. They rated each speaker on one scale of social distance and on three vocational measures: the number of jobs the speaker was perceived as being able to handle; the degree of prestige associated with those jobs; and the degree of public contact entailed in those jobs. Half the subjects were provided with simple information about laryngectomized speakers prior to judging the films or tapes.

Gilmore (1974) determined that the esophageal speakers were per-ceived as being able to hold significantly fewer positions, entailing sig-nificantly less prestige and significantly less social contact, than the nonlaryngectomized speakers. They were also relegated to significantly more distant social positions than the nonlaryngectomized speakers. Provision of information improved laryngectomee acceptability for the social distance, number of jobs, and job prestige criteria, but it had no effect on the degree of public contact associated with those jobs. The public contact criterion may be the measure having the greatest social and speech significance, since it reflects both social access and opportu-nities to speak. The differences favoring the nonlaryngectomized speak-ers prevailed across all three manners of presentation, indicating that they resulted from both audible and visible attributes of the esophageal speakers. Gilmore called for increased public education as well as elimi-nation of visible and audible stigmata during speech training.

Natvig (1984) observed that unexpected reactions from the public and friends had frequently been experienced as hurtful by his 189 Norwegian subjects, resulting in withdrawal from social ties. Many felt that increased public education regarding their disability would have been advantageous. Natvig indicated that public reactions may vary from pity, curiosity, attention, and thoughtlessness to anxiety and disgust. He suggested that patients need to be taught to deal with those possible reactions.

Killarney and Lass (1979) explored the knowledge and attitudes of 127 speech pathologists, social workers, and rehabilitation counselors toward laryngectomees. Speech pathologists had significantly higher knowledge scores than the other two groups, who did not differ from each other. Speech pathologists also had the greatest exposure to laryngectomized persons (80 per cent), followed by rehabilitation counselors (55 per cent) and social workers (40 per cent). Attitudes did not differ among the professions. Laryngectomees were considered different from individuals having larynxes, and they were perceived as being ashamed, feeling sorry for themselves, and requiring special attention. Social workers and counselors felt that they had annoying speech and that others felt uncomfortable with them. Social workers and speech pathologists felt uncomfortable with them. Social workers and speech pathologists felt that they were less confident and happy than nonlaryngectomized individuals. Speech pathologists and counselors felt that they were more easily upset than nonlaryngectomized people. Social workers felt that they were more aggressive, worried more, and tended to get discharged more easily than nonlaryngectomized people. All three groups felt that they strongly resembled nonlaryngectomized people in that they can be successful employees, can care for themselves, and have personalities no different from nonlaryngectomized persons. The authors concluded from their study that social workers and counselors must learn about the particular problems of the laryngectomized during their training and that continuing professional education is needed for all rehabilitation workers regarding associated vocational, social, psychological, and sociological problems.

In summary, both the needs and rewards for communication are based in social interacting. The social concomitants of being laryngectomized can be widespread, involving spouse, family, friends, and the community at large. Although family dissolution is atypical, problems do occur, including those related to impaired communication, sexual adjustment, financial burdens, and to changes in social contact, occupation, and attitudes and behaviors. Withdrawal and social inactivity may result. Rejection and social stigma can impede social and vocational acceptance. The need for early and frequent counseling for the patient and family has been expressed by both parties as well as by contributors to the literature. Professionals are also in need of greater training about problems faced by the laryngectomee.

Occupational Concomitants

Among the numerous changes potentially requiring adjustment by the laryngectomized are the ways in which time may be occupied. The two major activities occupying time are vocational, relating to the individual's gainful employment, and avocational, relating to time spent in recreation.

Many of the physical changes described earlier, especially loss of speech, have occupational significance. For instance, early retirement in this population with a mean age in the mid-fifties is not infrequent. Also, breathing through the stoma may necessitate a job change to avoid such irritants as dust, fumes, or sprays (Levin, 1967), or speech disabilities may jeopardize teaching, practicing law, or safety on a construction job. A listing of jobs held by 209 Veterans Administration subjects (Johnson, 1960) indicated that 57 per cent held positions in which exposure to dust, paint, or other irritants and to noisy environments might affect employment: 25 per cent were farm related workers; 12 per cent, construction workers; 10 per cent, carpenters; 10 per cent, machinists. Similarly, hobbies such as water sports and wood working, and recreations such as dinner parties and card playing, may be significantly restricted or precluded.

Changes in vocation and avocation may result in reductions in income, reward, recognition, satisfaction, status, and self-esteem. Financial problems or reliance on the spouse to fill vacant time may disturb marital or familial stability or both. These and a host of related problems may threaten psychological stability.

Changes in Employment.   A relatively large number of writers and researchers have explored the employment status of the laryngectomized. This interest probably reflects the implications for financial, familial, and social status associated with having a job or not and with income. Vocational rehabilitation is a significant component of total rehabilitation. It probably also reflects the importance of "the work ethic" on both society's and the individual's estimate of a person's value and "moral fiber." Richardson's (1983) and Natvig's (1983d) findings regarding increasing numbers accepting disability benefits or retirement suggests, however, that there may be changes occurring in these attitudes.

The significance of employment for the laryngectomized individual has been stated by several authors. Hudson (1967) established that it was an important element of motivation, which in turn was a significant determinant of esophageal speech learning in her 16 Veterans Administration patients. Ranney (1975) stated that although speech is the most important aspect of rehabilitation, re-employment is second, and that most other aspects—financial security, family relations, community life, social and recreational activities, and emotional stability—are dependent on employment. Barton (1965) found that in his 50 private patients, concern for losing their jobs was among the major postoperative traumas. King and colleagues (1971) suggested that the need for employment may act as both a stimulus to rehabilitative effort and a source of anxiety. Parvulescu (1970), however, cautioned that resumption of the former occupation might be a problem.

Employment Status.   Several writers have explored employment status, determining that a sizable number of individuals either lost or changed positions or retired postoperatively. Of the 3,366 subjects studied by Horn (1962), the percentage of retired doubled from 12 per cent to 24 per cent, and the percentage unemployed rose from 2 to 18 per cent. Only 4.4 per cent reported any vocational training. Twenty-two per cent reported their present occupation or work situation to be less satisfying; 6 per cent, more satisfying; 27 per cent, the same; and 45 per cent omitted the question. Twenty-five per cent attributed the change in the workplace or occupation to their laryngectomy; an equal percentage did not. Occupational changes were less frequent among professionals, semiprofessionals, and unskilled labor and greatest in managerial, sales, clerical, skilled, and semiskilled occupations. Horn concluded, "It is clear that problems of occupational change, loss of income, and loss of job situation loom large among the problems faced by the laryngectomee" (p. 7).

A review of the literature led King and colleagues (1968) to cite a range of employment figures from 46 to 94 per cent. Their series of 138 subjects from the Portland, Oregon, Veterans Administration Hospital revealed that only 5.5 per cent were employed full-time and 22 per cent part-time. Matched for sex and age, over twice as many Veterans Administration amputees as laryngectomees contributed to their own support. The authors concluded that the proportion of employed laryngectomees was extremely low.

Amster and associates (1972) determined that presurgically, 14 of their 20 veterans were retired owing to age or disability, 2 were unemployed, and 4 were employed, whereas postsurgically, 7 of those previously retired worked full- or part-time. Employment status remained essentially the same over the 3 year follow-up period. DeBeule and Damsté (1972) found that 27 per cent of their subjects retired because of the operation and 22 per cent changed occupations.

Of Gilchrist's (1973) 40 British subjects, 55 per cent returned to their preoperative employment, many to jobs requiring good voice or strenuous physical effort. Five modified their positions, 5 changed work places, and 5 ceased work as a result of their surgery, and 5 changed for reasons unrelated directly to their surgery. Ranney's (1975) study of 1,229 laryngectomees, of whom 1,087 were employed at surgery, revealed that 76 per cent retained their jobs, 18 per cent were dismissed, 40 per cent were demoted, and 2 per cent quit. Of the 239 dismissed or demoted, 23 per cent felt that they could do the job as well as before; 49 per cent of the 192 dismissed felt that they could do as good a job at the same place but in another position. Only 43 per cent of those retired by the company were close to retirement age, and 57 per cent were forced to take early retirement. Only 19 per cent of those dismissed agreed with the employer, and 20 per cent never found another job. Sixty-two per cent of those demoted took severe pay reductions.

Fifty-three of Sako and associates' (1974) 85 subjects from Buffalo, New York, were gainfully employed outside their home presurgically, but only 21 (25 per cent) returned to the same job, and 1 took another job. Wallen and Webb (1975) found that 60 per cent of their 100 male subjects and 44 per cent of their 100 female subjects retired. Of Goldberg's (1975) 62 subjects, 39 per cent (24) returned to work, and 1 subject returned to homemaking, and 60 per cent (37) were unemployed.

Reports from Kommers and Sullivan's (1979) study of 45 wives indicated that 75 per cent of those husbands employed at time of surgery returned to their previous occupations full- or part-time, 79 per cent of them within 3 months of surgery. One fourth of those not returning to former jobs found other employment. Johnson and co-workers (1979) determined that most of their preemployed 25 New York state subjects, all of whom had a satisfactory means of communication, either returned to work or retired because of age.

Blanchard (1982) surveyed 115 laryngectomized individuals from around the United States, all with 12 or fewer months elapsed since surgery, and found 29 per cent employed, 58 per cent retired, and 12 per cent unemployed. Gates and associates (1982b) found that employment status was unchanged for 64 per cent of their 53 prospectively studied and 69 per cent of their 40 retrospectively studied subjects. Six per cent had to take lesser paying jobs postoperatively, and 1 subject was unable to find work although physically capable of working. A fourth of the prospective subjects were disabled by their illness and unable to work. Income losses averaging $1,035 were reported by 26 per cent of the prospective subjects.

A review of the literature led Richardson (1983) to conclude that laryngectomized patients experience greater difficulty than other cancer patients in retaining jobs or finding new ones. Of the 60 Los Angeles subjects she studied, 22 per cent worked full-time, 10 per cent worked part-time, 43 per cent were retired or not working for reasons related to health, and 25 per cent were retired or not working for reasons unrelated to health. Thirty-three per cent of the esophageal speakers, 35 per cent of the artificial larynx users, and 29 per cent of those communicating by writing or mouthing worked full- or part-time. Forty-three per cent of the esophageal speakers, 35 per cent of artificial larynx users, and 60 per cent of writers or mouthers were retired or not working owing to health problems. Many patients, particularly those between 55 and 64, considered the cancer-related illness an acceptable basis for not working and took early retirement or received disability payments.

One hundred ten of Natvig's (1983d) 189 Norwegian subjects who were operated prior to 65 years of age were gainfully employed at the time of surgery. Sixty-three per cent of those of occupational age were employed full- or part-time postoperatively, 34 per cent ceased work and received disability pensions, and 3 per cent were engaged in active rehabilitation programs with favorable re-employment outlooks. Average ages of surgery were 53 years for the employed and 55.8 years for the unemployed, indicating that the employed group tended to be younger. The median time from surgery to re-employment was 4.5 months, suggesting that return to work occurred relatively quickly. Fifty-five per cent were still employed at interview, and 45 per cent had ceased work after a mean occupation time of 6 years.

Factors Related to Employment.   Several of the writers explored the factors related to whether or not laryngectomized individuals resumed employment. Having intelligible speech appears to be a major factor. Gardner (1961) wrote that the desire to return to work was one of the strongest motivating factors for learning speech and also that the deprivation of speech may precipitate reluctance to return to work. Approximately 25 per cent of the 224 patients studied by Heaver and Arnold (1962) lost their jobs because they could not talk. A few found jobs, but usually with reduced income, ego-satisfaction, and prestige. Gardner (1966) determined from his female subjects that return to work was closely related to regaining speech. Good speech was regained by 84 per cent who returned to work but by only 66 per cent of those who did not.

King and co-workers (1968) determined that one half of their employment-eligible patients who communicated with esophageal speech alone had some form of employment, while none of those without esophageal speech were employed. Three of Gilchrist's (1973) 13 subjects who changed or ceased work did so owing to inadequate voice. The reason given by Natvig's (1983d) subjects for not resuming employment included speech or stomal problems or both in 27 cases and various reasons unrelated to the laryngectomy in 13 instances. The reasons for ceasing employment included reaching pensionable age in 17 subjects, laryngectomy-related reasons in 8 subjects, and other reasons in 6 subjects.

Among other reasons cited in the literature for limitations on the work that can be done, or for failure to return to or maintain work, were: a dusty atmosphere, an inability to climb heights, and an inability to wear a required high collar comfortably (Gilchrist, 1973); both physical and psychological factors (King et al., 1968); the need to avoid the risk of submersion or of airborne irritants because of the tracheostoma; inability to communicate above noise or to warn of hazards by shouting; inability to do heavy lifting because of trapezius paralysis following radical neck dissection or the absence of glottic fixation (King et al., 1971); disability due to illness (Gates et al., 1982a); health (Richardson, 1983); and occupations having a premium on speech, or dust, fumes, any sort of air pollution, or cold or dry air (Natvig, 1983d). Natvig also indicated that a number of his subjects held positions involving these factors as well as heavy physical effort nevertheless. Additionally, King and colleagues (1971) suggested that many older patients might seek a pension rather than economic competition.

Kommers and Sullivan (1979) determined from their study of 45 wives that approximately 7 per cent felt their husbands' not working was related to the psychological effects of the laryngectomy and 22 per cent to its medical effects. Two failed to return to their jobs because of feeling awkward and inadequate. The most frequent reason for inability to work among the nonretired was medical problems.

In a study of factors related to employment in 25 subjects, Nahum and Golden (1963) found no statistical difference in social function among those working full- or part-time, those not working owing to health, or those who were retired. They concluded that failure to return to work did not result in social impairment in other areas involving social interaction. They also determined that postoperative employment status was not correlated with higher educational level, white collar status, or using esophageal versus artificial larynx speech, although people using writing were less likely to be employed. They found that the decision to retire early often preceded adoption of a particular communication mode, which they felt suggested that learning esophageal speech was not a causal factor in employment.

Goldberg (1975) undertook a study of home, social, and vocational adjustment of 62 subjects, 5 of whom were women. He determined that the best predictors of vocational adjustment were predisability measures of the patient's vocational plans and household activities and postdisability measures of motivation to survive and cope with the disability, irrespective of the severity of the laryngeal cancer. Persons having realistic plans prior to disability accepted greater responsibility for work and had a better chance of becoming employed. Those with greater optimism, realism, and motivation for survival were more likely to resume work, household, and social activities. No significant differences were found among the clinical stages of cancer with regard to vocational adjustment.

Re-employed subjects in Natvig's (1983d) study received significantly higher scores than the unemployed in all three categories of factors explored for relationships with return to work: preoperative work factors, type of work or employment, and postoperative work factors. Employment status was found to be positively related to high social group, education beyond junior secondary level, living in urban areas, and time elapsed since surgery. Most of Natvig's subjects who succeeded in re-employment returned to work within 9 months of surgery, usually before sickness benefits were discontinued. Subjects demonstrating low stress vulnerability and good preoperative adaptation patterns resumed work significantly more frequently, and these variables had the greatest predictive value.

Employment status was unrelated in Natvig's subjects to having children under 15 years old, age at surgery, physical demands or air pollution at preoperative employment, or having socially acceptable speech. Individuals demonstrating alcohol abuse gave up work more easily.

Discrimination in Employment. Ranney (1975) concluded from his study of 1,229 laryngectomized subjects that discrimination existed, some caused by fellow employees as well as employers. This conclusion is supported by the findings of Gilmore (1974), who found esophageal speakers to be acceptable to captive audiences of business and professional men in fewer and less prestigious positions and in ones having significantly less public contact. Ranney (1975) called upon physicians to help overcome the fear of contagion and upon Lost Chord Clubs to serve as public advocates.

Following her study of 60 subjects, Richardson (1983) concluded that discrimination in postsurgical employment appeared to be secondary to the individual's own desires and decisions about returning to work. Although often considered indicative of general rehabilitation success after disabling illness, Richardson contended that her study did not support employment status as a yardstick of all adjustment, since there were no significant differences between the employed and unemployed groups in other areas explored.

King and colleagues (1971) perhaps summarized the vocational problem when they indicated that about 70 per cent of laryngectomees could return to their former employment but that this would require support from the rehabilitation team members as well as maintaining contact with and reassuring the employer.

Changes in Avocation. Few writers have explored recreational changes following laryngectomy. Some, as indicated earlier, commented on restrictions in water sports because of the stomal opening; in strenuous sports because of reduced strength or endurance; in dinner parties because of difficulties with eating, drinking, and speaking simultaneously; and in interaction with friends who may have hearing losses related to aging. Certainly hobbies involving dust or noxious fumes might also be restricted, as would singing, playing wind instruments, and acting. In some cases, ambivalence or rejection on the part of previous friends or the general public, or the individual's self-consciousness and embarrassment, may curtail diversional activities.

King and co-workers (1968) determined that half of their 61 veteran patients were never out of their homes socially, and over half (58.9 per cent) had no hobbies. These were largely the same individuals. They stated that this withdrawal appeared to be more frequent with older individuals and those who had neither esophageal nor artificial larynx speech. Snidecor (1970) reported that over half the 155 laryngectomees responding to his questionnaire experienced changes in social, religious, and recreational activities. King and colleagues (1971) stated, "Many laryngectomees will remain virtually isolated, with no outside personal contacts, interests or hobbies" (p. 117).

Kommers and Sullivan (1979) determined from their survey of 45 wives that, with the exception of some "realistic" changes (for example, no boating), 64 per cent reported no changes in their husbands' hobbies postoperatively. Some reported that new hobbies were undertaken.

Gardner (1966) noted that being unable to swim was the one activity reported by his optimistic female respondents as being deleted. Darvill (1983) also commented on restrictions in swimming but acknowledged the development in 1974 of an inflatable cuff swimming aid. Darvill indicated that early preoperative coughing fits, or reduced stamina, might restrict activity in sports requiring strenuous physical activity.

In summary, changes in employment and employment status were reported frequently enough to cause concern. Often they reflected physical changes resulting from the surgery; occasionally they reflected the stigma attached by the community or the attitudes and motivation of the laryngectomized individual. Having acceptable speech was generally related to both return to and success in work. Avocational changes may also occur. Changes in how the individual occupies his time, whether in work or recreation, may involve reductions in rewards, status, and ego-satisfaction.

Psychological Concomitants

Removal of the larynx precipitates a number of physical, social, and occupational changes, described earlier. These sudden and extensive changes result in a series of crises in identity and in consequent stress as the individual struggles to cope and to adjust to them. Indeed, King and co-workers (1968) acknowledged that "the psychological blow of laryngectomy, both to the patient and [to] his family, is tremendous, and for some it may be overpowering'' (p. 201). Another writer suggested, ''An experience of the traumatic intensity of a laryngectomy, by its very nature, has the potential of a disturbing effect upon the patient's sense of belonging, his self-concept, his attitudes, and many other aspects of his phenomenologic field'' (p. 551) (Beamer, 1954, cited in Stoll, 1958).

The resulting emotions, attitudes, and behaviors constitute the psychological concomitants of being laryngectomized. Not only do these emotions and behaviors reflect the physical, social, and occupational concomitants of laryngectomy; they may also have significant impact *upon* each of those domains. For instance, depression and withdrawal can have significant effects on family, friends, job, and even health. In particular, a number of writers and researchers have explored the relationship between the psychological status of the laryngectomized individual and postoperative acquisition of speech.

Understanding and management of psychological concomitants can reduce the distress felt by patients and the people with whom they interact. It also releases time, funds, and psychic energy for use in reducing other disability problems, which should facilitate psychological adjustment and rehabilitation in general.

Psychological Impact.   Psychic factors play a vital role in laryngectomee rehabilitation, and they become operative at the moment of diagnosis or before, according to J. Greene (1947). Cancer results in fear of death, loss of speech, and loss of jobs and friends; some even contemplate suicide (Gardner, 1971). Levin (1967) suggested that

> Emotional disturbances of varying degrees occur in nearly all the patients. While the introverted person suffers more in proportion, even the extrovert is depressed when he finds himself entirely speechless. These reactions are to be expected, because the patient has undergone a major operation after confirmation of a serious diagnosis; on discharge from the hospital he must return to his community, with all the economic and social problems involved and where loss of speech is a serious defect; and he has a fear of recurrence of cancer. (p. 760)

Several writers analyzed the psychological impact of a laryngectomy according to a temporal frame. The following psychological traits were found by J. Greene (1947) among the 70 respondents to his questionnaire: fear, anxiety, depression, sensitivity, ego-deflation, apprehension, suicidal tendencies, job-retention fear, seclusiveness, irritability, and ''philosophic resignation'' (passivism). Fear, apprehension, and anxiety occurred initially in 19 subjects at the onset of hoarseness and in 10 after it persisted. Fifty-one became acutely depressed and apprehensive on hearing the diagnosis and being told they would lose the larynx, with at least 3 considering suicide. A number felt unprepared for surgery and indicated that a paucity of information contributed greatly to their anxiety and apprehension. Their lowest point of depression occurred after surgery when they tried to talk, with 63 of the 70 subjects reporting extreme depression at that time. One third indicated that worry about retaining their jobs added to the depression, that they felt "desolated" and "just about went insane."

After surgery, when attempting to resume interpersonal relations and old associations, more than half reported being depressed, sensitive, becoming reclusive, and avoiding even best friends. Some reported that using an artificial larynx even increased their sensitivity and that they "felt like a freak." Learning they could talk again led to a "resurgence of hope and optimism." It is at this stage of rehabilitation, when the patient comes to training in order to develop a substitute voice, that Greene believed the influence of psychic features to be the most apparent. At this point "they can actually and very definitely hamper treatment." The patient who is abnormally depressed, sensitive and anxious, Greene contended, has much greater difficulty in developing a substitute voice.

Heaver and colleagues (1955) determined from their study of 224 patients that on hearing the diagnosis of cancer and hearing that speech would be lost, almost all experienced various degrees of severe emotional trauma, chiefly depression. The most frequent emotional reactions before and after operation were fright, anxiety, confusion, self-pity, fear of death, and insomnia. Two patients attempted suicide; 32 seemed euphoric. The emotional trauma was compounded for most by consequent disruption of economic security.

The laryngectomee receives three blows to his equanimity, according to Gardner (1971): (1) the news that he has cancer; (2) a mental and physical impression immediately postoperatively that centers around the frustration associated with loss of communication, except for writing; and (3) the necessity of appearing before the public as a laryngectomee, with a hole in his neck, feeling embarrassed, frustrated, inferior, and a social and economic failure.

Sanchez-Salazar and Stark (1972) identified four moments of crisis for the laryngectomee: (1) when the patient first learns he has cancer and must have a laryngectomy; (2) after surgery, when the patient fully appreciates what has taken place; (3) at the time of discharge from the protective atmosphere of the hospital; and (4) weeks after surgery, when the patient has convalesced and friends and family are not so attentive.

A review of the literature concerning the psychology of the laryngectomee was done by Locke (1966). He divided the topic into three major, essentially temporal, areas: psychological reaction to the disease itself; psychological factors involved in rehabilitation; and psychological considerations in the use of esophageal voice versus an artificial larynx. Locke stated that the psychological trauma related to the disease is equally as serious as the physical trauma and that a marked decompensation in personality may result, often leading to excessive use of alcohol and weakening or break-up in the family structure. Many patients, he claimed, view the procedure as a form of castration. Fears and anxieties abound regarding surgery, death, and loss of voice, security, and friends. These are accompanied by insomnia, confusion, self-pity, devitalization of the patient's psychic energy, and severe reactive depression. Postoperative fears include those related to recurrence and death, the physiological changes, old age, and uselessness due to speech loss. Often these reactions are aggravated by loss of earning power, inability to re-establish interpersonal relationships, and anticipated failure to learn speech.

The psychological factors involved in rehabilitation, according to Locke (1966), include motivation (which is the most vital), severe depression, sensitivity, anxiety, and perhaps seclusiveness and withdrawal.

Concerning the controversy over the use of esophageal voice versus an artificial larynx, Locke (1966) stated that no area generates more conflict and that the argument has important psychological implications. He summarized the literature dealing with the advantages and disadvantages of voice prostheses: He appeared to lean away from them and toward esophageal speech, indicating that patients find them unacceptable for purely psychological reasons. These reasons included the constant reminder to self and others of the disability, embarrassment, possible objectionable characteristics for the listener, and the more "human" nature of esophageal voice.

More recent literature (Gates et al., 1982b; Gates et al., 1982c; Lauder, 1968; Lauder, 1970; Salmon and Goldstein, 1978), however, has begun to dispute the substantially negative attitudes toward use of artificial larynxes and to recognize their psychological values in decreasing frustration and despair and in permitting oral exchange and catharsis while learning esophageal speech. Additionally, the implied failure and onus of being poorly motivated, passive, dependent, and not persevering are being replaced by a pragmatic approach stressing intelligibility regardless of mode, the advantages of dual modes, and the individual's right of choice. These changes suggest that conflict associated with artificial larynxes will be reduced in the future.

One laryngectomee described her own feelings and reactions during her first two years according to her preoperative and postoperative responses (Nicholson, 1975). Preoperatively she felt shock and numbness immediately, a sense of loss related to having traded her voice for a "makeshift," gratefulness for family support, fear of the surgery, and repulsion for the disfigurement. Postoperatively, she felt the "relentless impact of voicelessness" as though she was "imprisoned by silence," defeat due to failure to develop satisfactory esophageal voice, a "love-hate relationship" with her artificial larynx, and annoyance and embarrassment with her inability to laugh aloud, sing, swim, smell, suck up soup from a spoon, blow out birthday candles, and call out for help in danger. She indicated that her most grievous loss was a "forfeiture of personality," which she attributed to communicating so poorly, being "bereft . . . of repartee with others," and "infrequent cruelties, such as when strangers hang up on the phone or laugh thinking it's a joke." She stated, "There are still times of depression, but fewer as time goes by," and concluded, ". . . I shall adjust to the brokenness and deprivations inherent in may present status" (p. 2158).

Premorbid Personality Traits.   Several writers have suggested that the laryngectomized individual's personality prior to surgery is a major factor contributing to reactions following surgery. J. Greene (1947) stated that ". . . among the principal factors influencing the patient's psychology, and, hence, his adjustment to the loss of his larynx and his responses to voice training, are his personality and vocation before the operation, as well as his social and economic status."

Levin (1940), discussing the influence of psychological factors on rehabilitation, indicated that

> Another great difficulty which must be overcome is the mental attitude of these patients. The ease with which they learn is dependent in a measure on their personalities and make-up. The aggressive extrovert goes after the problem of learning in a direct business-like way . . . he has the attitude of a good student. The emotionally unstable and introverted type, not having recovered from the psychic trauma incidental to the diagnosis of cancer and the subsequent radical operation and hospitalization, finds it difficult to concentrate and learn anything new . . . requires constant prodding, encouragement and the influence of the stronger will of the teacher. A few give up the struggle easily and quit after a few days. . . ." (pp. 309–310)

In a later article, Levin (1967) suggested that the introverted person suffered more than the extrovert.

Bisi and Conley (1965) classified the laryngectomized population into three psychological groups relative to speech attainment. The first included the 70 per cent of the population who master and accept esophageal speech as a satisfactory communication means, whom the authors indicated have the "emotional status . . . adequate for the demands of adaptation imposed by loss of the voice-producing organ" (p. 1073). The second group included the 15 per cent who accept an artificial larynx, whose emotional status may prove adequate or inadequate with respect to adaptation. The third group included the 15 per cent of persons who fail to acquire esophageal speech and reject the artificial larynx, choosing to communicate by writing, lip movement, whispering, and gesture.

In summarizing the literature, Snidecor (1975) commented on findings suggesting that laryngectomees have personalities reflecting amorous and aggressive needs and tendencies toward withdrawal and self-concealment as well as repression and internalization.

Three research articles were uncovered that explored preoperative personality traits. Webb and Irving (1964) studied 77 laryngectomized patients' pre- and postoperative responses to the Szondi projective test. They concluded that there is a specific behavioral pattern that differentiates laryngectomized patients from those having other cancer types or loci. That behavioral pattern is manifested by an oral triad of excessive speaking, drinking, and smoking along with associated signs and tendencies toward aggressiveness, instability, and abnormal drive tensions. The authors felt that addictive tendencies to drinking and smoking, found in over half their subjects, reflected a psychoanalytic factor of orality in the genesis of laryngeal cancer.

Webb and Irving (1964) stated that the emotional trauma resulting from the laryngectomy was temporary and reactive, and that it constituted only a minor factor in the personality patterns characteristic of the laryngectomee. They indicated that the trauma involved concern about bodily disfigurement and consequent social rejection; withdrawal tendencies and self-effacement; increased dependency needs, indicated by excessive demands for individual attention; and a reactive depression, so severe it could lead to suicide (there were three suicides and seven suicide attempts in their 77 patients).

Sako and associates (1974) concluded from their study of 85 patients that the emotional problems present before surgery were magnified by the new situation and its attendant trauma and by awareness of disease, inability to accept a new voice, lack of motivation, lack of practice, living alone, and reluctance to call attention to self and disability. They indicated that together these constituted the psychological concomitants of laryngectomy.

An extensive study of 188 Norwegian subjects was performed by Natvig (1983a) who utilized data obtained from interview responses to investigate a number of variables, including the relationships between premorbid adjustment patterns. Of his subjects, 43.5 per cent were judged as having either proven or indicated successful preoperative adjustment; 37.8 per cent were considered well adjusted but without clearly discernable preoperative adjustment patterns (e.g., had overcome alcoholism, were good spouses); 14.4 per cent had patterns of maladjustment (e.g., poor relations with neighbors, inability to support the family, alcohol abuse, and anxiety); and 4.3 per cent showed mixed preoperative adjustment patterns. Patients with good premorbid adjustment patterns often showed lower vulnerability to stress than did the patients judged as maladjusted and were better able to master the laryngectomy event. The explanation given by Natvig for some of those having good premorbid adjustment patterns but insufficient mastery of the laryngectomy event was "undoubtedly that normal voice and appearance were essential factors for their self-image, and their lack could not be accepted" (p. 161).

Specific Psychological Responses. A broad array of specific responses to the laryngectomy and its physical, social, and occupational concomitants have been discussed in the literature. The initial response to both the diagnosis and the surgery is usually emotional shock and trauma and often denial (Fontaine and Mitchell, 1960; Gates et al., 1982c; Heaver and colleagues, 1955; Lerman, 1966; Webb and Irving, 1964). Gates and co-workers (1982a) concluded that denial was common postoperatively. The found substantial denial in 47 per cent of their prospectively studied subjects and "distorted perceptions of reality" in another 35 per cent 6 months posttreatment. Fifteen per cent of their retrospectively studied subjects demonstrated substantial denial, and 49 per cent distorted perceptions of reality.

Associated with the shock are anxiety, worry, withdrawal, and depression (Fontaine and Mitchell, 1960; Green, 1979; J. Greene, 1947; Heaver and Arnold, 1962; Heaver and colleagues, 1955; Meyers et al., 1980; Webb and Irving, 1964). Gilchrist (1973) determined that nearly all of his 50 patients admitted some early anxiety and depression, lasting 6 months in most cases. Nine suffered severe depression lasting up to 12 months, but none required psychiatric referral. Johnson and co-workers (1979) found that the psychological profiles of the 25 subjects they interviewed revealed high degrees of depression and frustration.

Depression is the most common state encountered in rehabilitation failures, according to Bisi and Conley (1965). Associated with it are resentment of the stoma (mucus, crusts, and its offensiveness to esthetic feelings); distress from changes in eating and swallowing habits; loss of self-esteem, feelings of inferiority, and corollary feelings of rejection; fear of loss of friends, job, money, and prestige, and the associated fear of isolation; loss of interest in the world and self; and perhaps the abandonment of efforts to obtain speech training. In the late postoperative period, according to Morrison (1941), the patient is likely to suffer from mental depression because of social and economic barriers and burdens imposed by aphonia.

The most frequent factor related to depression has been speech. Loss of speech and failure to acquire speech readily or satisfactorily have been acknowledged as major causes of depression. Moreover, failure in speech acquisition has often been viewed as a result of depression.

Among those indicating speech loss and failure to acquire speech as causes of depression are Haase (in Drummond, 1967), who reported depression in 19 of 40 preoperative patients, due primarily to anticipated voice loss. Levin (1967) stated that the sudden silence is often very depressing unless patients have been adequately prepared for it preoperatively. Green (1979) maintained that a period of mental depression commonly follows laryngectomy but that it diminishes when the patient learns to compensate for the lost vocal function in one way or another. Bagshaw (1967) maintained that a delay in speech therapy may have such profound psychological effects, for example withdrawal and depression, that it becomes difficult to encourage the patient to obtain voice. The likelihood of depression and frustration resulting from failure to obtain esophageal voice was indicated by Bisi and Conley (1965).

A number of authors have suggested that depression is a significant determinant of speech acquisition and proficiency. (The discussion of this literature can be found in the section on emotional status and success in speech acquisition.) Gates and associates (1982a) also determined that depression, assessed by denial, poor self-image, and life attitude, was an adverse factor for successful overall rehabilitation (effective communication regardless of mode), a life style equivalent to pretreatment, and adequate psychological adjustment to disability in their 47 prospectively studied subjects.

Along with depression, which may occur at various times throughout an individual's adjustment to laryngectomy, other fluctuations in temperament may be found. A study of 40 German subjects (Haase, cited by Drummond, 1967) reported that the most frequent postoperative psychological reaction was increased affective irritability, thought to result from deprivation of the cathartic function of speech. Additionally, 17 patients had other reactions, including depression, jealousy, suspicion, and inferiority feelings.

Warner (1971) described certain temperamental differences among psychological factors that hamper speech acquisition. These included tension and overanxiety, which jeopardize speech through inability to relax physically; and mood changes, including anxiety, depression, and frustration, which accompany both the inability to communicate and the consequent social, work, and family problems resulting from that inability.

Reports from wives (Kommers and Sullivan, 1979) indicated that 58 per cent of the 45 husbands were more irritable after their surgery. When asked to specify personality and attitude changes following laryngectomy, approximately 36 per cent of the wives reported none, but 24 per cent reported depression and 27 per cent irritability. Frustration, especially with the inability to communicate or to develop esophageal speech, was specified by Fontaine and Mitchell (1960), Gardner (1971), and Bisi and Conley (1965) and was indicated as a prominent component in the psychological profile of the laryngectomee (Johnson et al., 1979).

Fears, anxiety, and worry occupy a relatively large portion of the literature concerned with the psychological responses of laryngectomized individuals. Usually they reflect concerns associated with the physical, social, and occupational concomitants of being laryngectomized, and often they were discussed as sources of depression. Among the specific fears, anxieties, and worries mentioned in the literature are recurrence of cancer, death, and survival; changes in anatomy and physiology, and their consequences; inability to speak; appearance and disfigurement; embarrassment and feelings of inferiority; loss of jobs, friends, prestige, and ego status; and old age and isolation.

Stoll (1958) suggested that certain personality changes can logically be expected, which he attributed to anxieties related to an array of fears associated with being laryngectomized. His array of preoperative fears included fear of the word "cancer" and its many semantic implications; of death, probably the paramount fear; and of permanent loss of voice. According to Stoll, the person's entire pattern of interpersonal relationships is threatened, and he worries about job loss, security, friends, and so forth. Stoll's catalogue of postoperative fears included recurrence of cancer and death; fears due to new physiological changes, involving lifting, stomal breathing, coughing, impaired senses of smell and taste, and cosmetic liabilities of the tracheostoma; fears of old age, aggravated by feelings of uselessness resulting from speech loss and often a root of depression; fear of inability to re-establish old interpersonal relationships; and fear associated with anticipation of failure to learn a new method of speaking.

Bagshaw's (1967) study of 123 laryngectomized subjects in Toronto indicated their major fears to be cancer and its threat of death, lost ability to communicate, and economic and social consequences. Bagshaw also suggested that patient reactions varied with their premorbid personalities but that they could be helped greatly by a rehabilitation program involving the surgeon, speech clinician, and family.

A study of 60 patients done by Minear and Lucente (1975) determined that their greatest preoperative fears included learning to speak again, cosmetic appearance, and being able to breathe adequately. Fear of death was admittedly the greatest fear, but this observation was offered by the subjects only after a while and circuitously.

Recurrence, death, and survival have probably constituted the most frequently acknowledged specific fears in the literature (Fontaine and Mitchell, 1960; Gardner, 1971; J. Greene, 1947; Heaver et al., 1955; Levin, 1967; Meyers et al., 1980; Webb and Irving, 1964; and others). Drummon (1967) claimed that the recently laryngectomized patient's first anxiety concerns survival. Beukelman and associates (1980) maintained that "the psychological impact of major surgery and fear of serious disease is present in all patients" (p. 717). Laguaite (1957) contended that "the very diagnosis of cancer often paralyzes the patient and he gives up completely with an attitude of 'what's the use' " (p. 86). Wallen and Webb (1975) established from 100 male and 100 female respondents, sampled from 2,000 returned questionnaires, that 38 per cent of the females and 33 per cent of the males were indeed worried about cancer recurrence.

Changes in anatomy and physiology and their consequent physical restrictions have been discussed in an earlier section. Among the authors who have acknowledged the psychological implications of these changes are Laguaite (1957), Bisi and Conley (1965), Levin (1967), King and colleagues (1971), and McNeil and co-workers (1981). They noted the increased need for caution and meticulous care, unnaturalness of functions, restrictions in activities and occupations, and associated adjustment problems accompanying these changes.

Lack of speech, the major physical concomitant of laryngectomy, has frequently been recognized in the literature as a primary source of anxiety. Stoll (1958) acknowledged this fact, stating that the rehabilitation program is entirely dependent on speech acquisition. Heaver and colleagues (1955) found anxiety related to speech loss and acquisition was expressed by all 224 patients they surveyed and that it pervaded the patient who could no longer talk.

Patient concerns about appearance and disfigurement have included both how they look and how they sound. Meyers and associates (1980) found disfigurement to be a fear that was documented by the literature; Thawley and associates (1983) suggested that the lack of development of good speech combined with cosmetic deformity, especially the permanent tracheostoma, tended to affect the psychological well-being of laryngectomized patients.

Bisi and Conley (1965) characterized laryngeal excision as representing a mutilation in both the strict physical sense and in its consequent deprivation of many important psychological functions. Along with numerous other writers, they also recognized the unnatural sound of esophageal voice as a source of consternation.

Gardner (1966) determined not only that many of his 240 female respondents were dismayed by the sound of their esophageal voices but that 50 per cent were also horrified by their surgical scars. Bagshaw (1967) contended from her study of 123 British patients that women tended to be more emotionally involved regarding their operations, because of being more affected by mutilation, highly aware of voice loss, and conscious of sounding like men. Bagshaw suggested that reassurance is needed if female subjects are to accept this difference.

Snidecor (1975) contended that laryngectomy is a cosmetic handicap for both male and female patients. He was supported by Wallen and Webb (1975), who determined that 52 per cent of their 100 female respondents and 29 per cent of their 100 male respondents, sampled from a pool of 2,000 questionnaires, reported worrying about how they looked.

Closely related to feelings of attractiveness and disfigurement are the acknowledgments in the literature of the sexual significance of being laryngectomized. Moses (1958) considered the larynx a secondary sex organ and discussed the castration complex he felt most men underwent after a laryngectomy. Parvulescu (1970) commented that surgical removal of the larynx has been viewed by many as a form of castration. Case histories were cited by Fontaine and Mitchell (1960) that they suggested indicated feelings of impotence in family roles and threats to masculinity. Such feelings have been substantiated more recently by questionnaire studies of wives (Kommers, et al., 1977; Kommers and Sullivan, 1979) and of laryngectomized subjects. Wallen and Webb (1975) found that only 44 per cent of their 100 female respondents and 38 per cent of the 100 male respondents considered themselves sexually attractive. Moreover, 8 per cent of the female respondents and 23 per cent of the male respondents expressed concern about their sexual lives. Thirty-three per cent of the 48 subjects studied by Meyers and co-workers (1980) indicated that their sex lives had changed since the operation; 40 per cent wished things could be different, and 18 per cent indicated that they felt less attractive.

Additional support for concerns regarding disfigurement was provided by Brouwer and associates (1979), who studied 50 European subjects, 50 per cent of whom reported their operations to be much worse than expected with regard to their speech disabilities and bodily mutilation. A significant implication of the Brouwer and co-workers study is that fear, worry, and anxiety may be due in part to inadequate patient preparation and counseling. Seven of these 50 subjects reported being unsatisfied with their preparation for the physical changes and speech changes, 2 of whom had received no preparation, and only 24 had discussed the results with their surgeons.

Embarrassment and feelings of disfigurement, both closely related to feelings about appearance and disfigurement, have also been cited frequently in the literature (Bagshaw, 1967; Bisi and Conley, 1965; Gardner, 1961, 1966, 1971; J. Greene, 1947; Haase, reported in Drummond, 1967; Heaver et al., 1955; Johnson et al., 1979; Nahum and Golden, 1963; Nicholson, 1975; Webb and Irving, 1964; and others). With regard to speech, Wallen and Webb (1975) found that 23 to 53 per cent of their subjects reported embarrassment with phoning and in speaking in front of groups and embarrassment with the sound of their voice, the percentages expressing embarrassment varying between men and women. J. Greene (1947) suggested that people dependent on voice for vocation suffered greater ego-deflation. Gates and colleagues (1982a) found self-image poorer postoperatively in 69 per cent of their subjects and attitudes to life poorer in 59 per cent.

Several writers have mentioned family oversolicitousness and overprotection, which to some extent probably reflect their awareness of the patient's changed status and possibly their own embarrassment and rejection. Johnson and colleagues (1966) indicated that their survey uncovered family reactions to physical changes in the patient and social embarrassment due to speech, stoma, and coughing, which they considered major unanticipated difficulties. Lerman (1966) suggested that depression and helplessness may be exaggerated and reinforced by an oversolicitous family. Laguaite (1957) stated that "probably the greatest psychological problem with which the speech therapist has to deal is the development of feelings or attitudes of fear, self-pity, or overprotection by the family" (p. 86). It seems logical to assume that attitudes of family members toward the acceptability of the changes resulting from a laryngectomy will significantly influence the attitude of the laryngectomized individual.

Fears regarding loss of jobs, friends, prestige, and ego status and those concerned with old age and isolation have generally been handled in the literature as components in an array of sources of depression and anxiety. Exemplary summaries were presented earlier in this section and in the sections dealing with the social and occupational concomitants of laryngectomy. The presence and significance of these fears have been affirmed by such clinical writers as J. Greene (1947), Stoll (1958), Fontaine and Mitchell (1960), Gardner (1961, 1971), Heaver and Arnold (1962), King and colleagues (1971), Meyers and co-workers (1980), and Davis (1981). Research substantiation in the form of interview and questionnaire responses by laryngectomees and their spouses have been provided by Horn (1962), Gardner (1966), Bagshaw (1967), Wallen and Webb (1975), Kommers and associates (1977), Kommers and Sullivan (1979), Brouwer and co-workers (1979), and Johnson and colleagues (1979).

Psychological Factors and Speech Proficiency. Many clinicians and researchers have attempted to explain why only approximately 60 to 70 per cent of laryngectomized individuals achieve readily intelligible and fluent speech (Snidecor, 1975) and what differentiates the 15 per cent who will have excellent intelligibility from the 55 per cent who are average speakers (Murry, 1974).

Assuming cancer control, two factors appear to be involved in speech acquisition following laryngectomy: (1) physiological alterations, which include the type and extent of surgery; postoperative physiological changes; amount and timing of pre- and postoperative radiation therapy; and the patient's postoperative physical status and other concomitant physical or medical problems (see section on Physical Concomitants); and (2) psychological alterations and psychosocial adjustment

(Gates et al., 1982a, 1983b; Schaefer and Johns, 1982). Inability to establish underlying anatomical or physiological factors to account for failure to develop speech in a number of patients and ascertainment that some patients are able to talk expertly with extensive surgical removal including most of the pharynx and portions of the tongue as well as the larynx (Putney, 1958; Ogura and Gershon, 1976) have led many to conclude that psychological factors may be more significant than organic factors as causes of failure.

Perhaps the most compelling support for this psychological view has been Diedrich and Youngstrom's (1966) conclusion, based on their own extensive anatomical and physiological data as well as those of other researchers, that ". . . esophageal speech skill following laryngectomy was not related to morphological function of the reconstructed hypopharynx and pharyngoesophageal junction. These results support those who believe that psychological factors are probably more important to the development of good speech than anatomical factors" (p. 61). Diedrich and Youngstrom suggested further that "the unknown variables of personality, motivation, family environment, and aspiration levels . . . may be more important than the physical variables in explaining why one-third of the laryngectomee population does not learn esophageal speech" (1966, p. 61).

Gardner (1971) proposed that there are two divisions of psychological factors influencing speech acquisition, emotional problems and motivation. Under emotional problems, he included introversion, brooding, withdrawal, depression, anxiety, and feelings of inferiority, rejection, and loss of self-esteem. He wrote that well-adjusted individuals may be expected to have fears and anxieties about the unknown. Regarding motivation, Gardner suggested that the need to make a living for the family, the desire to succeed in speech in order to regain prestige among friends and business associates, and seeking rather than avoiding friends portended a better likelihood of regaining speech. Gardner's insights were supported by Goldberg's (1975) conclusions following his study of the vocational, home, and social adjustment of 62 subjects: "The laryngectomee with greater motivation to return to work, with greater realistic assessment of his disability in relation to his interests, and with greater optimism about the future makes a better candidate for acquisition of intelligible speech" (p. 6).

The section dealing with psychological factors and speech proficiency reflects Gardner's (1971) dual categories of factors influencing speech acquisition, motivation, and emotional status. It modifies that orientation somewhat by acknowledging the personality and social variables often explored concurrently with emotional variables.

A number of writers have discussed the *importance of motivation for speech success* and its lack of significant contribution to failure. Morrison (1931, 1941), Brighton and Boone (1937), Levin (1940, 1952), Damsté, Van den Berg, and Moolinaar-Bijl (1956), Stoll (1958), Putney (1958), Horn (1962), Bisi and Conley (1965), Locke (1966), and Gardner (1966) considered motivation, including "willingness to learn," "self-discipline," "determination," "perseverance," "effort," "fortitude," "energy," and "industry" essential for esophageal speech mastery and the chief factor determining intelligibility.

Self-confidence and motivation to communicate again, according to Laguaite (1957, 1962), may be determined by feelings, attitudes, fears, and other tensions associated with laryngeal cancer. Poor motivation was considered by Griglione (1981) to be among the complicating factors that delay or hinder esophageal speech learning. Even with patients having internal shunts, Stallings (1981) felt that those who were not motivated were not likely to cooperate to the extent necessary for long-term voice restoration.

Several authors, notably MacComb (1966), have proposed a reduction in motivation associated with age as a factor in failure, suggesting that with approaching retirement individuals will not exert as great an effort. This idea was supported by DiBartolo (1971), who reasoned that the significantly lower age at surgery in his above-average speaker group reflected the heightened need to speak and its consequent "profound" motivation among those with longer life expectancies. Sako and associates (1974) also found that patients under 60 years of age were more likely to master esophageal speech and that retired patients did more poorly. Levin (1940) maintained that emotionally unstable and introverted patients required "constant prodding, encouragement, and the influence of the stronger will of the teacher" (p. 310). Horn (1962) felt that "someone must encourage, inspire, and literally drive" (p. 8) the laryngectomized individual to practice.

Among the writers reporting descriptive studies, lack of motivation and drive was considered by Warner (1971) to be a major deterrent to speech acquisition in her subjects, along with temperamental differences and social problems. Gilchrist (1973) felt that a lack of motivation, which might result from introversion, retirement from work, living alone, failure to persist when speech was not acquired rapidly, an overprotective wife, and insufficient fortitude or industry, was the most important factor among his 50 patients in failure to obtain good speech. Sixteen of the 21 patients of Gray and Konrad (1976) were unable to learn esophageal speech, 5 of whom "demonstrated disorganized mental status and/or poor motivation" (p. 142). Gardner (1966) determined that of his 240 female respondents, 91 per cent of those highly motivated to talk did so, whereas only 40 per cent of those who rejected esophageal speech developed it.

Two studies of motivation and speech proficiency involved controlled investigations utilizing psychological measures. Goldstein and Salmon (1978) found significantly higher mean scores on the Hutt Adaptation of the Bender-Gestalt Test (HABGT) Adience-Abience Scale, a measure of an individual's motivation to adapt to new experiences or to be inhibited from adapting, in their 15 esophageal speakers than in their 15 artificial larynx speakers. They also demonstrated a significant relationship between the motivation scores and judged speech proficiency in the artificial larynx and combined alaryngeal speaker groups but not in the esophageal speaker group alone. The lack of relationship to esophageal speech proficiency was thought possibly to reflect the smaller range of proficiency ratings obtained by that group. The authors concluded that the study demonstrated that a psychological variable contributing to differentiating alaryngeal speaker groups is also related to verbal communication proficiency.

Dabul and Lovestedt (1974) utilized both a questionnaire and a test battery (including the Gordon Personality Profile) to assess differences in ascendency, responsibility, emotional stability, attitudes, and other variables between a group of 16 "good" and 14 "poor" esophageal speakers. Neither the questionnaire as a whole nor its individual items, nor the four scales of the personality profile, differentiated between the two speaker groups. The authors concluded that they were unsuccessful in their attempts to isolate motivational, social, and personality differences between the groups.

Finally, a significant comment made by Natvig (1983c) and made earlier by Martin (1963) implies a need for caution regarding the relationship between speech acquisition and motivation: "Personal 'drive and motivation' indisputably influence acquisition of esophageal speech although many patients in possession of these qualities fail to achieve it" (Natvig, 1983c, p. 322).

Like that pertaining to motivation, the literature concerning *emotional, personality, and social status and success in speech acquisition* contains relatively few controlled studies. For the most part, the emotions, attitudes, and behaviors described in the sections on psychological impact, premorbid personality traits, and specific psychological responses were acknowledged as sources of speech delay or failure by the authors cited in those sections, usually on the basis of clinical experience, speculation, retrospective reviews of files, or interviews. As indicated by Salmon (1979), ". . . despite the numerous psychological characteristics that have in the past been suggested as related to esophageal speech rehabilitation, only a few have been shown to have such a relationship'' (p. 508).

The array of psychological factors associated by Sako and co-workers (1974) with speech rehabilitation and the importance placed on them by these authors appear to be fairly representative of the observations and speculations occurring throughout the literature. After discussing the physical factors established as important to speech acquisition by their review of 85 consecutive patients, they acknowledged a probably greater importance of the psychological factors revealed: psychological trauma concomitant with laryngectomy, awareness of the disease, inability to accept a new voice, lack of motivation, lack of practice, living alone, and emotional problems present before surgery but magnified by the new situation. They also indicated that the failure of some patients to use artificial larynxes was often related to reluctance to reveal their being disabled.

Additional factors impeding speech reported from patient series or questionnaire studies have included ''profound psychological effects of failure to obtain early therapy'' (p. 62), for example, withdrawal and depression (Bagshaw, 1967); fixed emotional attitudes, especially in women, including esthetic oversensitivity, fear that the new voice makes them conspicuous, and avoidance of attracting attention to themselves (Putney, 1958); loss of prestige and ego-satisfaction, frustration, embarrassment, and discouragement (Gardner, 1961, 1966); apathy about self and surroundings, loss of self-esteem, inferiority feelings, fear of rejection, passivity, and dependence (Bisi and Conley, 1965); and fear of recurrence, hypochondria, obsessive-compulsive reactions, paranoid reactions, and lack of self-confidence (Laguaite, 1962).

Two articles (Laguaite, 1962; Bisi and Conley, 1965) acknowledged secondary gains associated with failure to develop effective speech, which enable the individual to escape responsibility and fulfill needs associated with dependency, fear, aggression, insecurity, masochism, and self-pity. These would mediate against speech acquisition. One article (Locke, 1966) suggested that an extroverted personality, an outlook geared to the future, and involvement in professional and social activities made speech retraining easier.

Two relatively recent studies, one using retrospective review of case files (Volin, 1980) and the other extensive interviews (Natvig, 1983c) (but both subjecting their data to statistical analysis) were designed to relate speech acquisition and proficiency to psychosocial variables.

Volin (1980) explored 24 variables (14 of which could be classified as psychosocial) ascertained from the medical records of 59 New York City Veterans Administration patients to establish relationship with (1) achievement of socially functional conversational speech, either esophageal or artificial laryngeal and (2) achievement of esophageal as opposed to artificial laryngeal speech. Negative values of five variables that could be considered psychosocial, the first three of which were actually socioeconomic, related significantly to failure to regain functional speech: preoperative employment status, adequacy of income planning for hospitalization needs, dependency status in living arrangements, extrafamilial relationships, and consistency of attendance in therapy. Only one variable, motivation for therapy, differentiated between the esophageal and the artificial laryngeal speakers. No variable distinguished differences in both speech outcome and voice type. The following variables were not related to either criterion: alcohol consumption, tobacco consumption, history of alcohol abuse, history of psychological disorder, self-care (grooming and stoma care), and familial relationships.

Natvig (1983c) explored the relationship between three personal and behavioral variables (preoperative adjustment patterns, present mastery of laryngectomy event, and assumed vulnerability to stressful events), certain situational and social variables, and esophageal speech acquisition in 188 Norwegian subjects. Ratings of these and other variables were made by the author during structured interviews in the subjects' homes that lasted an average of 3.5 hours. Seventy per cent of the subjects had esophageal speech (63 per cent rated as "socially acceptable" and seven per cent as "poor"), 27.5 per cent had no esophageal speech, and 2.5 per cent had tracheoesophageal shunt speech. Acquisition of "socially acceptable esophageal speech" (speech that was reasonably easily understood at interview) was significantly more frequent among younger patients and those having assumed lower vulnerability to stressful events. Preoperative maladjustment and insufficient mastery of the laryngectomy event significantly reduced the capability for acquiring acceptable speech, but alcohol consumption, education, and marital status of time of surgery had no effect.

Eight controlled studies using psychological measures and statistical analysis of data have explored the personality and socioemotional characteristics of laryngectomees and related these traits to speech.

Barton and Hejna (1963) investigated the effects of motivation (determined from a written questionnaire regarding time spent in practice, frequency of lessons, and feelings regarding therapy) and personality (responses to the California Test of Personality) in 16 subjects, none of whom had physical factors preventing esophageal speech. Eight of the subjects were rated as very successful esophageal speakers and eight as unsuccessful. The two groups differed greatly on two self-adjustment factors from the personality measure: self-reliance and sense of personal worth. Differences were also found in family relations, occupational relations, community relations, mental ability, and social standards, the last variable being the only one on which the unsuccessful group had a higher mean. The authors concluded that patients who displayed better overall personality adjustment, who were more greatly motivated, were more intelligent, and did not hold to excessively high social standards, were more successful in speech acquisition than those possessing opposite attributes.

Shames, Font, and Matthews (1963) studied 108 esophageal and 35 artificial larynx speakers using a test of 15 normal personality needs (The Edwards Personality Preference Schedule), a questionnaire exploring personality and social behavior, and five measures of speech proficiency. The esophageal speakers had significant correlations involving nine personality needs and four speech measures; and the artificial larynx speakers had three significant correlations involving two needs and three speech measures. All 14 of these coefficients were low (.54 or less) and no patterns were obvious to the reviewer or discussed by the authors. Three correlations between personality-social questionnaire responses and speech measures were significant, but only in the artificial larynx group: difficult adjustment for family, speech problem as a source of embarrassment, and length of time of social withdrawal. These suggested that speech and social contingencies that were present to a greater extent in the speech appliance users may have been important in their electing the appliance over esophageal speech. The esophageal speakers showed a greater need to conform and to influence others and less need to persist with a task, but these could not be established as either presurgical or posttherapy personality traits and hence were not interpretable.

Webb and Irving (1964) analyzed past recollections, demographic data, and Szondi psychological profiles from 77 laryngectomized patients and compared them with similar measures from normal persons, institutionalized veterans, and emphysematous patients. Their conclusions regarding the personality of laryngectomees have been described in the earlier section on premorbid personality traits. Regarding speech rehabilitation, they concluded that the personality difficulties of laryngectomees rendered them atypical students in need of a holistic approach, with rehabilitation being more a psychotherapeutic problem than a pedagogical one.

Studying 94 male subjects divided into above-average, average, below-average, and nonesophageal speaker groups, DiBartolo (1971) determined that the average and above speakers had significantly higher self- and body-concepts and that the below-average speakers had higher anxiety levels and lower defensive distortion for maintaining self-esteem. Of particular interest was the finding that the scores of the nonesophageal speakers were more similar to those of the average and above esophageal speakers than to those of the below-average group on a number of measures. DiBartolo suggested that this finding reflected the higher communication capacity resulting from use of artificial laryngeal devices by some of the nonesophageal but none of the below-average esophageal speakers. No difference was found among the groups on two measures: integration of self-concept and overt-covert anxiety ratio (a measure of defensiveness).

Amster and associates (1972) completed a two-phase study. The first involved 20 laryngectomized speakers, 10 nonlaryngeal malignancy surgical patients, and 8 subjects without history of malignancy, all male veterans. Psychological status (including social service assessment of social adjustment, intelligence, anxiety, level of aspiration, and frustration tolerance) and speech intelligibility (words and sentences) were assessed. The second phase occurred 3 years later and involved 18 of the original laryngectomized subjects whose speech intelligibility and social adjustment were reassessed, and who indicated whether their speech had improved, regressed, or remained the same. Phase One revealed no psychosocial variables that clearly differentiated either among the three subject groups or among the laryngectomized subjects with respect to speech intelligibility. Although significant positive correlation coefficients were obtained between speech intelligibility scores and achievement motive, anxiety level, and verbal intelligence, they were of insufficient magnitude to be considered predictive. Phase Two results indicated only a moderate relationship between speech intelligibility and months postsurgery, with no significant gains after 24 months and no marked changes in social adjustment.

Keith and colleagues (1974) found that the only psychological factor that correlated significantly with the Wepman Scale ratings of speech proficiency of their 49 male subjects at their initial 3 month check-up was the MMPI (Minnesota Multiphasic Personality Inventory) depression scale. The authors concluded that patient reactions to their illness and operation may influence esophageal speech learning negatively, but that the correlation ($r = 0.31$) indicated that the relationship was not high. Some may learn speech in spite of depression, and some having only mild depression may have difficulty. They suggested that their findings indicated that the importance of psychological factors may not be as great as indicated in the literature.

Using 58 subjects receiving speech therapy at the same New York City center, Blake (1974) explored relationships between MMPI scores, obtained before and 4 months after initiation of therapy, and esophageal speech proficiency. Four personality measures related significantly to speech: hypochondriasis, social introversion, schizophrenia, and a scale used to predict patient acceptance of the therapeutic situation (F scale). Subjects scoring lower on these scales prior to therapy tended to achieve higher speech proficiency. Stepwise regression analysis indicated that the F scale, lie score, depression, psychasthenia, and schizophrenia measures were most influential, all relating negatively. Although no significant changes in personality traits occurred as therapy progressed, significant increases in speech proficiency occurred as K scale (a scale assessiguardedness and defensiveness) and psychopathic deviate scale scores decreased. Analysis of the 23 subjects who "dropped out" of therapy before 4 months revealed higher pretherapy MMPI scores across all traits, significantly so for depression, psychopathic deviate, schizophrenia, hysteria, and hypochondriasis.

Blake (1974) concluded that the poor speakers tended to be more socially withdrawn, have less self-confidence, lack the drive and motivation necessary to learn esophageal speech, and worry more about their health, the last of which might diminish the degree and the duration of drive required to learn esophageal speech. He thought that personality plays an important role in successful acquisition of esophageal speech, and that the lack of personality trait changes across time reflected concentration on teaching motor patterns rather than on changing attitudes, perceptions, and feelings. Blake indicated that changes in attitudes, perceptions, and feelings would be relevant additions to teaching esophageal speech.

Gates and colleagues (1982b) found only one psychological test item that differentiated between their 12 subjects who acquired speech and the 35 who did not, Factor I of the Sixteen Personality Factor Questionnaire, which indicated that the esophageal speakers were more tender minded than those not achieving esophageal speech. No differences were evident in Bender Gestalt, Attitude to Disabled Persons, and Fundamental Interpersonal Orientations tests, nor in 18 existential concerns, attitudes toward life, self-images, social lives, or uses of denial.

The 26 persons who were considered "successfully rehabilitated" (had effective communication regardless of method, returned to a life style equivalent to their preoperative condition, and had adequate psychological adjustment to their disability) demonstrated significantly greater denial; reported significantly more declines in social life, self-image and life attitudes; and were more imaginative, more independent, and more self-assured than their counterparts. All 12 esophageal speakers were included in the rehabilitated group. Depression, as indicated by denial, poor self-image and life attitudes, and decreased social activity, affected rehabilitation adversely.

Psychological Abnormality Versus Phases of Adjustment to Disability

The review of the literature regarding the psychological concomitants of being laryngectomized gives rise to a concern for statements and findings that may imply that laryngectomees constitute a psychologically abnormal population. References to failure reflecting dependency, weakness, inability or unwillingness to assume responsibility for life or to cope with misfortune, and to premorbid personality deficits, are scattered through the literature. As suggested earlier, an assumption underlying this implication is probably the one that presumes a psychogenic cause when physiological explanations for failure cannot be isolated.

As suggested by Green (1979), although it is easy to blame a lack of motivation for the failure to develop esophageal speech, there is a lack of both objective data supporting the hypothesis and instances of highly motivated individuals having difficulty with speech acquisition. Some writers have maintained that psychological "problems" are not consistent predictors of speech success. Keith and co-workers (1974) proposed that many depressed individuals do achieve speech and many without acute signs of depression do not. Natvig (1983d) proposed the same with regard to motivation.

Gates and associates (1982c) took issue with the literature's suggestion that laryngectomees typically are helpless, unwilling to assume responsibility for their own care, and dependent on spouse and therapist and that these traits develop from inability to communicate, postoperative depression, and a basic personality of the laryngeal cancer patient that is passive and dependent on cigarette smoking and other habits for a sense of well-being. They suggested that

> rather than project such negative feelings upon the patient, it would be more appropriate to recognize the period of grief that the patient must work through, the substantial psychic trauma that must realistically occur after loss of a major body part, and the deprivation of a lifetime's habit of verbal communication. To ascribe an authentic helplessness to a presumed personality deficit may be inaccurate as well as counterproductive to the rehabilitation process. Although some cancer patients do indeed have characteristics of the passive-dependent person, it would be too simplistic to extend this generalization to all laryngeal cancer patients; nor would it be useful to do so. (p. 98)

A more positive and productive approach has been presented by Athelstan (1981), who stated that

> considering the many negative effects of disability, it is only natural that the onset of a major disability will often be accompanied by significant emotional reactions. A useful way of describing the reactions that can occur is to examine the response to crises occurring over time. (p. 15)

Shontz (1965) has proposed a stage formulation involving a series of five phases of adjustment: shock, realization, defensive retreat, acknowledgment, and adaptation: "Each of these phases is accompanied by a characteristic emotional experience, and the predominant emotional reaction changes as a person progresses through the phases of adjustment."

Specific applications of stage formulation (i.e., stages of grief) to speech disorders are discussed by Potter and Schneiderman (1979) and by Tanner (1980).

SUMMARY AND CONCLUSIONS

The literature concerning the physical concomitants of being laryngectomized indicates that the percentage of patients acquiring esophageal speech varies considerably. In general, 60 to 70 per cent learn to speak esophageally, but the degree of proficiency within that group also tends to vary. The extent to which this variability is accounted for by physical or by psychological factors is an enigma.

A wide variety of physical problems other than speech compound the rehabilitation problems faced by the laryngectomee. These include impaired nonspeech communication, sensation, and biological functions; physical limitations; and problems associated with age and illness.

The social concomitants of being laryngectomized can be widespread, involving spouse, family, friends, and the community at large. Family problems relate to communication impairment, sexual adjustment, financial problems, changed social relationships, occupation, attitudes, and behaviors. Social stigma is a significant component of the social domain.

The occupational concomitants of being laryngectomized may involve changed employment and employment status. These changes may reflect physical changes, stigma, and patient attitudes or motivation. Changes may also occur in recreational pursuits. Both the vocational and the recreational changes may result in reductions of rewards, status, and ego-satisfaction.

The literature regarding the psychological concomitants of being laryngectomized describes an array of emotions, personality traits, and behaviors. Different authors describe different arrays. It appears that psychological responses to a laryngectomy vary as a function of time, reflecting two major periods. The initial period can be considered "perisurgical," commencing with suspicion or confirmation of laryngeal cancer and extending through completion of medical treatment of the cancer. The major focus at this time is on preserving life, acknowledging obvious physical changes (loss of speech, inability to breathe nasally, and so on) and perhaps vaguely acknowledging occupational, social, and psychological consequences. The psychological reactions of this period may include shock, fear, denial, depression, avoidance, embarrassment, anxiety, and problems associated with personal identity and ego crisis.

The second period is "postsurgical," commencing essentially after medical management of the tumor and extending through long-range adaptations to some physical changes and many increasingly explicit and complex speech, social, occupational, and psychological changes. This period is completed when the individual is rehabilitated (has achieved effective communication, a life style equivalent to pretreatment, and adequate psychological adjustment to his disabilities). The postsurgical period is characterized by many of the same psychological reactions that occurred presurgically, notably anxiety, denial, depression, withdrawal, embarrassment, and reduced motivation.

Contributions to the psychological literature can be viewed as having taken two primary forms. The first involved descriptions of responses by laryngectomees to their presurgical and postsurgical experiences and of psychological characteristics presumed overtly or covertly to be characteristic of the population. These articles relied heavily on observations made informally in the clinic or systematically with interviews and questionnaires. Many of the conclusions were speculative, a few were based on descriptive statistics, and occasionally probabilities were assessed. Controlled studies are lacking.

The second group of psychological articles consisted of attempts to establish factors preventing, impeding, or facilitating rehabilitation. The majority of these explored esophageal speech acquisition. Factors relating to social and vocational rehabilitation have been studied infrequently, and usually only with items constituting part of a questionnaire. These prognostic articles were also dominated by clinical interview, questionnaire observations, and speculation. Only eight controlled studies relating to speech acquisition were uncovered across a 23 year period.

Several articles have discussed the influence of premorbid personality traits on both psychological responses and on success in speech acquisition. For the most part these have been speculative.

None of the emotions, personality traits, and behaviors discussed in the literature have been consistently or conclusively found to typify the responses of the laryngectomized population to their circumstances or to explain why they do or do not succeed in adjusting, notably in acquiring speech.

This literature review suggests some problem areas, notably in the psychological domain.

1. Much of the work is old and based on subjective observations. Where applied, statistical analyses have relied primarily on correlation, and the coefficients obtained have generally been low. Many of the original assumptions continue to be expressed. It appears that some have almost become dogma. For example, failure implies problems with motivation; people "demonstrating" reduced motivation fail; depression prevents successful rehabilitation; use of an artificial larynx is reserved only for people who fail to learn esophageal speech and introduced only after prolonged periods of unsuccessful attempts to develop esophageal speech; use of an artificial larynx inhibits or precludes learning esophageal speech; premorbid personality traits are the primary determinants of success. Accepting the dogma may increase clinical failure by precluding explanation of other physical or psychosocial factors that are blocking progress. It

may increase the number of unrejected null hypotheses in the literature by precluding appropriate research designs. For example, client expectations may be significant determiners of depression or motivation, and failure to establish levels and controls for these variables may obscure significant findings. Both better-trained clinicians and more controlled research are needed.

2. Consistent psychological profiles describing the laryngectomized group as a whole or differentiating among successfully rehabilitated patients and "failures" have not been established. Some research findings are contradictory. These may reflect a number of research problems.

    a. Many of the psychological factors explored are ambiguous, subjective, and defined differently by different investigators. For example, motivation was defined as a score on a test of adience-abience by Goldstein and Salmon (1978) and inferred from attendance at therapy or even from successful acquisition of esophageal speech by Levin (1940, 1952).

    b. Psychological responses may be highly susceptible to management procedures. For example, surgical procedures facilitating rapid voice acquisition may increase success and motivation and reduce depression and withdrawal. Patients managed by integrated rehabilitation teams may be more successful than those handled otherwise, as suggested in the literature (e.g., Natvig, 1983d).

    c. Psychological measures, when they have been used in controlled studies, have tended to be those appropriate for assessing individuals having clinically significant psychological problems. It may be that the problems of the laryngectomee are more superficial and transitory. This possibility was suggested by Webb and Irving's (1964) conclusion that the associated emotional trauma is temporary and involves general posttraumatic depression usually following major surgery. It is also suggested by the five phases of adjustment proposed by Shontz (1965).

    d. Sample sizes have often been small, and samples have been drawn from restricted geographical areas and from single practices or agencies (e.g., Veterans Administration hospitals). Responses have often not been substantiated. For example, descriptions of procedures designed to assure reliable and valid responses to questionnaires or interviews have not been described. Most studies have been retrospective and the subjects tend to have been "long-term" survivors. Problems encountered by terminal patients and their families have not generally been reflected. Inferential statistics and multivariate analyses have rarely been used. The designs used have not permitted establishment of the "multiple co-existing factors which interact in a complex manner to facilitate or hinder the development of esophageal speech" (Martin, 1976, cited in Salmon, 1979, p. 509).

   e. It appears that there may be an implicit assumption that the laryngectomized population is a homogeneous group. For instance, although the literature suggests that age may be a significant determiner of motivation and of success, few of the eight "controlled studies" reviewed in the section on psychological factors took age into consideration, and none controlled for it. As suggested earlier, rapidity of success may also be a significant variable to be controlled when exploring psychological variables.

Homogeneity is an important clinical concept, as well. Recognition of individual differences is an essential prerequisite for responsible clinical management.

QUESTIONS

1. How do Gates and his co-workers (Gates and Hearn, 1982; Gates et al., 1982a, 1982c) explain their recent finding of a lower per cent of patients who did well in speech rehabilitation compared to patients in earlier studies?
2. Compare the overall success rates of TEP patients using prostheses with those of standard esophageal voice production.
3. What four uncertainties about the future contribute to King, Marshall, and Gunderson's (1971) "nightmare" effect?
4. How might the male spouse's reaction to the female patient's using esophageal voice (Gardner, 1966) differ from female spouse's reactions to a male esophageal speaker?
5. What do Heaver and Arnold (1962) and Ogura and Gershon (1976) suggest to lessen the effects of postoperative depression and isolation of laryngectomees?
6. List some social symptoms of reduced hearing function that might flag the clinician's suspicion that hearing decrement might be causing retarded rates of learning esophageal voice in his or her patients.
7. What is one possible explanation as to why laryngectomees may have problems lifting heavy weights?
8. What evidence suggests that laryngectomized patients' marriages are not disturbed by the surgical event?
9. Elaborate on the statement "Postoperative financial status influences life style for laryngectomized patients."

10. What programs might you as a clinician institute to help ward off negative biases in business and professional men, found by Gilmore (1974), about employing laryngectomized individuals?
11. List behaviors a clinician might adopt to build a client's self-image regarding physical appearance and another list of behaviors to build a sense of success in rehabilitation.
12. How might the four domains considered in this chapter (physical, social, occupational, and psychological concomitants of laryngectomy) contribute separately and interactively to the psychosocial status of a given patient?

REFERENCES

✓Amster, W., Love, R., Menzel, O., Sandler, J., Sculthorpe, W., and Gross, R. (1972). Psycho-social factors and speech after laryngectomy. *J. Commun. Dis., 5,* 1–18.

Athelstan, G. (1981). Psychosocial adjustment to chronic disease and disability. In W. Stolov and M. Clowers (Eds.), *Handbook of severe disability* (13–18). Washington, DC.: U.S. Dept. of Education, Rehabilitation Services Administration.

Bagshaw, M. (1967). Rehabilitation of post-laryngectomy patients. *Brit. J. Dis. Commun., 2,* 54–63.

Barton, J., and Hejna, R. (1963). Factors associated with success and non-success in acquisition of esophageal speech. *J. Speech Hear. Res., 4,* 19–20.

✓Barton, R. (1965). Life after laryngectomy. *Laryngoscope, 75,* 1408–1415.

? Beamer, M. W. (1954). A qualitative study of the personality adjustment of laryngectomized subjects. Unpublished master's thesis, Texas State College for Women, Denton.

Berlin, C. (1964). Hearing loss, palatal function, and other factors in post-laryngectomy rehabilitation. *J. Chron. Dis., 17,* 677–684.

Beukelman, D., Cummings, C., Dobie, R., and Weymuller, M., Jr. (1980). Objective assessment of laryngectomized patients with surgical reconstruction. *Arch. Otolaryngol., 106,* 715–718.

✓ Bisi, R., and Conley, J. (1965). Psychologic factors influencing vocal rehabilitation of the post-laryngectomy patient. *Ann. Otol. Rhinol. Laryngol., 75,* 1073–1078.

? Blake, I. (1974, November). Relationship between personality and esophageal speech proficiency. Paper presented at annual convention of the American Speech-Language and Hearing Association, Las Vegas, NV.

✓ Blanchard, S. L. (1982). Current practices in counseling of the laryngectomy patient. *J. Commun. Dis., 15,* 233–241.

Blom, E., Singer, M., and Hamaker, R. (1985). An improved esophageal insufflation test. *Arch. Otolaryngol., 111,* 211–212.

Brighton, G., and Boone, W. (1937). Roentgenographic demonstration of method of speech in cases of complete laryngectomy. *Am. J. Roentgen., 38,* 571–583.

✓ Brouwer, B., Snow, G., and Van Dam, F. (1979). Experiences of patients who undergo laryngectomy. *Clin. Otolaryngol., 4,* 109–118.

Cogswell, B. (1967). Rehabilitation of the paraplegic: Processes of socialization. *Sociology Inquiry, 37,* 11–26.

Coyne, J. M., Stram, J., Payton, O., Klein, G., and Gressler, J. (1968). The laryngectomee and lifting. *Arch. Otolaryngol., 88,* 80–83.

Dabul, B., and Lovestedt, L. (1974). Prognostic indicators of esophageal speech. *J. Surg. Oncol., 5,* 461–469.

Damsté, P. H. (1975). Methods of restoring the voice after laryngectomy. *Laryngoscope, 85,* 649–655.

Damsté, P., Van den Berg, J., and Moolinaar-Bijl, A. (1956). Why are some patients unable to learn esophageal speech? *Ann. Otol., 65,* 998–1105.

Darvill, G. (1983). Rehabilitation—not just voice. In Y. Edels (Ed.), *Laryngectomy: Diagnosis to rehabilitation* (pp. 192–217). London: Aspen Systems Corp.

Davis, P. (1981). Rehabilitation after total laryngectomy. *Med. J. Australia, 1,* 396–400.

DeBeule, G., and Damsté, P. (1972). Rehabilitation following laryngectomy: Results of a questionnaire study. *Brit. J. Disord. Commun., 7,* 141–147.

DiBartolo, R. (1971). Psychological considerations in the attainment of esophageal speech. *J. Surg. Oncol., 3,* 451–466.

Diedrich, W., and Youngstrom, K. (1966). *Alaryngeal speech.* Springfield, IL: Charles C Thomas.

Drummond, S. (1967). Vocal rehabilitation after laryngectomy. *Brit. J. Disord. Commun., 2,* 39–44.

Erskine, M. (1979). Treatment of the laryngectomy patient. *Ear, Nose, and Throat J., 58,* 82–83.

Fontaine, A., and Mitchell, J. (1960). Esophageal voice: A factor of readiness. *J. Laryngol. Otol., 74,* 870–876.

Gardner, W. (1961). Problems of laryngectomees. *Rehab. Record., 2,* 15–18.

Gardner, W. (1966). Adjustment problems of laryngectomized women. *Arch. Otolaryng., 83,* 31–42.

Gardner, W. (1971). *Laryngectomee speech and rehabilitation.* Springfield, IL: Charles C Thomas.

Gates, G., and Hearne, E. (1982). Predicting esophageal speech. *Annals Otol. Rhinol. Laryngol., 91,* 454–457.

Gates, G., Ryan, W., Cantu, E., and Hearne, E. (1982b). Current status of laryngectomee rehabilitation: II. Causes of failure. *Am. J. Otolaryngol., 3,* 8–14.

Gates, G., Ryan, W., Cooper, J., Lawlis, G. F., Cantu, E., Hayashi, T., Lauder, E., Welch, R., and Hearne, E. (1982a). Current status of laryngectomee rehabilitation: I. Results of therapy. *Am. J. Otolaryngol., 3,* 1–7.

Gates, G., Ryan, W., and Lauder, E. (1982c). Current status of laryngectomee rehabilitation: IV. Attitudes about laryngectomee rehabilitation should change. *Am. J. Otolaryngol., 3,* 97–103.

Gibbs, H., and Achterberg-Lewis, J. (1979). The spouse is facilitator for esophageal speech: A research perspective. *J. Surg. Oncology, 11,* 89–94.

Gilchrist, A. (1973). Rehabilitation after laryngectomy. *Acta Otolaryngol., 75,* 511–518.

Gilmore, S. I. (1961). Rehabilitating laryngectomees. *J. Rehab., 26,* 28–29.

Gilmore, S. I. (1974). Social and vocational acceptability of esophageal speakers compared to normal speakers. *J. Speech Hear. Res., 17,* 599–607.

Goldberg, R. T. (1975). Vocational and social adjustment after laryngectomy. *Scand. J. Rehab. Med., 7,* 1–8.

Goldstein, L., and Salmon, S. (1978). The relationship between adience-abience scale scores and judged communication proficiency of alaryngeal speakers. *Laryngoscope, 88,* 1855–1860.

Gray, S., and Konrad, H. (1976). Laryngectomy: Post-surgical rehabilitation of communication. *Arch. Phys. Med. Rehab., 57,* 140–142.

Green, G. (1979). Esophageal speech: Why the failures? A literature review. *Australian J. Commun. Dis., 7,* 51–62.

✓Greene, J. (1947). Laryngectomy and its psychologic implications. *N.Y. State J. Med., 47,* 53–56.

Greene, J. (1949). Speech rehabilitation following laryngectomy. *Am. J. Nursing, 49,* 1–2.

? Greene, J., and Faulkner, W. B. (1940). Objective esophageal changes due to psychic factors, an esophagoscope study. *Am. J. Med. Sci., 130,* 796–803.

Greene, M. C. L. (1967). Management of aphonia after surgical treatment of carcinoma of the larynx, pharynx and esophagus. *Brit. J. Disord. Commun., 2,* 134–145.

Griglione, D. (1981). Nonsurgical restoration of communication for the laryngectomee. *Ear, Nose, Throat J., 60,* 286–289.

Hamaker, R., Singer, M., Blom, E., and Daniels, H. (1985). Primary voice restoration at laryngectomy. *Arch. Otolaryngol., 111,* 182–186.

Heaver, L., and Arnold, G. (1962). Rehabilitation of alaryngeal aphonia. *Postgrad. Med., 32,* 11–17.

Heaver, L., White, W., and Goldstein, N. (1955). Clinical experience in restoring oral communication to 274 laryngectomized patients by esophageal voice. *J. Am. Geriat. Soc., 3,* 687–690.

Horn, D. (1962, August). *Laryngectomee survey report summary.* Presented at the 11th annual meeting of the International Association of Laryngectomees, Memphis, TN.

Hudson, A. (1967). An approach to the rehabilitation of the laryngectomized veteran. *Brit. J. Disord. Commun. Dis., 2,* 45–53.

Hunt, R. (1964). Rehabilitation of the laryngectomee. *Laryngoscope, 74,* 382–395.

Jackson, C., and Jackson, C. L. (1937). *The larynx and its diseases.* Philadelphia: W. B. Saunders.

Jesberg, N. (1956). Speech after laryngectomy. *Med. Times, 84,* 1312.

Johnson, C. (1960). A survey of laryngectomee patients in Veterans Administration Hospitals. *Arch. Otolaryngol., 72,* 768–773.

Johnson, J., Casper, J., and Lesswing, N. (1979). Toward the total rehabilitation of the alaryngeal patient. *Laryngoscope, 89,* 1813–1819.

Kashima, H., and Kalinowski, B. (1979). Taste impairment following laryngectomy. *Ear, Nose, Throat J., 58,* 88–92.

Keith, R., Ewert, J., and Flowers, C. (1974). Factors influencing the learning of esophageal speech. *Brit. J. Disord. Commun., 9,* 110–116.

Keith, R. L., and Shanks, J. C. (1983). Laryngectomee rehabilitation: Past and present in speech and language. *Advances in basic research and practice, Vol. 9* (pp. 103–152). New York: Academic Press.

Killarney, G., and Lass, N. (1979). A comparative study of the knowledge, exposure and attitude of speech pathologists, rehabilitation counselors and social workers toward laryngectomized persons. *J. Rehab., 44,* 34–38.

King, P., Fowlks, E., and Pierson, G. (1968). Rehabilitation and adaptation of laryngectomy patients. *Am. J. Physical Med., 47,* 192–203.

King, P., Lewis, F., Weddle, J., and Fowlks, E. (1973). Effect of radical neck dissection on total rehabilitation of the laryngectomee. *Am. J. Phys. Med., 52,* 1-17.

King, P., Marshall, R., and Gunderson, H. (1971). Management of the older laryngectomee. *Geriatrics, 26,* 112-118.

√ Kommers, M., and Sullivan, M. (1979). Wives' evaluation of problems related to laryngectomy. *J. Commun. Dis., 12,* 411-430.

Kommers, M., Sullivan, M., and Yonkers, A. (1977). Counseling the laryngectomized patient. *Laryngoscope, 87,* 1961-1965.

Laguaite, J. (1957). Techniques of therapy for the laryngectomized patient. *Southern Speech J., 23,* 79-86.

√ Laguaite, J. (1962). Psychological and social problems of the laryngectomized individual. ASHA Short Course on Esophageal Speech, New York, NY.

Lauder, E. (1968). The laryngectomee and the artificial larynx. *J. Speech Hear. Dis., 33,* 146-157.

Lauder, E. (1970). The laryngectomee and the artificial larynx—a second look. *J. Speech Hear. Dis., 35,* 62-65.

Lerman, J. W. (1966). Alaryngeal voice production. *Connecticut Med., 29,* 271-272.

Levin, N. (1940). Teaching the laryngectomized patient to talk. *Arch. Otolaryngol., 32,* 299-314.

Levin, N. (1952). Speech rehabilitation after total removal of the larynx. *J. Am. Med. Assoc., 208,* 1281-1286.

Levin, N. (1967). Rehabilitation after total laryngectomy. *Eye, Ear, Nose, Throat Monthly, 46,* 756-762.

Levy, J., and Abramson, A. (1983). Immediate verbal communication following laryngectomy. *Bull, N.Y. Acad. Med., 59,* 306-312.

√ Locke, B. (1966). Psychology of the laryngectomee. *Military Med., 131,* 593-599.

Lowry, W. (1975). Alcoholism in cancer of the head and neck. *Laryngoscope, 85,* 1275-1280.

MacComb, W. (1966). Cancer of the larynx. *Cancer, 19,* 149-156.

Martin, D. E. (1976). The relationship between esophageal speech proficiency and selected measures of auditory function. In *Proceedings of the Laryngectomy Rehabilitation Seminar: A Supplement.* Rochester, MN: Mayo Clinic.

Martin, D., Hoops, H., and Shanks, J. (1974). Relationship between esophageal speech proficiency and selected measures of auditory function. *J. Speech Hear. Dis., 17,* 80-85.

Martin, H. (1963). Rehabilitation of the laryngectomee. *Cancer, 16,* 823-841.

McDonald, E. (1949, June). The rehabilitation of the laryngectomized. A.M.A. Scientific Exhibit, Atlantic City, NJ.

√ McNeil, B., Weichselbaum, M., and Pauker, S. (1981). Speech survival tradeoffs between quality and quantity of life in laryngeal cancer. *New Engl. J. Med., 305,* 982-987.

Meyers, A. D., Aarons, B., Suzuki, B., and Pilcher, L. (1980). Sexual behavior following laryngectomy. *Ear, Nose, Throat J., 59,* 327-329.

√ Minear, D., and Lucente, F. D. (1979). Current attitudes of laryngectomy patients. *Laryngoscope, 89,* 1061-1065.

Morrison, W. (1931). The production of voice and speech after total laryngectomy. *Arch. Otolaryngol., 14,* 413-423.

Morrison, W. (1941). Physical rehabilitation of the laryngectomized patient. *Arch. Otolaryngol., 34,* 1101-1112.

Moses, P. (1958). Rehabilitation of the post-laryngectomized patient; the vocal therapist and contributions to the rehabilitation program. *Ann. Otol., 67,* 538–543.

Murry, T. (1974). In P. Alberti and P. Bryce (Eds.), Biophysical requirements for new and projected procedures and devices for voice rehabilitation after total laryngectomy. *Centennial conference on laryngeal cancer* (pp. 585–586). New York: Appleton Century-Crofts.

Nahum, A., and Golden, J. (1963). Psychological problems of laryngectomy. *J. Am. Med. Assoc., 186,* 1136–1138.

Natvig, K. (1983a). Laryngectomees in Norway, Study No. 1. Social, personal and behavioral factors related to patient mastery of the laryngectomy. *J. Otolaryngol., 12,* 155–162.

Natvig, K. (1983b). Laryngectomees in Norway, Study No. 2. Preoperative counseling and postoperative training evaluated by the patients and their spouses. *J. Otolaryngol., 12,* 249–254.

Natvig, K. (1983c). Laryngectomees in Norway, Study No. 3. Pre- and postoperative factors of significance to esophageal speech acquisition. *J. Otolaryngol., 12,* 322–328.

Natvig, K. (1983d). Laryngectomees in Norway, Study No. 4. Social, occupational, and personal factors related to vocational rehabilitation. *J. Otolaryngol., 12,* 370–376.

Natvig, K. (1984). Laryngectomees in Norway, Study No. 5. Problems of everyday life. *J. Otolaryngol., 13,* 16–22.

Nicholson, E. (1975). Personal notes of a laryngectomee. *Am. J. Nursing, 75,* 2157–2158.

Ogura, J., and Gershon, J. (1976). The Larynx. In T. F. Nealon (Ed.), *Management of the patient with cancer* (2nd ed.) (pp. 206–238). Philadelphia: W. B. Saunders Co.

Parvulescu, N. (1970). Care of the surgically speechless patient. *Nursing Clin. N.A., 5,* 517–525.

Pitkin, Y. (1953). Factors affecting psychological adjustment in a laryngectomized patient. *Arch. Otolaryngol., 58,* 38–49.

Potter, R., and Schneiderman, C. (1979). Understanding death, dying, and the critically ill: A concern for speech-language pathologists. *J. Commun. Dis., 12,* 495–501.

Putney, F. (1958). Rehabilitation of the post-laryngectomized patient. *Ann. Otolaryngol., 67,* 544–549.

Ranney, J. (1975). Rehabilitation through employment. *Laryngoscope, 85,* 674–676.

Richardson, J. (1983). Vocational adjustment after total laryngectomy. *Arch. Phys. Med. Rehab., 64,* 172–175.

Robbins, J. (1984). Acoustic differentiation of laryngeal, esophageal, and tracheoesophageal speech. *J. Speech Hear. Res., 27,* 577–585.

Robbins, J., Fisher, H., Blom, E., and Singer, M. A. (1984a). A comparative study of normal esophageal and tracheoesophageal speech production. *J. Speech Hear. Dis., 49,* 202–210.

Robbins, J. A., Fisher, H., Blom, E., and Singer, M. (1984b). Selected acoustic features of tracheoesophageal, esophageal and laryngeal speech. *Arch. Otolaryngol., 110,* 670–672.

Ryan, W., Gates, G., Cantu, E., and Hearne, E. (1982). Current status of laryngectomee rehabilitation: III. Understanding of esophageal speech. *Am. J. Otolaryngol., 3,* 91–96.

Sako, K., Cardinale, S., Marchetta, F., and Shedd, D. (1974). Speech and vocational rehabilitation of the laryngectomized patient. *J. Surg. Oncology, 6,* 197–202.

Salmon, S. (1979). Factors that may interfere with acquiring esophageal speech. In R. Keith and F. Darley (Eds.), *Laryngectomee rehabilitation* (pp. 501–512). San Diego: College-Hill Press.

Salmon, S., and Goldstein, L. (1978). *Artificial larynx handbook.* New York: Grune and Stratton.

Sanchez-Salazar, V., and Stark, A. (1972). The use of crisis intervention in the rehabilitation of laryngectomees. *J. Speech Hear. Dis., 37,* 323–328.

Schaefer, S. D., and Johns, D. F. (1982). Attaining functional esophageal speech. *Arch. Otolaryngol., 108,* 647–649.

Shames, G., Font, J., and Matthews, J. (1963). Factors related to speech proficiency of the laryngectomized. *J. Speech Hear. Dis., 28,* 273–287.

Shapiro, M., and Vadakkencherry, R. (1982). Trachea stoma vent voice prosthesis. *Laryngoscope, 92,* 1126–1129.

Shedd, D., Schaaf, N., and Weinberg, B. (1976). Technical aspects of reed fistula speech following pharyngolaryngectomy. *J. Surg. Oncol., 8,* 305–310.

Shontz, F. (1965). Reactions of crisis. *Volta Review, 67,* 364–370.

Singer, M. I. (1983). Tracheoesophageal speech: Vocal rehabilitation after total laryngectomy. *Laryngoscope, 93,* 1454–1465.

Singer, M., and Blom, E. (1980). An endoscopic technique for restoration of voice after laryngectomy. *Ann. Otol., Rhinol., Laryngol., 89.* 529–533.

Singer, M., Blom, E., and Hamaker, R. (1981). Further experience with voice restoration after total laryngectomy. *Ann. Otol., 90,* 498–502.

Singer, M., Blom, E., and Hamaker, R. (1983). Voice rehabilitation after total laryngectomy. *J. Otolaryngol., 12,* 329–334.

√ Snidecor, J. (1970). The family of the laryngectomee. In S. E. Gerber (Ed.), *The family as supportive personnel in speech and hearing remediation* (pp. 12–30). Santa Barbara, CA: University of California Press.

Snidecor, J. C. (1975). Some scientific foundations for voice reconstruction. *Laryngoscope, 85,* 640–648.

Snidecor, J., and Curry, E. (1960). How effectively can the laryngectomee speak? *Laryngoscope, 70,* 62–67.

Stallings, J. O. (1981). Surgical voice restoration—a 20th century reality. *Ear, Nose, Throat J., 60,* 250–253.

√ Stoll, B. (1958). Psychological factors determining the success or failure of the rehabilitation program of laryngectomized patients. *Ann. Otol., Rhinol., Laryngol., 67,* 550–557.

Stolov, W. C. (1981). Comprehensive rehabilitation: Evaluation and treatment. In W. C. Stolov and M. R. Clowers (Eds.), *Handbook of severe disability.* Washington, DC: U.S. Department of Education, Rehabilitation Services Administration.

√ Tanner, D. (1980). Loss and grief: Implications for the speech-language pathologist and audiologist. *Asha, 22,* 916–928.

Thawley, S., Fuller, D., and Setzen, S. (1983). Voice restoration after total laryngectomy. *Missouri Med., 80,* 752–775.

Timiras, P. (1978). Biological perspectives on aging. *Am. Scientist, 65,* 605–613.

Volin, R. (1980). Predicting failure to speak after laryngectomy. *Laryngoscope, 90,* 1727–1736.

√ Wallen, V., and Webb, B. (1975). A survey of background characteristics of 2000 laryngectomees: A preliminary report. *Military Med., 140,* 532–534.

Warner, J. (1971). Vocal rehabilitation following total laryngectomy. *J. Laryngol. Otol., 85,* 577–582.

Webb, M., and Irving, R. (1964). Psychologic and anamnestic patterns characteristic of laryngectomees: Relation to speech rehabilitation. *J. Am. Geriat. Soc., 12,* 303–322.

Weinberg, B., and Bennett, S. (1971). A study of talker sex recognition of esophageal voices. *J. Speech Hear. Res., 14,* 382–390.

Weinberg, B., Horii, Y., Blom, E., and Singer, M. (1982). Airway resistance during esophageal phonation. *J. Speech Hear. Dis., 47,* 194–199.

Weinberg, B., and Moon, J. (1984). Aerodynamic properties of four tracheoesophageal puncture prostheses. *Arch. Otolaryngol., 110,* 673–675.

Weinberg, B., Shedd, D., and Horii, Y. (1978). Reed-fistula speech following pharyngolaryngectomy. *J. Speech Hear. Dis., 43,* 401–413.

Wetmore, S., Grueger, K., and Wesson, K. (1981). The Singer-Blom speech rehabilitation procedure. *Laryngoscope, 91,* 1109–1117.

Wolfe, R., Olson, J., and Goldenberg, D. (1971). Rehabilitation of the laryngectomee: The role of the distal sphincter. *Laryngoscope, 81,* 1971–1978.

Appendix. Final Exam

INSTRUCTOR EXAMINATION

Enter the letters before the items of your choice in the blanks provided.

Theoretical Issues

_______ 1. Approximately
(a) 3,000
(b) 4,000
(c) 5,000
(d) 6,000
(e) 7,000
new laryngectomies are performed each year.

_______ 2. For a Ti-M0-N0 lesion of the false vocal fold, the likelihood of treatment by total laryngectomy is
(a) none
(b) hardly any
(c) 50–50
(d) fairly likely
(e) assured

_______ 3. By and large, the consequences of radiation therapy of the larynx and perilaryngeal area on communication are
(a) identical
(b) similar
(c) less affective
(d) somewhat greater
(e) more devastating
than those associated with laryngectomy.

_______ 4. Selection of an intraoral artificial larynx for use by a laryngectomee just 3 or 4 days after the operation may be more desirable than a neck device because
(a) of swelling in the neck area
(b) pulmonary support is inadequate after surgery
(c) patients are too weak to hold the device to the neck
(d) neck types are unintelligible
(e) the cost of a neck type is too great

_______ 5. Identify two electric neck-type artificial larynxes from the group listed:
  (a) Memacon
  (b) Tokyo
  (c) Aurex
  (d) Western Electric
  (e) Speechmaster

_______ 6. The
  (a) Western Electric
  (b) Aurex
  (c) Servox
  (d) Cooper-Rand
  (e) Tokyo
  is the least expensive of those indicated.

_______ 7. Pitch and intensity variation within a phrase might best be accomplished by the use of a
  (a) pneumatic
  (b) electric neck-type
  (c) electric intraoral
  (d) modified electric necktype
  (e) none of the foregoing
  artificial larynx.

_______ 8. The least significant factor influencing esophageal voice production is changes in
  (a) atmospheric pressure
  (b) intraoral air pressure
  (c) PE segment tension
  (d) esophageal air pressure
  (e) pressure in the stomach

_______ 9. For accomplishment of an air charge, it is essential that
  (a) air pressure above the PE segment exceeds atmospherical pressure
  (b) pressure in the lumen of the PE segment be less than pressure above the PE segment
  (c) pressure within and below the lumen of the PE segment be less than that above the segment
  (d) the person must have no "gas" in the stomach
  (e) the person inhales before attempting insufflation

_______ 10. The item that is least important for erucation of esophageal sound is
  (a) pressure below the PE segment which exceeds that above the segment
  (b) no tension in the PE segment
  (c) the mouth being open
  (d) strong contraction of the abdominal muscles
  (e) air flowing through the PE segment

_______ 11. The 5 year cure rate of laryngeal cancer is best described as
  (a) 51 to 60 per cent
  (b) 61 to 70 per cent
  (c) 71 to 80 per cent
  (d) 81 to 90 per cent
  (e) 91 to 100 per cent

_____ 12. A lump in the neck often is associated with laryngeal cancer because
(a) the cancer spreads to the lymph glands through the blood system
(b) the cancer grows outside of the larynx to the adjacent tissues
(c) the cancer invades the lymph nodes through the lymphatic channels
(d) the cancer infects the tonsils, which swell
(e) none of the above

_____ 13. Laryngeal pathologies most unlikely to be associated with malignancies are
(a) papillomatosis and Reinke's edema
(b) leukoplakia and hyperkeritosis
(c) Reinke's edema and vocal cord nodules
(d) leukoplakia and vocal cord nodules
(e) squamous cell granuloma and Reinke's edema

_____ 14. Differences between esophageal voice and laryngeal voice probably are most influenced by
(a) irregularity of vibration of the PE segment compared with that of the vocal cords
(b) pitch of the voices
(c) loudness of the voices
(d) interphrase pause time
(e) consistency of phonation

_____ 15. The mean fundamental frequency of esophageal voice for men compared with women is
(a) higher for the men
(b) too unpredictable to compare
(c) higher for the women
(d) the same for men and women
(e) not reported in the literature

_____ 16. Rate of speech using standard esophageal voice production methods is, on the average
(a) 85 words per minute
(b) 115 words per minute
(c) 140 words per minute
(d) 175 words per minute
(e) four times slower than for users of laryngeal voice

_____ 17. The major problem that speakers with standard esophageal voice might experience in terms of intelligibility is that
(a) the vowels are often not heard as intended
(b) voiceless-voiced consonant confusions are experienced
(c) voice is not loud enough to be understood
(d) the problems are no different than for users of laryngeal voice
(e) there is insufficient air available to produce plosives

_____ 18. Compared with poor speakers, good speakers using standard esophageal voice production probably will have greater pressures in the
(a) oral cavity
(b) esophagus
(c) PE segment
(d) stomach
(e) trachea
than poorer speakers.

_______ 19. Compared with good speakers, poorer users of esophageal voice will probably have greater pressures in the
(a) oral cavity
(b) esophagus
(c) PE segment
(d) in the stomach
(e) in the trachea
than good speakers.

_______ 20. The prosthesis with a resistance of 35 cm H_2O/LPS is the
(a) Mueller Blom-Singer Duckbill
(b) Bivona Blom-Singer Duckbill
(c) Panje Button
(d) Bivona flapper valve
(e) Panje flapper valve

Clinical Issues

_______ 21. A 65 year old male laryngectomee suffered a stroke shortly after his operation, which left his tongue, lips, and palate weak. The method of air charge most likely to be successful is
(a) injecting with production of /p/
(b) glossal press
(c) glossopharyngeal press
(d) inhalation
(e) a combination of techniques

_______ 22. (a) ch, p, n
(b) ch, n, o
(c) t, ch, n
(d) p, t, ch
(e) ch, n, t
might be the most effective set for consonant injection.

_______ 23. Of the items below, that which does not relate to the degree of acceptability of an esophageal speaker is
(a) stomal noise
(b) multiple air charges
(c) klunk
(d) 120 words per minute
(e) voicing the voiceless consonants

_______ 24. A 57 year old laryngectomized carpenter who cannot produce esophageal voice because of esophageal spasms would seem to be a candidate for
(a) a Panje button
(b) a Tokyo artificial larynx
(c) a myotomy
(d) a Western Electric intraoral artificial larynx
(e) a Cooper-Rand artificial larynx

_______ 25. Which three items would be most effective in decreasing stomal noise?
(1) enlarging the stoma
(2) attempting to decrease vocal intensity

     (3) covering the stoma with sponge rubber
     (4) ignoring the problem, believing that eventually it will go away
     (5) implementing relaxation procedures

_____ 26. For air to flow into the esophagus via the inhalation method, pressure in the oral cavity must
     (a) be less than pulmonary air pressure
     (b) be higher than atmospheric presure
     (c) be less than 12 psi
     (d) be more than air pressure in the esophagus
     (e) be increased to over 15 psi

_____ 27. The method to decrease PE tonicity during phonation that probably would give the most immediate desired results is
     (a) teaching the patient relaxation techniques
     (b) head positioning
     (c) imagining the act of swallowing a sword during insufflation
     (d) modifying the diet to exclude soft foods
     (e) using less effort on eructation

_____ 28. For a person who complains of too much "gas in the stomach" the clinician might best consider
     (a) recommendation of a change in diet
     (b) whether the client is "swallowing" as a form of air charge
     (c) suggesting exercise after practicing speech
     (d) encouragment of a shorter Latency I
     (e) recommendation that the client talk softer

_____ 29. Effecting louder phonation probably would be accomplished best by
     (a) digital pressure
     (b) covering the stoma
     (c) head positioning
     (d) increasing air volume per insufflation
     (e) changing air charge methods

_____ 30. With the first attempts at esophageal voice, the activity that might lead to the desired results with less confusion on the client's part is to ask that client to
     (a) burp on purpose
     (b) say "out"
     (c) say /t/ followed by "ah"
     (d) say "tie"
     (e) cover the stoma during air intake before attempting eructation

Enter "T" for statements that are true and "F" for statements that are false.

_____ 31. Currently, there are more male laryngectomees than female by a ratio of approximately 8 to 2.

_____ 32. Good esophageal speakers will utter 20 to 25 syllables per air charge.

_____ 33. There are no electrical artificial larynxes on the market today that allow the user to vary pitch prosodically by manipulation of a switch.

_____ 34. Laryngectomees can develop the ability to appreciate odors by pumping air from the mouth upward through the velopharyngeal area and out through the nostrils.

_____ 35. A laryngectomee saying *bed* for *Ed* demonstrates the concept of intrusive consonants.

_____ 36. Uttering *gate* for *Kate* is a potential risk associated with inhalation type of air charges.

_____ 37. Consonant Injection, Glossopharyngeal Press, and Inhalation are three methods of eructating esophageal air.

_____ 38. Most laryngectomees will produce a voice with a fundamental frequency of around 40 Hz.

_____ 39. Stomal noise reduction may be accomplished by holding a whistle over the stoma or a strip of tissue in front of the stoma to help the person talk softer.

_____ 40. Having the client hold up a finger to indicate his anticipation of successful voice production helps the clinician to assess the client's monitoring of air insufflation.

_____ 41. Generally speaking, clients should not be requested or encouraged to use esophageal voice production in words until the client achieves a duration of voice that exceeds 2 seconds.

_____ 42. Latency II is more likely with a "swallow" air charge than with "Consonant Injection."

_____ 43. Elimination of the "klunk" may be facilitated by suggesting the client take in more air on an air charge and do it quicker.

_____ 44. The laryngectomee who also has had a partial glossectomy probably will not be successful using inhalation air charge.

_____ 45. Multiple attempts to charge air will probably be associated with longer "Latency I" times than "Latency II's" in most clients.

Please identify the following items, designated 46 to 51, by placing their respective numerals appropriately on the diagram on the following page.

46. The structure that functions to keep sound out of the nose.
47. The windpipe.
48. The air reservoir for producing esophageal voice.
49. The sound-producing mechanism.
50. Site from which the sounds *m, n,* and *ng* exit the vocal tract.
51. Site where a prosthesis, such as the Panje button, might be inserted.

52. Describe how *consonant injection* is accomplished.

53. Describe how insufflation by *inhalation* is accomplished.

54. What instructions might you give to a person who fails to "burp" voluntarily that would help him or her to charge the esophagus by a "pumping" action other than by the method of Consonant Injection. (Use the back of this page if necessary.)

Answers: 1, c; 2, a or b; 3, c; 4, a; 5, c or d; 6, e; 7, a; 8, a; 9, c; 10, c; 11, d; 12, c; 13, c; 14, b; 15, d; 16, a; 17, b; 18, d; 19, c; 20, c; 21, d; 22, d; 23, e; 24, c; 25, a, b, and e; 26, d; 27, a; 28, b; 29, a; 30, a; 31, T; 32, F; 33, T; 34, T; 35, T; 36, F; 37, F; 38, F; 39, T; 40, T; 41, F; 42, T; 43, F; 44, F; 45, T.

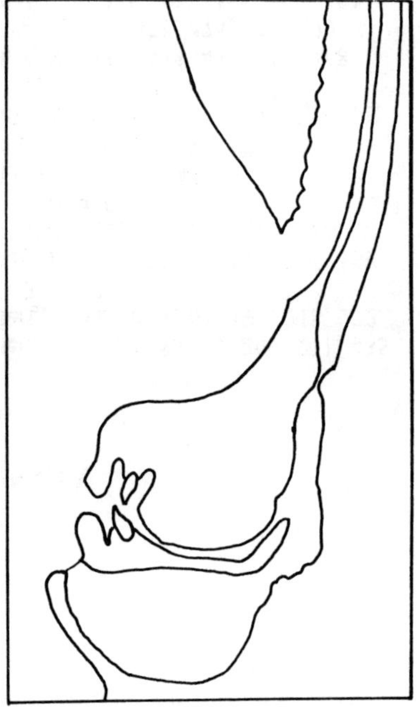

Page numbers in *italics* refer to illustrations.

SUBJECT INDEX

Page numbers in *italics* refer to illustrations; (t) indicates tables.